# Mild Head Injury

# Mild Head Injury

Edited by

HARVEY S. LEVIN, Ph.D.

HOWARD M. EISENBERG, M.D.

ARTHUR L. BENTON, Ph.D.

New York   Oxford
OXFORD UNIVERSITY PRESS
1989

for Robert L. Moody,
a distinguished public citizen

Oxford University Press

Oxford   New York   Toronto
Delhi   Bombay   Calcutta   Madras   Karachi
Petaling Jaya   Singapore   Hong Kong   Tokyo
Nairobi   Dar es Salaam   Cape Town
Melbourne   Auckland

and associated companies in
Berlin   Ibadan

Published by Oxford University Press, Inc.,
200 Madison Avenue, New York, New York 10016

Oxford is a registered trademark of Oxford University Press

Library of Congress Cataloging-in-Publication Data
Mild head injury.
Based on a conference held at the University
of Texas Medical Branch at Galveston on Mar. 20–21, 1987.
Includes bibliographies and index.
1. Head—Wounds and injuries—Congresses.
2. Head—Wounds and injuries—Complications and sequelae—Congresses.
3. Brain—Concussion—Complications and sequelae—Congresses.
I. Levin, Harvey S.   II. Eisenberg, Howard M.   III. Benton, Arthur Lester, 1909–
[DNLM: 1. Brain Injuries—congresses.
WL 354 M641 1987]   RD521.M55 1989   617'.51044
88-12569   ISBN 0-19-505301-X

9 8 7 6 5 4 3 2 1
Printed in the United States of America
on acid-free paper

# Preface

Despite the extensive documentation of postconcussion symptoms following apparently mild head injury in clinical reports and other publications during the period of industrialization in Western countries which is described in Benton's historical sketch (Chapter 1), the full magnitude of the problem in terms of medical care and social costs has only recently been appreciated. The prospective collection of population-based epidemiological data reviewed by Kraus and Nourjah (Chapter 2) has disclosed that mild head injury accounts for about two-thirds to three-fourths of all hospital admissions for head trauma. Extrapolation to the U.S. population of 250 million from the overall incidence of 130.8 patients per 100,000 population reported by these authors leads to an estimate of more than 325,000 new cases of mild head injury annually. Given the number of individuals hospitalized for mild head injury, the cost of their medical care, the burden on health services, and the social and economic consequences of their relatively brief periods of disability are enormous. Moreover, as Jennett (Chapter 3) points out, approximately five cases of mild head injury are treated on an outpatient basis in emergency rooms for every one that is admitted to a hospital.

As discussed by Benton and Rutherford in Chapters 1 and 14, respectively, definitions of mild head injury require further clarification despite recent efforts using the Glasgow Coma Scale. Although the Glasgow Coma Scale is unquestionably useful and represents the state-of-the-art for monitoring the clinical course and prognosticating survival after severe head injury, it was designed primarily to evaluate depth of coma rather than to quantitate relatively mild disturbance of consciousness and manifestations of posttraumatic amnesia following mild injuries. Loss of consciousness is typically brief in mild head injury, and measuring its duration often depends on information obtained from untrained observers. Mild head injury is not synonymous with mild brain injury nor is it clear whether either term implies concussion. The relationship of neurological deficit and postconcussion symptoms during the early stages of recovery to long-term sequelae is discussed by Rutherford in Chapter 14.

Advances in the neurosurgical management of mild head injury have enabled us to identify patients at high risk for neurological deterioration after an apparently mild head injury. Dacey (Chapter 6) reports a major prospective study of hospital admissions for apparent mild head injury that characterizes the clinical features of patients whose delayed deterioration often requires

urgent neurosurgical intervention. He also compares the relative costs and efficiency of different approaches to neurosurgical management of mild head
injury including the use of skull x-rays and computed tomography (CT). An
international perspective on the clinical management of mild head injury is
provided by Jennett (Chapter 3) who discusses differences between European
and American centers with regard to outpatient treatment in the emergency
room as opposed to hospital admission. General surgeons and other medical
specialists are involved in the management of mild head injury in Britain and
other European countries, in contrast to the predominant role of neurosurgeons in the care of these patients in North America. Eisenberg and Levin
(Chapter 8) describe recent studies on the use of magnetic resonance imaging
(MRI) in patients sustaining mild to moderate injury that indicate the presence
of parenchymal abnormalities in most cases with normal CT scans. However,
MRI revealed that most of these intracranial lesions or edematous areas
resolved over a period of one to three months in parallel with marked
improvement in neurobehavioral functioning. Preliminary findings described
by Eisenberg and Levin indicate that the localization of parenchymal abnormalities by MRI is related to the early pattern of neurobehavioral deficits in
patients with mild to moderate head injury. Similarly, Schoenhuber and Gentilini (Chapter 9) describe neurophysiological abnormalities (e.g., evoked
potentials) detected initially after mild head injury which tend to resolve over
the first three months.

Experimental models of head injury described by Povlishock and Hayes
and their co-workers (Chapters 4 and 5) have elucidated the neuropathological
and neurochemical alterations produced by mild head injury. The microscopic
changes in the parenchyma produced by the fluid percussion model are
remarkably similar to the neuropathological findings in published reports of
patients sustaining mild head injury who died from other causes. Recent experimental studies by Povlishock and co-workers indicate that early intervention
may prevent complete tearing of partially injured axons. Using the fluid percussion model, Hayes and his coauthors describe alterations in the cholinergic
system following injury. These results support the view that neurotransmitter
changes may mediate the impairment of consciousness and neurobehavioral
sequelae of mild head injury. It is possible that pharmacological therapy
involving receptor blockade or other manipulation of neurotransmitters may
prevent neurological deterioration and reduce morbidity in those patients who
suffer acute mild head injury. Further studies with varied dosages, timing of
intervention, and end-point measures are needed to evaluate the efficacy of
drug therapy. It is clear from the work by Povlishock, Hayes, and their colleagues that experimental models of head injury have considerable potential
for improving the treatment of patients who suffer mild head injury.

Neurobehavioral sequelae, postconcussional symptoms, and the stress
associated with increased mental effort constitute the major source of disability
and of secondary problems (e.g., depression) in most patients sustaining mild
head injury. Differentiating the effects of primary neurological injury from secondary psychosocial problems is often difficult for clinicians and engenders
controversy. Given the unremarkable physical appearance of many patients

after recently sustaining a mild head injury and their typically normal findings on conventional neurological examination, the basis of their persistent postconcussional complaints if often disputed. This enigma is especially apparent when medicolegal issues arise in cases of mild head injury in which equivocal neurological findings are difficult to reconcile with persistent complaints.

Attention and efficiency of information processing are typically impaired during the initial hospitalization and early weeks of convalescence after mild head injury, but substantial recovery is found by the end of the first month. Findings on the Paced Auditory Serial Addition Test (PASAT) are reported by Gronwall (Chapter 10), whereas Gentilini and co-workers (Chapter 11) describe other recently developed measures of attention that appear to be highly sensitive to sequelae of mild head injury as compared with conventional neuropsychological assessment techniques. Moreover, Gronwall has documented slower recovery of information processing on the PASAT following a second mild head injury, which suggests that the effects are cumulative. Although Ruff and his colleagues (Chapter 12) describe impairment of memory for verbal information and geometric designs in patients studied within one week of mild head injury at three university hospitals, these patients improved to a level of performance similar to that of uninjured comparison subjects over a period of one to three months. Dikmen and co-workers (Chapter 15) confirm substantial neurobehavioral recovery by one month in patients with uncomplicated mild head injury; yet their preliminary data indicate that concomitant multiple trauma can prolong disability and cognitive deficit.

Perhaps the most impressive evidence for resolution of cognitive impairment and postconcussional complaints derives from the study of concussed college football players reported by Barth et al. (Chapter 17). The opportunity to evaluate these players before and after sustaining a mild head injury and to compare the results with data obtained from their uninjured teammates provides strong documentation of neurobehavioral recovery within two weeks. Whether the findings from these sports injuries are strictly comparable to those from injuries sustained in motor vehicle accidents and other situations remains to be seen.

The overall incidence of head injury in the pediatric age range (i.e., 185 for boys and 132 for girls per 100,000 population) closely approximates the annual number of new cases in adults (see Chapter 13 by Levin, Ewing-Cobbs, and Fletcher). Similarly, mild head injury accounts for more than 80% of head trauma admissions in children and adolescents. Notwithstanding the implications of these incidence data for child development, education, and health, few studies have serially examined children after mild head injury in any systematic way. Snoek (Chapter 7) presents a detailed and insightful discussion of the assessment and management of apparently mild head injury in children, its clinical manifestations, and the problem of delayed deterioration. Maturational issues, including the possibility that delayed effects of mild head injury depend upon the developmental level of specific cognitive skills at the time of injury, are discussed by Levin, Ewing-Cobbs, and Fletcher (Chapter 13). Although the available evidence supports a generally good prognosis for neurobehavioral recovery from mild head injury in children, the possibility of increased risk for a second injury suggests that subtle, remote consequences may not be detected by neurobehavioral assessment techniques in current use. An alternative interpretation is that accident-prone children tend to have multiple injuries.

Education of the patient and family concerning the stages of recovery from mild head injury and the importance of gradual resumption of activities is increasingly recognized as part of the postacute management to mitigate distress and facilitate the resolution of postconcussional symptoms. In Chapter 16, Wrightson discusses interventions such as patient groups and counseling of selected patients at risk for persistent sequelae. He also describes the organization and management of a postconcussion clinic. Finally, Marshall and Ruff (Chapter 18) remind us of the limitations of currently employed neurobehavioral methods designed to characterize the outcome of mild head injury. Patients report cognitive and emotional difficulties in coping with occupational and educational situations that require attention to two or more tasks under sustained pressure for rapid performance, a condition that might not be adequately simulated by currently employed assessment techniques. The dissociation between improved scores on conventional neuropsychological tests and some persistent postconcussion complaints (see Chapter 15 by Dikmen et al. and Chapter 18 by Marshall and Ruff) remains an enigma. Although investigators and clinicians have advanced understanding and treatment of mild head injury, further research and dissemination of information are needed for society to fully appreciate the consequences, mitigate the sequelae, and improve prevention.

In summary, this volume presents detailed observations that reflect the advances made in recent years in the understanding, treatment and management of mild head injury. At the same time, it calls attention to the serious gaps in our knowledge and to the questions that future investigation must address if continued progress is to be achieved. We hope that our effort will prove to be of value both to practicing clinicians and to researchers.

H.S.L.
H.M.E.
October, 1988                                                              A.L.B.

# Acknowledgments

This volume is based on a conference concerning mild head injury which was held at the University of Texas Medical Branch at Galveston on March 20–21, 1987. Support for the conference and preparation of this volume was generously provided by the Moody Foundation of Galveston. Research by the editors that is described in this volume was supported by National Institutes of Health Grant NS 21889, Javits Neuroscience Investigator Award, Moody Foundation Grant 84-152A and by NINCDS Contract NS 9-2314, Comprehensive Central Nervous System Trauma Center. The editors are indebted to Sarah A. DeLosSantos, Julie A. Sifuentes, and Liz Zindler for their secretarial assistance in preparing the manuscript, to Lynn Burke for assistance in searching the literature, to Inci A. Bowman, Ph.D. for providing the cover illustration, and to Jeffrey House of Oxford University Press for his editorial advice and encouragement.

# Contents

# Contributors

WAYNE M. ALVES, PH.D.
Division of Neurosurgery
University of Pennsylvania
3400 Spruce Street
Philadelphia, PA 19104

GAY ARMSDEN, PH.D.
Department of Rehabilitation Medicine
University of Washington
Seattle, WA 98195

JEFFREY T. BARTH, PH.D.
Neuropsychology Laboratory
Department of Behavioral Medicine
    and Psychiatry
University of Virginia School of Medicine
Charlottesville, VA 22908

ARTHUR L. BENTON, PH.D.
Department of Neurology
University of Iowa Hospital and Clinics
Iowa City, IA 52242

THOMAS H. COBURN
Department of Anatomy
Medical College of Virginia
Virginia Commonwealth University
Box 709 MCV Station
Richmond, VA 23298-0709

RALPH G. DACEY, JR., M.D.
Department of Neurological Surgery
University of North Carolina at Chapel
    Hill
Chapel Hill, NC 27599-7060

SUREYYA S. DIKMEN, PH.D.
Departments of Rehabilitation Medicine,
    RJ30,
Neurological Surgery, and Psychiatry
    and Behavioral Services
University of Washington
Seattle, WA 98195

HOWARD M. EISENBERG, M.D.
Division of Neurosurgery
The University of Texas Medical Branch
Galveston, TX 77550

LINDA EWING-COBBS, PH.D.
Department of Psychiatry and Behavioral
    Science
University of Texas Health
    and Science Center at Houston
P.O. Box 20708
Houston, TX 77225

JACK M. FLETCHER, PH.D.
Department of Psychology
University of Houston
4800 Calhoun Road
Houston, TX 77004

MASSIMO GENTILINI, M.D.
Clinica Neurologica
Università di Modena
Largo del Pozzo 71
41100 Modena, Italy

DOROTHY GRONWALL, PH.D.
Concussion Clinic
Auckland Hospital
Park Road
Auckland, 1, New Zealand

RONALD L. HAYES, PH.D.
Division of Neurological Surgery
Virginia Commonwealth University
MCV Station
P.O. Box 508
Richmond, VA 23298-0001

WALTER M. HIGH, JR., PH.D.
Division of Neurosurgery
University of Texas Medical Branch
Galveston, TX 77550

JOHN A. JANE, M.D., PH.D.
Department of Neurological Surgery
University of Virginia School of Medicine
Charlottesville, VA 22908

LARRY W. JENKINS, PH.D.
Division of Neurological Surgery
Virginia Commonwealth University
MCV Station
P.O. Box 508
Richmond, VA 23298-0001

BRYAN JENNETT, M.D., F.R.C.S.
Institute of Neurological Sciences
Glasgow, G51 4TF
Scotland

JESS F. KRAUS, M.P.H., PH.D.
Division of Epidemiology
UCLA School of Public Health
Los Angeles, CA 90024-1772

HARVEY S. LEVIN, PH.D.
Division of Neurosurgery
The University of Texas Medical Branch
Galveston, TX 77550

BRUCE G. LYETH, PH.D.
Division of Neurological Surgery
Virginia Commonwealth University
MCV Station
P.O. Box 508
Richmond, VA 23298-0001

STEPHEN N. MACCIOCCHI, PH.D.
Neuropsychology Section
Division of Behavioral Medicine
Northeast Georgia Medical Center
743 Spring Street, N.E.
Gainesville, Georgia 30505

LAWRENCE F. MARSHALL, M.D.
Division of Neurological Surgery
University of California Medical Center
225 Dickinson Street
San Diego, CA 92103

STEVEN MATTIS, PH.D.
The New York Hospital
Cornell Medical Center
21 Bloomingdale Road
White Plains, NY 10605

WILLIAM E. NELSON, M.D.
Division of Sports Medicine
University of Virginia Medical School
Charlottesville, VA 22901

PAOLO NICHELLI, M.D.
Clinica Neurologica
Università di Modena
Via del Pozzo 71
41100 Modena, Italy

PARIVASH NOURJAH, M.S.
Division of Epidemiology
UCLA School of Public Health
Los Angeles, CA 90024-1772

JOHN T. POVLISHOCK, PH.D.
Department of Anatomy
Medical College of Virginia
Virginia Commonwealth University
Box 709 MCV Station
Richmond, VA 23298-0709

REBECCA W. RIMEL, R.N., M.B.A.
The Pew Charitable Trusts
Three Parkway, Suite 501
Philadelphia, PA 19102

RONALD M. RUFF, PH.D.
Department of Psychiatry, UCSD
Gifford Mental Health Clinic
3427 Fourth Avenue
San Diego, CA 92103

WILLIAM H. RUTHERFORD, O.B.E.,
   M.B., F.R.C.S.ED., F.R.C.S.E.
34 Malone View Road
Belfast, BT9 5PH
Northern Ireland

THOMAS V. RYAN, PH.D.
Neuropsychology Laboratory
Department of Behavioral Medicine
   and Psychiatry
University of Virginia School of Medicine
Charlottesville, VA 22908

RUDOLF SCHOENHUBER, M.D.
Clinica Neurologica
Università di Modena
Largo del Pozzo 71
41100 Modena, Italy

J. W. SNOEK, M.D.
Department of Neurology
University Hospital Groningen
P.O. Box 30.001
9700 RB Groningen
The Netherlands

KAMRAN TABADDOR, M.D.
159 East Dunhill Road
Bronx, NY 10467

NANCY TEMKIN, PH.D.
Departments of Neurological Surgery
    and Biostatistics, ZA-50
University of Washington
Seattle, WA

PHILIP WRIGHTSON, M.A., M.B.,
    F.R.A.C.S.
Department of Neurology
    and Neurosurgery
Auckland Hospital
Auckland, New Zealand
18 Crocus Place
Remuera, Auckland 5
New Zealand

# I
# History and Epidemiology

# 1

# Historical Notes on the Postconcussion Syndrome

## ARTHUR L. BENTON

To begin with, perhaps a capsule definition of the postconcussion syndrome is in order. It is generally understood to refer to a condition in which a person who has sustained a concussion complains of a variety of somatic, cognitive, emotional, motor, or sensory disabilities which he or she ascribes to the concussion. At the same time, convincing historical and clinical evidence of significant brain injury cannot be elicited. The typical history indicates that at the time of the accident and shortly thereafter, the person was comatose for only a very brief period if at all, and showed practically no retrograde amnesia and very little posttraumatic amnesia. After examination and treatment at the emergency unit, the patient may be sent home unless there are complicating factors such as drunkenness or limb fracture, in which case he or she may be hospitalized for a day or two.

Weeks or months after the accident, the patient will voice one or more complaints which, in their totality, have come to be called the *posttraumatic symptom-complex* or *syndrome*. Prominent features of the syndrome include headache, impairment in attention and concentration, poor memory, depression and emotional instability, lowered tolerance of frustration, sleep disturbances, loss of sexual drive, and intolerance to alcohol (Benton, 1979; Binder, 1986; Levin, Benton, and Grossman, 1982). The net effect of these impairments often (but by no means always) is to render the person significantly handicapped from a social and economic standpoint. However, at this time, clinical examination discloses very little cognitive, motor, or sensory deficit that can be reasonably ascribed to brain injury, and, in the opinion of the examining physician, the findings are essentially negative. Thus there is a striking discrepancy between the presumably "subjective" complaints of the patient and the presumably "objective" findings of the physician; this almost inevitably leads to an uncomfortable state of cognitive dissonance in both parties and sometimes to open conflict between them.

Of course, the dire behavioral consequences that may ensue from traumatic head injury have been known since time immemorial. In fact, much of what was learned about brain–behavior relationships before the nineteenth century came from clinical observations of head-injured patients. Thus almost all the very early descriptions of aphasic disorder deal with patients who had sustained either penetrating or closed head injuries (Benton and Joynt, 1960). The first case report of a pure alexia without agraphia (by Mercuriale in the sixteenth century) concerned a printer who had struck his head in a fall and who lost the capacity to read and, although he could write, "could no longer read what he had himself had written" (Meunier, 1924). The relative neglect of the cerebral hemispheres, which was so characteristic of the early attempts of clinicians to localize functions in the brain and which seems so odd to us today, was also conditioned at least in part by the circumstance that traumatically injured patients formed a large part of the case material from which they drew their inferences. Thus, the eighteenth-century French surgeon, La Peyronie, having observed that different regions of the hemispheres could be traumatized without apparent loss of mental capacity, concluded, "from the facts and by way of exclusion," that the corpus callosum was the seat of intellectual functions (Soury, 1899).

Early clinicians were also well aware that apparently mild head injuries, as indicated by the history, could have the most serious long-term consequences. Trimble (1981) cites a number of eighteenth-century and early nineteenth-century case reports describing patients who suffered minor injury with no immediate untoward effects but who later became progressively incapacitated until early death. Postmortem examination of these cases disclosed widespread cerebral pathology that was ascribed to the original injury. In retrospect, it is not clear that the inference was always correct, but, in any case, it was an opinion that was widely held.

However, this view that mild head injury could have late consequences of the most serious import is, of course, quite different from the concept of the postconcussional symptom-complex, which attained prominence only in the later decades of the nineteenth century. As is well known, the rapid development of railway transportation, which evidently was accompanied by a frightfully high frequency of collisions, derailments, and sudden stops, was a major factor in this respect. Occupational injuries were also a major producer of the posttraumatic syndrome. Social and political changes coincident with the progressive expansion of industry and finance, such as the establishment of private and governmental insurance schemes, the passage of legislation providing for workers' compensation, the rise of labor unions, and the increasingly strong insistence on workers' rights, created a setting in which the authority of employers and their physicians could be challenged. There was a rapid rise in the number of cases of real or factitious posttraumatic disability that could not be diagnosed in a fully satisfactory way. Unsympathetic observers called it an "epidemic"—a designation that was supported by statistics. Rigler (1879) was able to document a dramatic increase in invalidism after railway accidents in the years immediately following the passage in 1871 of a law in Prussia providing for compensation for injuries in such accidents.

John Erichsen, a London surgeon, whose writings are described in detail by Trimble (1981), was a major figure in this early period. He insisted that apparently slight concussions, twists, and wrenches of the spine could and did cause serious injury not only to the spine but to other parts of the body, the outcome being severe disability. The underlying pathology, according to Erichsen, consisted of "molecular disarrangement" and /or anemia of the spinal cord. And, although Erichsen himself was largely concerned with spinal injuries, his views were extended to brain injuries as well. His book entitled *On Concussion of the Spine: Nervous Shock and Other Obscure Injuries of the Nervous System in Their Medico-legal Aspects* (Erichsen, 1882) was widely influential in the legal arena as well as in medical circles. Trimble (1981) remarks that "few cases, it seems, were taken to court without the book appearing and being cited."

Erichsen's views received a mixed reception from his fellow physicians and surgeons. There were some who were sympathetic to his basic conceptions although they might or might not agree with his specific formulations about the nature of the underlying pathology. However, they did believe that the myriad complaints of patients suffering from what was then called "railway spine" could have an organic basis. But other physicians were more than skeptical; they firmly opposed the notion that these postaccident complaints, which defied validation, were due to obscure, undemonstrable organic changes. Instead, they ascribed the symptoms to the effects of the traumatic event on an inherently unstable person or to frank malingering for financial gain. Some clinicians took a judicious middle position, stating that some cases did in fact have an organic basis whereas others were "psychological" in origin. Oppenheim (1889) employed the term "traumatic neurosis" to reflect his belief that the sequelae of mild traumatic head injury represented an interaction of structural and functional factors.

With the rise of modern medical psychology, preeminently represented by the development of psychoanalysis, a new dimension was added to the picture. The Freudian concepts of the far-reaching effects of early psychic trauma and of the defensive mechanisms of repression, regression, and symptom-formation could be readily applied to the physical trauma of concussion and its subsequent effects. The casualties of World War I provided ample case material for this approach which emphasized the role of subconscious factors, such as perceived threats to the integrity of the patient as a person and regression to a state of dependency, as determinants of the symptoms exhibited after concussion or even after a frightening experience that did not involve physical injury. Although these views of the psychoanalysts were often derided, they did have a significant effect on the thinking of many clinicians who now enlarged the scope of their evaluation to include consideration of life history and situational factors as possible contributors to the clinical picture.

Nevertheless, the controversy between those who saw the postconcussional syndrome as purely "psychological" (if not outright malingering) and those who believed that it had a real, if obscure, organic basis continued throughout the 1920s and 1930s. A variety of minimal signs alleged to be indicative of organic brain disease were described, but, given the lack of systematic study and especially observations on control subjects, their validity remained very questionable (Strauss and Savitsky, 1934).

World War II and its aftermath brought more effective methods of evaluation and management along all fronts: neuropathology, neuroradiology, neurosurgery, clinical neurology, neuropsychology, and (of increasing importance) social psychology, and sociology. There was a steady accumulation of information indicating that in fact the disabilities of patients who had sustained a mild head injury were very likely to be based on cerebral dysfunction, which in turn implied some type of structural alteration of the brain. At the same time, the problem of malingering, although always present, receded in importance. It also became evident that the clinical picture reflected a dynamic state of affairs to which physical, personal, social, and economic factors contribute in varying degrees and in a changing way. Factors such as, for example, the premorbid personality, alcoholism, the marital or familial situation, and whether or not there is a network of social support, were implicated as determining not only the nature and persistence of patients' complaints but also whether or not they find themselves able to return to work. Oddy, Humphrey, and Uttley (1978) found only a very weak positive relationship between these two factors; their sample included patients with multiple complaints who nevertheless returned to full-time employment and those with fewer complaints who did not return to work. In addition, they found no relationship between pending claims for compensation and delay in returning to work.

The thrust of post-World War II experience has been to confirm the reality of the postconcussional syndrome as a consequence of mild head injury. The concept that it is a congeries of symptoms and complaints that has multiple determinants—physical, psychological, and social—is now generally accepted. Moreover, increased concern with the occurrence of delayed deterioration following mild head injury, especially in children, has added another dimension to a complex picture (cf. Snoek et al., 1984).

However, we have yet to achieve reasonably precise definitions of many of these determinants, as well as an understanding of how they interact to produce symptoms and disability. Both types of information are required for more effective methods of evaluation and treatment. A variety of specific questions remain to be addressed. The contributors to this volume should provide at least provisional answers to some of these questions.

## REFERENCES

Benton AL. Behavioral consequences of closed head injury. *In* Odom GL (ed), Central Nervous System Trauma Research Report. Bethesda, MD: NINCDS, National Institutes of Health, 1979, pp 220–231.

Benton AL, Joynt RJ. Early descriptions of aphasia. Arch Neurol 3:205–221, 1960.

Binder, LM. Persisting symptoms after mild head injury: a review of the postconcussive syndrome. J Clin Exp Neuropsychol 8:323–346, 1986.

Erichsen JE. On Concussion of the Spine: Nervous Shock and Other Obscure Injuries of the Nervous System in Their Clinical and Medico-Legal Aspects. London: Longmans Green, 1882.

Levin HS, Benton AL, Grossman RG. Neurobehavioral Consequences of Closed Head Injury. New York: Oxford University Press, 1982.

Meunier M. Histoire de la médecine. Paris: LeFrançois, 1924.

Oddy M, Humphrey M, Uttley D. (1978). Subjective impairment and social recovery after closed head injury. J Neurol Neurosurg Psychiatry 41:611–616.

Oppenheim H. Die Traumatischen Neurosen. Berlin: Hirschwald, 1889.

Rigler J. Ueber die Verletzungen auf Eisenbahnen insbesondere der Verletzungen des Rueckenmarks. Berlin: Reimer, 1879.

Snoek JW, Minderhoud JM, Wilmink JT. Delayed deterioration following mild head injury in children. Brain 107:15–36, 1984.

Soury J. Le système nerveux central. Paris: Carré et Naud, 1899.

Strauss I, Savitsky N. Head injury: Neurologic and psychiatric aspects. Arch Neurol Psychiatry 31:893–955, 1934.

Trimble MR. Post-traumatic Neurosis: From Railway Spine to the Whiplash. New York: John Wiley, 1981.

# 2

# The Epidemiology of Mild Head Injury

JESS F. KRAUS
AND PARIVASH NOURJAH

It is surprising to find so little epidemiological information in the scientific literature on mild brain injury, an entity accounting for most of the head trauma in the United States and other industrialized countries of the world. There have been only four population-based studies of hospitalized patients with mild head injuries in the United States (Table 2–1; see also Frankowski et al., 1986). Annegers and colleagues (1980) studied head injuries among hospitalized residents of Olmsted County, Minnesota, from 1935 to 1974. The investigators defined mild head injury as injury resulting in loss of consciousness (LOC) or posttraumatic amnesia of less than one-half hour's duration without skull fracture. The investigators reported that 55% of male hospitalized patients and 61% of female hospitalized patients had mild head trauma.

Rimel (1981) and Jagger et al. (1984b) studied patients admitted, at least overnight, to the University of Virginia hospital in 1977–9; they were referred from 14 counties of north central Virginia. Their results showed that 49% had "minor" central nervous system (CNS) injuries or a Glasgow Coma Scale (GCS) of 12 or greater. This hospital is the major source for neurosurgical coverage for the region, and possibly persons with minor head injuries may not have been as readily referred to the university hospital as would more seriously injured patients.

The Glasgow Coma Scale was the basis for classification of brain injury severity for all hospital-admitted brain-injured residents in 1981 in San Diego County, California (Kraus et al., 1984). Those with a GCS of 13–15 were termed "mild" and included about 82% of the persons hospitalized with a brain injury.

Head trauma in the inner city was the subject of a report by Whitman and

**Table 2-1**  Epidemiological Features of Population-Based Studies of Mild Head Injury, United States, 1980–86

| Authors (year) | Place | Data year(s) | Rate of mild head injury per 100,000 | Percentage of all head injury | Definition of mild head injury |
|---|---|---|---|---|---|
| Annegers, et al. 1980 | Olmsted County, Minnesota | 1935–74 | 149 | 60 | LOC <30 min and no skull fracture |
| Rimel, 1981 Jagger et al., 1984b | north central Virginia | 1977–79 | not reported | 49 | GCS = 12–15 or chart notation |
| Kraus et al., 1984 | San Diego County, California | 1981 | 131 | 82 | GCS = 13–15 |
| Whitman et al., 1984 | Chicago area | 1979–80 | 120–284[a] | 80 | LOC <30 min plus "trivial" |

*Abbreviations:* GCS, Glasgow Coma Scale; LOC, loss of consciousness.
[a]Range in three communities.

colleagues (1984) in the Chicago area for 1979–80. The medical records on hospital discharges in the region selected were examined and those with a brain injury diagnosis were identified. Injuries in patients with loss of consciousness of less than 30 minutes were classified as "mild," whereas those in patients not moderately, severely, or fatally head-injured were called "trivial." About 80% of all patients identified in this study had either a mild or trivial head injury.

Results from the four population-based studies mentioned above are not comparable, even though mild or minor head (brain) injuries were specifically identified and tabulated. Even though LOC was the basis for head-injury severity classification, the wide differences in the proportion of mild head injuries between Olmsted County, Minnesota, and the Chicago area study may be accounted for by differences in times of the studies (1935–74 vs. 1979–80), reflecting differences in policies on hospitalization for mild brain injury between the study periods. In addition, case ascertainment procedures and/or whether or not accompanying skull fracture was an identifying feature of the head injury may have differed between these two studies.

The two studies (north central Virginia and San Diego County, California) that used the GCS for severity classification are not comparable either, but for different reasons. One difference might be the proportion of mild head injuries referred to the university hospital in the north central Virginia region where the injury took place, in contrast to San Diego where all hospitals were surveyed. A second reason for the differences in proportions is that in the north central Virginia study, patients were classified according to the chart notation *or* the GCS, whereas in the 1981 San Diego study, only the GCS was used for determining brain injury severity.

Because of the vast differences in study designs and definitions, conclusions from the four population-based studies must be guarded. The high proportion of such injuries among all brain-injured hospitalized patients combined with the high index of suspicion associated with possible unfavorable outcomes of mild trauma (Casey et al., 1986; Chadwick et al., 1981; Dacey et al., 1986; Gronwall and Wrightson, 1974; Jane et al., 1985; Klonoff et al., 1977; Levin and Eisenberg, 1979; Levin et al., 1987; Lidvall, 1975; McLean et al., 1983; Oppenheimer, 1968; Rimel et al., 1981; Rutherford et al., 1977; Symonds, 1962) suggest that a presentation of basic epidemiological factors associated with this level of brain injury is needed. For this purpose, data from the population-based study of brain injury in San Diego County have been analyzed, and findings on incidence, external cause, prehospital factors, diagnoses, alcohol use, and hospital treatment costs are presented. Little or no published information on these factors is published elsewhere.

## METHODS

Members of the study cohort were residents of San Diego County, California, in 1981 and were hospitalized during that year (1981) for brain injuries. Specific details of the study design, population description, case ascertainment, and methodology are reported elsewhere (Kraus et al., 1984), but certain relevant points are summarized here.

For purposes of this study, a mild brain injury is physical damage to, or functional impairment of, the cranial contents from acute mechanical energy exchange exclusive of birth trauma. This definition includes mostly concussion, but also contusion, hemorrhage, laceration, and other intracranial injury of the brain due to blunt or penetrating force. It does not include fracture of the skull or facial bones or injury to the soft tissues of the eye, ear, or face without concurrent brain injury. Information was ascertained on persons admitted to a hospital having a physician-diagnosed brain injury.

The Glasgow Coma Scale (Jennett and Teasdale, 1981) was used to assess the level of brain injury severity for people reaching a hospital emergency room. This scale, which was designed to assess impaired consciousness in persons with diffuse brain damage, was used consistently in all San Diego County emergency rooms during 1981 and was used on 100% of all patients with a mild brain injury. The GCS used for this report was measured upon or shortly after arrival at the emergency room. A mild brain injury included a GCS of 13–15 while the patient was in the emergency room and before hospital admission.

Mild brain-injury cases as defined among county residents were identified from emergency room and inpatient hospital records of acute-care general hospitals in the county and review of the discharge records of the nine major hospitals in the three counties bordering San Diego County.

Brain injury diagnoses were confirmed and abstracted by neurosurgical nurse data abstractors. The International Classification of Diseases (ICD) (clinical modification) diagnoses were abstracted as recorded in the medical record. Information on external cause of the injury was abstracted from hospital records and /or police reports. Information on data and time of injury and arrival at the emergency room, on date of discharge, and on method of emergency transport was obtained from the hospital medical record, paramedic, or private ambulance logs.

Blood samples for alcohol concentration were generally obtained while the person was in the emergency room, and results were abstracted as recorded in the hospital record, not based on police reports. Most hospitals used a gas chromatographic method to determine blood alcohol concentration.

Direct hospital-cost data in 1981 dollars by ICD diagnoses, length of hospital stay, and age group were provided by the San Diego and Imperial County Health Systems Agency. The costs are aggregate and include all in-hospital services and professional personnel charges for only those patients with a concussion (ICD-850) or other intracranial injury (ICD-854), because almost all persons with mild brain injuries had these diagnoses and very few of those with contusion or hemorrhage (ICD-851, 852, 853) were mildly brain-injured. Estimates of prehospital paramedic and private ambulance emergency transport were provided by pertinent county agencies. Indirect costs were not calculated, and total dollar costs were not discounted. Post-hospital charges for continuing care and costs for damage to property are not included in the cost figures.

## RESULTS

Over 72% of the 3,358 San Diego County residents with brain trauma identified from all record sources sustained a mild brain injury in 1981, an incidence rate of 130.8 per 100,000 per year. The proportion of mild brain injury among all *hospitalized* cases was 82%. The rate for males (174.7 per 100,000) was about twice as high as that for females (85.2 per 100,000) (Table 2–2). Figure 2–1 shows age-specific rates for males and females. Highest rates are seen for males at all ages (except 75 years and older), and peak rates are noted for males aged 15–24. Peak incidence for females is over age 75 years and less than 5 years.

Table 2–2  Number Injured and Rate of Mild Brain Injury per 100,000 Population by Gender, San Diego County, California, 1981

| Gender | Number injured | Number and rate, 1981 population | Rate per 100,000 |
|---|---|---|---|
| Males | 1,656 | 947,699 | 174.7 |
| Females | 779 | 914,147 | 85.2 |
| Total | 2,435 | 1,861,846 | 130.8 |

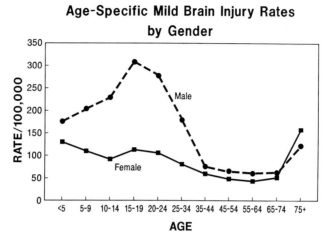

**Figure 2–1**  Age-specific mild brain injury rates by gender.

### Prehospital Factors: External Causes

Almost 42% of all mild brain injuries involved a motor vehicle crash, in which the injured person was an occupant of the vehicle (64%), a motorcyclist (20%), a pedestrian (10%), or a bicyclist (6%). Falls accounted for 23% of the cases, and the third most common cause was assaults (14%), which included three persons injured from firearms. Bicycle collisions not involving a motor vehicle, and sports and recreation activities accounted for 6% each. All other causes accounted for 8%.

Figure 2–2 shows age- and gender-specific mild brain injury rates for four

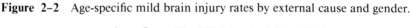

**Figure 2–2**  Age-specific mild brain injury rates by external cause and gender.

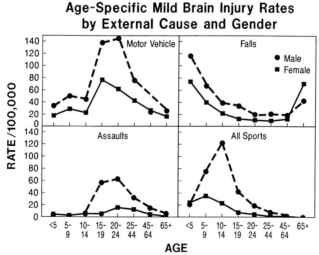

general categories of external causes. Rates are highest for causes related to motor vehicle crashes, with peak age of occurrence from 15 to 24 years. A similar pattern (but of lower magnitude) is observed for brain injuries from assaults. Persons brain-injured from falls showed peak incidence rates at extremes of the age range, with highest rates among children less than 5 years of age and among adults 65 years and over for both males and females—the youngest and oldest age groups. Brain injuries from recreation or sports activities are generally higher for males than for females, but the pattern is not the same for both genders. Rates for males peak at ages 10–14, whereas rates for females peak five years earlier, on the average.

## Type of Emergency Transport

Information on type of emergency transport was available for 2,261 of the 2,435 (93%) persons seen in an emergency room and subsequently admitted to a hospital for a mild brain injury. Almost 40% of the patients were transported by a paramedic unit, and an additional 17% by a private ambulance. A private vehicle (e.g., passenger car) was the method of transport for 35% of the cases. Transport by helicopter (2%), police vehicle (3%), or other methods (2%) accounted for the remainder. The method of transport of mildly brain-injured persons did not depend on severity (GCS score = 13, 14, or 15) or external cause but was related to age, with more than 65% of children under age 15 transported in private vehicles, compared to 17% of adults having similar severity of injuries.

Thirty-five percent of mildly brain-injured patients reached a hospital emergency room within 30 minutes of injury (Table 2–3), 62% arrived at an emergency room within one hour, whereas slightly over 12% did not arrive at an emergency room until four hours post injury.

## Brain Injury Diagnoses

The distribution of mild brain-injury diagnoses is given in Table 2–4. Over 80% of the patients had a concussion (including 7% with an accompanying

**Table 2–3** Number, Percentage, and Cumulative Percentage of Mildly Brain-Injured Patients by Time Interval from Injury to Arrival at the Emergency Room, San Diego, 1981

| Time interval from injury to ER arrival (min) | Number of patients | Percentage | Cumulative percentage |
|---|---|---|---|
| <30 | 580 | 35.3 | 35.3 |
| 30–59 | 442 | 26.9 | 62.2 |
| 60–119 | 251 | 15.3 | 77.5 |
| 120–179 | 119 | 7.2 | 84.7 |
| 180–239 | 52 | 3.2 | 87.9 |
| 240+ | 199 | 12.1 | 100.0 |

*Note:* Patients with unrecorded time of injury (i.e., 35%) are excluded.

**Table 2–4**  Number and Percentage of Mild Brain Injuries by ICD Diagnoses

| Diagnoses (ICD No.) | Number | Percentage |
|---|---|---|
| Contusion–laceration (851) | 109 | 4.5 |
| With fx[a] | (41) | (1.7) |
| Without fx | (68) | (2.8) |
| Hemorrhage (852–853) | 21 | 0.9 |
| With fx | (9) | (0.4) |
| Without fx | (12) | (0.5) |
| Other intracranial (854) | 351 | 14.4 |
| With fx | (24) | (1.0) |
| Without fx | (327) | (13.4) |
| Concussion (850) | 1954 | 80.2 |
| With fx | (172) | (7.1) |
| Without fx | (1782) | (73.2) |
| All diagnoses | 2435 | 100 |

[a]fx, fracture.

fracture of the skull or facial bones). Other intracranial injuries accounted for 14.4% of all mild brain injuries, with only 1% having concurrent skull or facial fracture. Contusion or hemorrhage accounted for 4.5% of all cases, of which about one-third had an accompanying fracture of skull or facial bones. When a fracture was present (in less than 10% of the cases), it involved one or more facial bones.

The distribution of patients with mild brain injuries by emergency room Glasgow Coma Scale (GCS) value and brain-injury diagnosis with and without

**Table 2–5**  Number and Percentage of Mild Brain Injuries by Glasgow Coma Scale and Diagnoses, San Diego County, California, 1981

| Diagnoses | GCS 13 No. | GCS 13 % | GCS 14 No. | GCS 14 % | GCS 15 No. | GCS 15 % | Total No. | Total % |
|---|---|---|---|---|---|---|---|---|
| Contusion | | | | | | | | |
| With fx[a] | 5 | 12.2 | 11 | 26.8 | 25 | 61.0 | 41 | — |
| Without fx | 5 | 7.5 | 17 | 25.4 | 45 | 67.2 | 67 | |
| Hemorrhage | | | | | | | | |
| With fx | 2 | 22.2 | 2 | 22.2 | 5 | 55.6 | 9 | — |
| Without fx | 1 | 8.3 | 1 | 8.3 | 10 | 83.0 | 12 | — |
| Other intracranial | | | | | | | | |
| With fx | 1 | 4.2 | 10 | 41.7 | 13 | 54.2 | 24 | — |
| Without fx | 19 | 5.9 | 77 | 23.8 | 227 | 70.3 | 323 | — |
| Concussion | | | | | | | | |
| With fx | 12 | 7.1 | 48 | 28.2 | 110 | 64.7 | 170 | — |
| Without fx | 92 | 5.2 | 322 | 18.3 | 1342 | 76.4 | 1756 | — |
| Subtotal | | | | | | | | |
| With fx | 20 | 8.2 | 71 | 29.1 | 153 | 62.3 | 244 | — |
| Without fx | 117 | 5.4 | 417 | 19.3 | 1624 | 75.3 | 2158 | — |
| Total | 137 | 5.7 | 488 | 20.3 | 1777 | 74.0 | 2402 | 100 |

[a]fx, fracture.

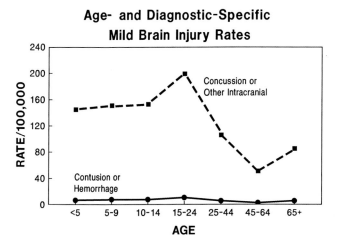

**Figure 2–3**  Age- and diagnostic-specific mild brain injury rates.

head fracture is shown in Table 2–5. Almost 75% of all hospital-admitted patients had a GCS of 15 (no impairment of verbal, eye, or motor response). The proportion with a GCS of 15 was less (62.3%) if a fracture of skull or facial bones was present. This finding was similar for all of the brain injury diagnoses, the greatest proportion with a GCS of 13–14 being found among those having hemorrhage or other intracranial injury.

Age-specific rates for persons with concussion/other intracranial injury showed peak occurrence from ages 15 to 24, and then declined until age 45, with a slight increase through ages 65 and older (Figure 2–3). There was no discernible age pattern in rates for those having a mild contusion or hemorrhage.

## Length of Hospital Stay

About two-thirds (64%) of all hospital-admitted mildly brain-injured patients stayed less than three days (Table 2–6). About 87% required hospitalization of less than a week, and 5% were hospitalized for two weeks or longer. Length of hospital stay may not necessarily relate specifically to observation or treatment of the brain injury since many patients had concurrent trauma to other body regions.

Length of stay by grouped ICD diagnoses is seen in Figure 2–4. Note that persons with mild brain-injury diagnoses of contusion or hemorrhage had a longer median length of stay than those with concussion or other intracranial injury. This pattern did not change appreciably for patients with or without associated fractures of the skull or facial bones.

Table 2–7 shows the cumulative percentage of hospital days by Glasgow Coma Scale. For patients with a GCS of 13–14, the median length of stay was almost three days, whereas for patients with an emergency room GCS of 15, the median length of stay was about two days.

**Table 2–6** Number and Cumulative Percentage of Mild Brain Injuries by Hospital Days

| Number of hospital days | Number of admissions[a] | Percentage | Cumulative percentage |
|---|---|---|---|
| <1 | 120 | 5.0 | 5.0 |
| 1–2 | 905 | 37.5 | 42.5 |
| 2–3 | 519 | 21.5 | 64.0 |
| 3–4 | 230 | 9.5 | 73.5 |
| 4–5 | 148 | 6.1 | 79.6 |
| 5–6 | 97 | 4.0 | 83.7 |
| 6–7 | 75 | 3.1 | 86.8 |
| 7–14 | 194 | 8.0 | 94.8 |
| 14–28 | 72 | 3.0 | 97.8 |
| 28+ | 53 | 2.2 | 100.0 |
| Total | 2413 | 100.0 | — |

[a]Excludes 22 persons with unknown hospital days.

### Time and Hour of Injury

Figure 2–5 shows the distribution of mild brain injuries by day of week. For all causes combined, the frequencies increase with the weekend days (Fridays, Saturdays, and Sundays). Brain injuries from falls and sports or recreational activities do not have the pronounced weekend excess, whereas injuries from motor vehicle crashes and assaults are most frequent on weekends.

Table 2–8 shows the percentage distribution of mild brain injuries by hour. More than one-half of all injuries occurred from 2:00 p.m. until 10:00 p.m., with 70% occurring in the 12-hour period of 2:00 p.m. until 2:00 a.m. Motor vehicle-related injuries are most frequent in all time intervals, with fall-

**Figure 2–4** Cumulative percent hospital days by grouped diagnoses and length of stay.

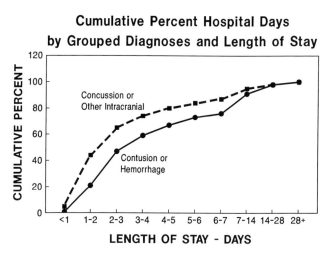

Cumulative Percent Hospital Days by Grouped Diagnoses and Length of Stay

**Table 2–7** Cumulative Percentage of Hospital Days for Mild Brain Injuries by Glasgow Coma Scale, San Diego County, California, 1981

| Hospital days | Glasgow Coma Scale | | |
|---|---|---|---|
| | 13 | 14 | 15 |
| <1 | 6 | 4 | 5 |
| 1–2 | 27 | 34 | 46 |
| 2–3 | 52 | 57 | 67 |
| 3–4 | 63 | 68 | 76 |
| 4–5 | 70 | 75 | 82 |
| 5–6 | 74 | 80 | 86 |
| 6–7 | 78 | 84 | 89 |
| 7–14 | 89 | 94 | 96 |
| 14–21 | 91 | 95 | 98 |
| 21–27 | 93 | 97 | 99 |
| 28+ | 100 | 100 | 100 |

related causes second in occurrence from 6:00 a.m. until 2:00 p.m. Assault-related causes are the second most common cause from 10:00 p.m. until 2:00 a.m. Sports and all other causes are second in frequency from 2:00 p.m. until 6:00 p.m.

## Alcohol Testing and Prevalence of Intoxication

Almost 30% of patients aged 15 and older who were admitted to a hospital with a mild brain injury were blood-tested for alcohol. Highest testing rates were seen for those aged 20–24, with lowest testing rate for those aged 75 years and

**Figure 2–5** Distribution of mild brain injuries by day of week and external cause.

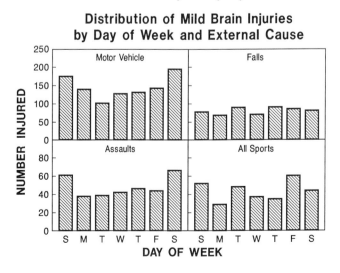

Distribution of Mild Brain Injuries by Day of Week and External Cause

**Table 2-8**  Percentage Distribution of Mild Brain Injuries by Hour of Occurrence and External Cause, San Diego County, California, 1981

| Hour of occurrence | All causes (100%) | Motor vehicle (%) | Falls (%) | Assaults (%) | All others (%) | Total (%) |
|---|---|---|---|---|---|---|
| 0200–0559 | 6.7 | 70 | 8 | 21 | 1 | 100 |
| 0600–0959 | 6.7 | 58 | 23 | 5 | 13 | 99 |
| 1000–1359 | 16.4 | 42 | 26 | 7 | 25 | 99 |
| 1400–1759 | 26.8 | 47 | 21 | 4 | 28 | 100 |
| 1800–2159 | 25.4 | 53 | 19 | 13 | 16 | 101 |
| 2200–0159 | 18.1 | 62 | 10 | 23 | 4 | 99 |

older (Table 2–9). Among those tested, two-thirds had a blood alcohol content (BAC) reading of 100 mg% or higher, which is the legal intoxication level in California. Over 85% of those aged 35–44 or 55–64 had high (i.e., ≥100 mg%) levels of blood alcohol readings.

The BAC testing rate (Table 2–10) was inversely related to Glasgow Coma Scale, with the highest testing rate (33.6%) in those with a GCS of 13. Only 20% of those with a GCS of 15 were tested for blood alcohol. Age adjustment did not change this finding appreciably. Among those tested, over 63% had a blood alcohol test result of 100 mg% or higher. The prevalence of elevated (≥100 mg%) blood alcohol levels was highest in those with a GCS of 14 and 13, as compared with those with a GCS of 15.

## Treatment Costs and Outcome

Total in-hospital costs in 1981 dollars for treatment of mild brain injuries in San Diego County was 6.3 million (dollars), with an average cost per admission of $2,774 (Table 2–11). Average costs per admission increased with length of hospital stay. Treatment costs were higher for patients with other intracranial injuries (excluding contusion, laceration, or hemorrhage), as compared with

**Table 2-9**  Number and Percentage of Blood-Alcohol-Tested Cases and Rate of BAC in Excess of Legal Limit by Age, San Diego County, California, 1981

| Age | Number injured | Percent tested | Rate per 100 tested with BAC ≥100 mg% |
|---|---|---|---|
| 15–19 | 388 | 19.3 | 48.0 |
| 20–24 | 459 | 39.4 | 64.2 |
| 25–34 | 451 | 34.8 | 72.6 |
| 35–44 | 158 | 29.1 | 87.0 |
| 45–54 | 97 | 29.9 | 65.5 |
| 55–64 | 86 | 31.4 | 85.2 |
| 65–74 | 106 | 9.4 | 60.0 |
| Total | 1812 | 27.8 | 68.8 |

Table 2–10  Number and Percentage of Blood-Alcohol-Tested Cases and Rate of BAC in Excess of 100 mg% by Glasgow Coma Scale, San Diego County, California, 1981

| Glasgow Coma Scale | Number of patients | Percent tested | Rate per 100 tested with BAC ≥ 100 mg% |
|---|---|---|---|
| 13 | 137 | 33.6 | 66.7 |
| 14 | 488 | 28.7 | 72.9 |
| 15 | 1777 | 20.1 | 58.3 |
| All "mild" | 2402 | 22.6 | 63.5 |

patients diagnosed with concussion. Data were not available by presence or absence of fractures to the head, but the dollar estimates show increased hospital costs for older as compared to younger patients having similar mild brain injury diagnoses.

The average cost of a paramedic or private ambulance transport in 1981 was about $160, adding about $210,000 to the $6.3 million in hospital costs.

Finally, all but 15 of the 2,435 mild brain injury cases admitted to the hospital were discharged alive without further planned medical contact. All but three of the 2,435 patients had a Glasgow Outcome Scale reading indicative of good recovery.

## DISCUSSION

The mild brain injury incidence rate in San Diego County in 1981 was 131 per 100,000 population. Extending this rate to the approximate population of the United States of 250,000,000 results in an annual incidence figure of about 325,000 cases of mild head injury per year. About half of these cases are caused by motor vehicle crashes, most specifically involving occupants of passenger vehicles. Males have twice the risk of females for mild head injury except for the very young and those past the age of 45, where the excess in rate diminishes. The mild brain injury rate is higher for females as compared with males past the age of 75, owing mostly to fall-related causes.

Table 2–11  Age-Adjusted In-Hospital Treatment Costs for Mild Brain Injuries by Grouped Diagnoses and Length of Hospital Stay, San Diego County, California, 1981

| Length of hospital stay | Concussion | | Other intracranial | | Total | |
|---|---|---|---|---|---|---|
| | Cost (× $1000) | Average ($) per person | Cost (× $1000) | Average ($) per person | Cost (× $1000) | Average ($) per person |
| 0–1 | 647 | 778 | 209 | 1,253 | 856 | 858 |
| 2–7 | 1,512 | 1,766 | 492 | 3,437 | 2,004 | 3,440 |
| 7–14 | 675 | 4,592 | 218 | 8,077 | 893 | 3,260 |
| 14+ | 2,146 | 21,035 | 439 | 36,578 | 2,585 | 22,675 |
| Total | 4,980 | 2,572 | 1,358 | 3,891 | 6,338 | 2,774 |

About half of all mild brain injury cases in the United States occur in persons between the ages of 15 and 34. This excess risk is found not only for mild brain injuries but also for severe and moderate brain injuries. The risk of injury of all kinds in this age group is an important public health problem that deserves far more attention than it currently receives.

Forty percent of all mild brain injury victims were transported to an emergency room in nonemergency vehicles. Although there is no evidence to support a deleterious outcome from this method of emergency transport, one must be concerned about the potential harm that may arise from improper emergency transport, particularly if, in addition to mild brain injuries, damage to other body parts is involved. This practice of emergency transport is most understandable when the victims are infants and small children; their parents, anxious over the perceived delay that may be associated with arrival of emergency treatment, may "scoop and run" the child to the closest emergency room for treatment. As mentioned earlier, the effects on the patient from nonprofessional emergency transport are unknown, particularly among mildly brain-injured patients. Potential harm should, however, be a focus of future research.

Although a substantial proportion of all brain-injured people arrive at the emergency room within one hour of the injury, the fact that 15% of these victims arrive after a delay of three hours or more is of concern and raises questions as to the reasons for such delay. Obviously, if the delays are occasioned by lack of availability of emergency medical transport, then closer scrutiny of the area's emergency medical system is needed. If, on the other hand, the delay is due to lack of perception of importance of the injury, then the approach must be more toward education to ensure that persons with evidence of mild brain injury seek out care sooner. There is no evidence that delays of three or four hours have resulted in any deleterious effects, yet occasionally a mildly brain-injured patient may, in fact, have more serious problems than originally observed (Dacey et al., 1986).

Eighty-five percent of all mildly brain-injured patients seen in hospitals have either a concussion or another intracranial injury. However, 15% of these mildly brain-injured patients with a Glasgow Coma Score of 13–15 were diagnosed as having a contusion, laceration, or hemorrhage of the brain. It may be that the diagnoses for these cases may be incomplete or inaccurate. It is difficult to believe that a patient diagnosed with a GCS of 13 or 14 and with a contusion or hemorrhage would have been discharged from the hospital in two to four days, yet, for purposes of this study, we abstracted verbatim not only the Glasgow Coma Score, but the actual diagnoses as recorded in the medical record. An important finding from this study is not so much the high proportion of concussion-diagnosed injuries, but the more significant proportion of injuries diagnosed as contusion or hemorrhage.

A significant proportion (14%) of hospitalized brain injuries had a diagnosis of "other intracranial injury." This definition lacks specificity, and greater attention to a more accurate clinical and classification description is needed.

This study used the Glasgow Coma Score for gauging brain injury severity. A GCS of 13–15 comprised the mild brain-injury group, yet on the basis of the diagnosis in the medical record and the length of hospital stay (which is subject to fewer vagaries of interpretation), the GCS may not be the most valid and sensitive indicator of a mild brain injury. A careful reexamination of the GCS in light of these findings for this particular group of patients is warranted. Although the outcome at hospital discharge, as measured by the Glasgow Outcome Scale, was almost always good or favorable, for mildly brain-injured patients a more sensitive instrument or measure may be needed because of the growing incidence (Levin, HS, et al., 1987; Levin, HS, and Eisenberg, HM., 1979; Lidvall, H., 1975; McLean, A. et al., 1983; Oppenheimer, R., 1968; Rimel, RW., 1981; Rimel, RW. et al., 1981; Rutherford, W. et al.,1977; Symonds, C., 1962.) of potential long-term deleterious effects in this group of patients. Much more research on this large group of brain-injured patients is needed to resolve the question of effects following mild brain injury.

That only about 28% of persons admitted to a hospital over the age of 15 for mild brain injury were blood-tested for alcohol must seriously compromise the utility of prevalence data on blood alcohol. Despite this shortcoming, it is noteworthy that about two-thirds of those tested had a BAC greater than or equal to 100 mg%—a disturbing proportion. If, in fact, there was no selection bias in those tested or not tested, a patient presenting evidence of mild brain injury must be considered for alcohol involvement. The relationship between the presence of alcohol at these levels and the ability to diagnose or interpret history and findings correctly may be of concern (see Jagger et al.,1984a). Blood alcohol has, of course, been shown in numerous earlier studies to be a risk factor for injury involvement, but also the examining physician must consider that alcohol could significantly interfere with the ability to diagnose even mild brain injury and possibly even interfere with normal recovery, as evidenced from animal data.

If the distribution of mild brain injury by age, diagnosis, and length of stay as determined for San Diego is similar throughout the United States, one can extrapolate from the San Diego County data and show that annual costs for mild brain injury in the United States were slightly over $900 million in 1981. This cost estimate is for hospitalized persons having at least a mild brain injury, but an unknown proportion of these patients may have other nonbrain injuries as well. Surely by 1987, the costs must have exceeded $1 billion, and if one considers the number of persons hospitalized, the length of hospital stay, the potential for future deleterious effects of mild brain injuries, and the cost of treatment, the burden of mild brain injury in the United States cannot be considered trivial. Far more attention must be given not only to preventive strategies but also to the potential for long-term sequelae in this group of patients.

## ACKNOWLEDGMENTS

The authors wish to thank Virginia Hansen for her editorial advice and suggestions. The data for this chapter were made possible by a grant from the Insurance Institute for Highway Safety, Washington, D.C. The opinions, findings, and conclusions expressed in this paper are those of the authors.

## REFERENCES

Annegers JF, Grabow JD, Kurland LT, Laws ER, Jr. The incidence, causes, and secular trends of head trauma in Olmsted County, Minnesota, 1935–1974. Neurology 30:912–919, 1980.

Casey R, Ludwig S, McCormick M. Morbidity following minor head trauma in children. Pediatrics 73:497–502, 1986.

Chadwick O, Rutter M, Brown G, Shaffer D, and Traub M. A prospective study of children with injuries II. Cognitive sequelae. Psychol. Med 11:49–61, 1981.

Dacey RG, Alves WM, Rimel RW, Winn R, Jane JA. Neurosurgical complications after apparently minor head injury. Assessment of risk in a series of 610 patients. J Neurosurg 65:203–210, 1986.

Frankowski RF, Annegers JF, Whitman S. The descriptive epidemiology of head trauma in the United States. *In* Becker D, Povlishock J (eds); Central Nervous System Trauma Status Report—1985. Bethesda, MD: NINCDS, National Institute of Health, 1986.

Gronwall D, Wrightson P. Delayed recovery of intellectual function after minor head injury. Lancet 2:602–609, 1974.

Jagger J, Fife D, Vernberg K, Jane J. Effect of alcohol intoxication on the diagnosis and apparent severity of brain injury. Neurosurgery 15:303–306, 1984a.

Jagger J, Levine JI, Jane JA, Rimel RW. Epidemiologic features of head injury in a predominantly rural population. J Trauma 24:40–44, 1984b.

Jane J, Steward O, Gennarelli T. Axonal degeneration induced by experimental noninvasive minor head injury. J Neurosurg 62:96–100, 1985.

Jennett B, Teasdale G. Management of head injuries. Philadelphia: FA Davis, 1981.

Klonoff H, Low MD, Clark D. Head injuries in children: a prospective five-year follow-up. J Neurol Neurosurg Psychiatry 40:1211–1219, 1977.

Kraus JF, Black MA, Hessol N, Ley P, Rokaw W, Sullivan C, Bowers S, Knowlton S, Marshall L. The incidence of acute brain injury and serious impairment in a defined population. Am J Epidemiol 119:186–201, 1984.

Levin HS, Eisenberg HM. Neuropsychological outcome of closed head injury in children and adolescents. Child's Brain 5:281–292, 1979.

Levin H, Mattis S, Ruff RM, Eisenberg HM, Marshall LF, Tabaddor K, High WM Jr. Neurobehavioral outcome following minor head injury: a three-center study. J Neurosurg 66:234–243, 1987.

Lidvall H. Recovery after minor head injury. Lancet 1:100, 1975.

McLean A, Temkin NR, Dikmen S, Wyler AR. The behavioral sequelae of head injury. J Clin Neuropsychol 5:361–376, 1983.

Oppenheimer R. Microscopic lesions in the brain following head injury. J Neurol Neurosurg Psychiatry 21:299–306, 1968.

Rimel RW. A prospective study of patients with central nervous system trauma. J Neurosurg Nurs 13:132–141, 1981.

Rimel RW, Girodani B, Barth JT, Boll TJ, Jane JA. Disability caused by minor head injury. Neurosurgery 9:221–228, 1981.

Rutherford W, Merrett J, McDonald J. Sequelae of concussion caused by minor head injury. Lancet 1:1–4, 1977.

Symonds C. Concussion and its sequelae. Lancet 1:1–5, 1962.

Whitman S, Coonley-Hoganson R, Desai BT. Comparative head trauma experiences in two socioeconomically different Chicago-area communities—a population study. Am J Epidemiol 119:570–580, 1984.

# 3

# Some International Comparisons

BRYAN JENNETT

Recognition that trauma is now the leading cause of death under the age of 45 and that some three-quarters of accidental deaths are due to head injuries has led to growing awareness over the past decade or so that head injuries constitute a major public health problem. Efforts to reduce mortality have naturally focused on severe injuries, for the management of which new methods of diagnosis (e.g., computerized tomography and magnetic resonance imaging) and of monitoring (of intracranial pressure and electrical activity) have been harnessed. These have led to some improvements in the outcome of the minority of head injuries who develop a surgically significant intracranial hematoma or some other remediable complication. For other severe injuries, various aggressive therapeutic regimes have been developed (e.g., steroids, osmotics, hyperventilation, and barbiturates). There is now reluctant recognition that the gains from these latter developments have been modest, chiefly because a good outcome is largely dependent on the amount of brain damage that has already been sustained by the time a patient reaches a specialist unit.

A substantial reduction in mortality and morbidity from head injuries as a whole therefore seems more likely to be achieved by directing more attention to the large number of injuries that are initially of mild or moderate severity. One goal of such a policy would be to minimize secondary brain damage due to complications that can result in more severe brain damage than was caused initially. The other would be to reduce morbidity from the sequelae of uncomplicated mild injuries. It is, however, much less easy to study mild injuries because they are so common that their care depends on a variety of medical disciplines (Jennett, 1975). Depending on organizational features in different countries, regions, and hospitals the disciplines involved may include emergency room physicians, general and orthopedic surgeons, pediatricians, and neurologists, and also primary-care or family physicians. Neurosurgical complications are rare when seen from the perspective of the vast number of mild injuries that present to these other disciplines. This can lead to the cynical view that the care of the mildly injured is of little significance, because almost all such patients make a satisfactory recovery no matter how *little* is done for them. There is also sometimes a suspicion that even the care of the severely injured may be less important than neurosurgeons claim because many of these patients do badly no matter how *much* is done for them. When reviewing mild injuries, it is therefore important to consider where they fit into the overall pattern of occurrence of trauma—and of mortality and morbidity—in order to determine how resources should be deployed in a comprehensive scheme for the care of all head injuries in a community.

Another problem with studying mild injuries is that of definition. The widespread adoption of the Glasgow Coma Scale has made it easier to classify severe injuries, but it was not intended as a means of distinguishing among different types of milder injury. Many of these patients are oriented by the time they are first assessed and therefore score at the top of the Glasgow scale. Yet some of these patients have had a period of altered consciousness, either witnessed or evidenced by their being amnesic for events immediately following injury. Impairment of consciousness is indicative of *diffuse* brain damage, but there can also be marked *local* damage without either alteration in consciousness or amnesia; this was so for 25% of one large series of patients with compound depressed fractures of the skull vault (Jennett and Miller, 1972). Scalp lacerations are frequent in mildly head-injured patients and may feature in the definition of a head injury when there is no evidence of brain damage.

The International Classification of Diseases (ICD) coding is unhelpful, not only because the terms used are ill-defined but also because there is wide variation in how they are used (Jennett and Teasdale, 1981). Some institutions code most mild injuries as concussion (No. 850); others prefer "unspecified intracranial injury" (No. 854); yet others use "unqualified skull fracture" (No. 803) without any serious regard to whether or not a fracture was diagnosed. The inclusion of patients with injuries limited to the face inflates some statistics.

Data are available in most places only for patients who were admitted to hospital. This was so for the four American studies reviewed in Chapter 2 as well as for that in Chapter 6; also for the studies in the Bronx (Cooper et al., 1983) and in three metropolitan U.S. counties (Frankowski, Annegers, and Whitman, 1985); also for the Australian surveys (Trauma Subcommittee, 1986) and for that conducted in Edinburgh (Miller and Jones, 1985). In the United States attempts have been made to discover the number of head-injured patients who are not hospitalized, by means of household surveys and by scrutiny of some emergency room records (Kalsbeek, McLaurin, Harris et al., 1980). Best estimates are that 20–40% of head-injured patients in the United States do not seek medical care but that 50–60% of those attending hospital are admitted (Frankowski et al., 1985). A survey of emergency-room attenders in one Vancouver hospital 20 years ago showed, however, that only one in five was admitted (Klonoff and Thompson, 1969)—the same proportion as in the survey of Scotland (Strang et al., 1978).

The Scottish Head Injury Management Study included all attenders and admissions, as well as deaths before hospital and secondary transfers to neurosurgery (Jennett and MacMillan, 1981). In that it takes account of all head injuries of all severities within a community, it is the only comprehensive study published thus far. The original Scottish survey for 1974 has been repeated for 1985; these two surveys, together with a number of studies in individual hospitals in the United Kingdom, make data available for many thousands of injuries managed in a health care system that allows equity of access for the whole population, subject only to the constraints of local geography. Recognizing that causes, clinical features, risk of complications, and management are different in children, the Scottish data have recently been analyzed separately for adults and children (aged 14 years or less).

## ATTENDERS AT ACCIDENT/EMERGENCY DEPARTMENTS IN SCOTLAND

Of more than 12,000 cases studied (Brookes et al., in press; Strang et al., 1978) 44% were under age 15; scalp lacerations occurred in 42%, being equally common in children and adults. Between 50% and 60% of adults and children had a skull x-ray in the accident department which showed a fracture in about 3% of each age group. Evidence of brain damage was found in 20% of all cases (26% of adults and 12% of children). Only 5% still had altered consciousness on arrival at the emergency department, but another 15% had recovered from an episode of altered consciousness. About 18% of all attenders were admitted to hospital, the rate being higher for adults (23%) than for children (11%). Attendance rates (per $10^5$ population) varied with age, sex, and cause (Table 3-1).

Evidence of recent ingestion of alcohol was noted in 22% of adult attenders at emergency departments after head injury in Scotland (Strang et al.,

**Table 3-1**  Attendance at Accident/Emergency
Departments (rate per $10^5$ population, Scotland, 1974)

|            | All causes | Road accident | Assaults |
|------------|-----------|---------------|----------|
| All cases  | 1778      | 314           | 244      |
| Males      | 2591      | 415           | 405      |
| Females    | 1024      | 216           | 94       |
| Age <15 yr | 3017      | 265           | 94       |
| 15–24 yr   | 2359      | 523           | 775      |
| 25–64 yr   | 1184      | 298           | 275      |
| ≥65 yr     | 829       | 202           | 12       |

*Source:* Jennett and MacMillan (1981).

1978). It was more commonly found after falls (53%) and assaults (34%) than after road accidents (16%); and it was recorded more than twice as often in injured pedestrians (26%) as in vehicle occupants (10%).

## CRITERIA FOR ADMISSION

It is no surprise that the percentage of admitted head injury cases that were classified as mild varied greatly in the American series reviewed in Chapter 2. The reason is that some of these series came from neurosurgical units and therefore included some secondary referrals from other hospitals. However, policies for *primary* admission to hospital also vary widely, making classification by admission an administrative rather than a biological definition of severity. Evidence for this is the much greater variation in death rates than in admission rates per unit of population both within and between countries, as reflected in the ratio of admissions to deaths (Table 3–2). The death rate for city blacks in Chicago most closely approaches the Australian rate, whereas that for the suburban whites in Chicago approaches the U.K. rate. Whether the striking difference between the admission/death ratios in the United States and the United Kingdom indicates that fewer mild injuries occur in the United States, or that fewer of these patients are admitted, cannot be determined because there are no U.S. data for the number of patients who came to hospital but were not admitted in those places from which series of admitted patients have been reported.

What is certain is that the incidence of serious injuries varies widely between countries, as reflected in deaths from head injuries; these tend to parallel variations in the death rates from all kinds of injuries ascribed to motor vehicle accidents (Jennett and Teasdale, 1981). However, as road accidents are

**Table 3–2**   Frequency of Head Injury in Various Cities and Countries

|  | Reference | Deaths/ $10^5$ | Admissions/ $10^5$ | Admissions/ deaths ratio |
|---|---|---|---|---|
| United States | Frankowski et al., 1985 | 25 | 200 | 8 |
| Olmstead | Annegers et al., 1980 | 22 | 193 | 9 |
| Bronx | Cooper et al., 1983 | 27 | 249 | 9 |
| San Diego | Kraus et al., 1984 | 30 | 180 | 6 |
| Virginia | Jagger et al., 1984 | 25 | 208 | 8 |
| Chicago | Whitman et al., 1984 |  |  |  |
| City black |  | 32 | 403 | 13 |
| Suburban black |  | 19 | 394 | 21 |
| Suburban white |  | 11 | 196 | 18 |
| Australia | Trauma Subcommittee, 1986 | 28 | 377 | 14 |
| England | Jennett and MacMillan, 1981 | 9 | 270 | 30 |
| Scotland | Jennett and MacMillan, 1981 | 9 | 313 | 35 |

much less dominant as a cause of less severe injuries, it may be that the incidence of head injuries at the two ends of the severity scale do vary independently. Another important variable is the different way that physicians in most countries deal with less severe injuries as compared with those in the United States: In the latter, both neurosurgeons and CT scanners are much more numerous and more widely distributed; moreover, a much larger proportion of the patients admitted to hospital after head injury are treated in a neurosurgical service. Furthermore, in many U.S. hospitals neurosurgical staff are available also to advise about doubtful cases in the emergency room (ER) and they may have the confidence to release some patients whom an ER physician would have admitted for observation. Cost is another possible disincentive to admission to the United States, because many of the mildly injured are underprivileged members of the community who may have inadequate insurance coverage.

In Europe and Australia, however, most head-injured patients are admitted initially to a general or community hospital; even where there is a neurosurgical unit in the hospital of first admission, in many hospitals all but the most severely injured first go to another surgical service, to emergency medicine, to pediatrics or—in some continental and Scandinavian countries—to neurology. In such a system, the management of mild and moderate head injuries poses a problem of triage, both for CT scanning and for neurosurgical consultation; where emergency scanning is available only at regional "neuro centres," these two aspects of triage coincide. In either event, referral often means transfer to another hospital by ambulance. If clinical deterioration has already occurred, suggesting an intracranial hematoma, then the hazards of delay and of transporting a patient in coma must be balanced with the limited prospects of success if the skull is opened by a local surgeon not trained in neurosurgery. Such operations are still not uncommon in some European countries and in parts of Australia.

In Britain, however, it is widely accepted that arrangements for the care of the mildly and moderately injured should be directed toward early identification of patients at risk of developing intracranial hematoma as well as of those with open injuries who are at risk of infection. The aim is to ensure the transfer of such patients to specialized facilities before complications have become evident, or at least as soon as there is any suspicion. That, in turn puts a premium on the identification of patients who are at risk—recognizing that these patients are only a small minority of those admitted to hospital and a tiny proportion of those who present at emergency rooms. It is, however, the fear of these complications that leads to the admission of large numbers of the mildly injured to hospital, even in Britain where resources for hospital care are more restricted than in many countries. The majority of these patients are discharged within 48 hours, but in aggregate they represent a considerable call on scarce resources, competing for beds that could be deployed with more benefit for the care of other patients. Moreover, patients unnecessarily admitted and their families are put to needless inconvenience (and often some expense); the admission of young children adds to the emotional trauma caused by injury the stress of separation from parents.

## ADMISSIONS TO HOSPITAL IN VARIOUS SERIES

There is no longer a shortage of data on head-injured patients admitted to hospital in various places. The difficulty is to compare like with like in regard to the source of the cases. Some are from what the Scottish study called "primary surgical wards" (PSWs), others are from neurosurgical units (NSU), and still others are from units that serve both purposes. The mix of cases in any service depends on local resources and policies. In most of the United Kingdom, only the more severe injuries are treated in NSUs—about 5% of all admitted injuries for the country as a whole. It is therefore in PSWs that the mild cases are found in Britain. In the United States, many mildly injured patients are admitted to NSUs, but the plurality of the health care system, with many hospitals competing in urban areas, means that few units can claim to have a population-based series of patients. Perhaps the two most comparable units on opposite sides of the Atlantic that have published surveys are each atypical of their own countries: the NSUs in Charlottesville, Virginia and in Edinburgh, Scotland. That in Charlottesville serves a mixed urban and rural area of northern Virginia, in which it is almost a monopoly supplier of neurosurgery (Jagger et al., 1984). All but the most trivial injuries are referred there, as well as more serious injuries from a wider population. The Edinburgh NSU is almost unique among U.K. NSUs in that it accepts all head-injured patients admitted from the accident department of the Edinburgh Royal Infirmary which deals with almost all trauma in that city (Miller and Jones, 1985). But in each of these two units, 15% of admissions are transfers of more seriously injured from further afield. By contrast, the Glasgow NSU takes only patients who have already been admitted to one of the 21 general hospitals in its catchment area (population ca. 2.7 million). Two-thirds come from the city of Glasgow, and the rest are from a wide area including the islands off the west coast of Scotland.

A further problem is the lack of uniformity in the definitions used in different reports. Even children cannot be identified by a consistent upper age limit. Severity of injury is increasingly classified by the Glasgow Coma Scale (GCS). Several recent American reports have been limited to patients whose GCS was $\geq 13$ on admission, and other reports have defined "moderately severe" injuries as those with a GCS score of 9–12. European reports include all the cases admitted, but a high proportion of these are mild.

Features that are available for a number of series are summarized in Table 3–3). In several series, over 80% of all hospital admissions were mild (GCS $\geq$ 13). In the Scottish PSW series, 82% were at this level by the time they were admitted—commonly at least a couple of hours after injury; but 44% had had altered consciousness from which they had recovered (Jennett and MacMillan, 1981). Only 55% of the patients in the NSUs in Virginia and Glasgow had GCS $\geq 13$ on arrival at those units; however, for most patients, that would be several hours after injury. But by then, some patients would have deteriorated as a result of raised intracranial pressure (ICP) and cerebral compression. In each of these units between one-fifth and one-quarter of patients had GCS $\leq 8$, whereas only 5% of admissions in Edinburgh and Norway comprised severely

**Table 3–3** Distribution of Severity and Clinical Features of Head-Injured Patients Admitted in Various Countries

| | Minnesota | San Diego | Virginia | Edinburgh | Scotland | Liverpool | Norway | Glasgow |
|---|---|---|---|---|---|---|---|---|
| Kind of unit | PSW | NSU | NSU | NSU | PSW | PSW | PSW/NSU | NSU |
| Selection | ≥13 | ≥13 | ≥13 | All | All | All | All | All |
| N | 333 | 2,435 | 610 | 1,919 | 1,181 | 11,837 | 1,220 | 572 |
| Age | | | | | | | | |
| <15 years | — | 26% | — | — | 36% | — | 31% | 24% |
| <20 years | 42% | 41% | — | — | 56% | | | |
| Road accident | 56% | 42% | 58% | 29% | 34% | 34% | 49% | 34% |
| EC injury | 19% | — | — | 20% | 16% | 16% | 16% | 13% |
| Skull fracture | 13% | 10% | 11% | 14% | 7% | 7% | 16% | 57% |
| Glasgow Coma Scale | | | | | | | | |
| 15 (of adm.) | | 61% | 48% | 80% | 80% | | | |
| ≥ 13 (of adm.) | 79% | 82% | 55% | 84% | | | | |
| ≤ 8 | | | 21% | 5% | 3% | | 5% | 24% |
| IC hematoma | 2% | 0.9% | 0.8% | 4% | 1% | | 4% | 34% |
| Hospital stay < 2 days | | 43% | 73% | 68% | 81% | 67% | 49% | 30% |

*Abbreviations:* adm, admissions; EC, extracranial; IC, intracranial; NSU, neurosurgical unit; PSW, primary surgical ward.

*Sources:* Minnesota: Fischer et al. (1981); San Diego: Kraus et al. (1984); Virginia: Jagger et al. (1984); Edinburgh: Miller and Jones (1985); Scotland: Jennett and MacMillan (1981); Liverpool: Jones and Jeffreys (1982); Norway: Edna (1983), Edna and Cappelen (1984); Glasgow: Jennett et al. (1979).

injured patients. Skull fractures were recorded in 7–16% of cases, except for the Glasgow unit where 57% had skull fractures. This difference reflects the policy in Glasgow of giving priority to the transfer of patients suspected of having an intracranial hematoma: 34% in that series had an operation for this complication. In other series the hematoma rate ranged from less than 1% to 4%. A major extracranial injury was recorded in 13–20% of cases in various series. Between about half and three-quarters of patients were discharged from hospital within two days. However, in the Glasgow unit, only one-third left as soon as this, and then it was often to return to their original hospital for further care as inpatients.

## AGE OF OCCURRENCE AND CAUSES OF MILD INJURIES

Children (<15 years) comprise a larger proportion of mild than severe injuries. They accounted for more than 40% of Scottish attenders, but for only about a third of admissions to hospital, a quarter of NSU transfers, and a fifth of severe injuries. In the three American series of admissions, road accidents accounted for 58%, 56%, and 42% of mild injuries whereas in Europe they accounted for 25–33% of all injuries. In the Scottish survey, road accidents were the precipitating factor for only 18% of attenders, but they accounted for 36% of cases admitted and 55% of severe injuries. Road accidents accounted for only 9% of attending children compared with 24% of adults. Sixty-six percent of children attending after road accidents were pedestrians and only 20% were car occupants, compared with 18% and 72%, respectively, for adults. Falls and assaults each accounted for about 20% of attenders, falls being more common in younger children and in adults over 65; assaults were more frequent in younger adults.

## COMPLICATIONS AFTER MILD INJURY

Less than 1% of mildly injured patients develop an intracranial hematoma, and about half that number present with a compound depressed fracture; a few others have dural tear of the base, and a few will develop raised ICP without having a clot. These proportions are so small that from the viewpoint of the emergency room or primary surgical ward it may seem as if time and resources are often wasted on the management of mild head injuries. There is indeed evidence that unnecessary admissions are common in some places, and that plain skull x-rays and CT scans are also overused by some physicians. Nevertheless, because mild injuries are so numerous they represent in aggregate a considerable proportion of complications, poor outcome, and prolonged hospital stay. Analysis of the Edinburgh series shows that injuries classified as mild on admission accounted for 72% of depressed fractures, for 30% each of cranial operations and of major complications in ICU, for 43% of patients who were vegetative or severely disabled on discharge, and for 48% of patients who stayed in hospital for more than one week.

The Glasgow NSU depends wholly on secondary referrals, but an analysis has been done on the initial severity of patients operated on for depressed fracture or for intracranial hematoma. Of 359 patients with compound depressed fractures, 44% were reported never to have lost consciousness (Jennett and Miller, 1972), and in a series of 825 cases 25% had no posttraumatic amnesia (PTA) at all. Because of the well-being of these patients (they were fully alert and had no focal signs), it is easy to overlook the significance of what can appear to be an innocent scalp laceration, especially since half the attenders at emergency departments who are sent home have a scalp laceration (Strang et al., 1978). Analysis of more than 1,000 cases of operated supratentorial hematomas in Glasgow shows that 57% of these patients had talked at some time after injury; 49% had GCS ≥ 13 when first seen; and 26% were reported to have been completely lucid at some stage (Teasdale and Murray, personal communication). However, only 15% of patients were found to have both an initially mild brain injury and no skull fracture; such a combination was twice as common in children with hematomas as in adults.

## MANAGEMENT OF MILD INJURIES

The frequency of occurrence of mild injuries makes it inevitable that the initial care of these patients will be widely dispersed within the health care system. Because so few of them develop complications, it would be wasteful of resources to advocate that all should have certain diagnostic procedures or that a large proportion should be admitted for observation, let alone be transferred to a neurosurgical service. Such policies would also precipitate needless inconvenience and anxiety in patients and their relatives, particularly since almost half of the mildly injured are children. As with most clinical decision-making, it is a question of balancing risks. Some clinicians are so fearful of the consequences of overlooking the possibility that an intracranial hematoma might develop—and of the probable delay in its diagnosis and treatment if the patient were to deteriorate at home—that they insist on admitting all patients who have been briefly unconscious or who have demonstrated even a few minutes of amnesia. Almost two-thirds of admissions and one-third of occupied bed days attributed to head-injured patients in primary surgical wards in Scotland were for patients who were fully alert and without neurological signs when admitted; and none had an extracranial injury that would have required admission (Jennett and MacMillan, 1981). No doubt some of these admissions were justified by the lack of any caring relative or by some other social or medical uncertainty, but the scale of this apparent misuse of resources is considerable.

Indications for admission was one topic addressed by a nationally representative group of neurosurgeons in the United Kingdom who met to devise guidelines for the initial management of adult head injuries. Other topics include indications for skull x-ray, for CT scanning and for neurosurgical consultation and transfer (Group of Neurosurgeons, 1984). Hospitals that have adopted these guidelines report significant reductions in admission rates (Brocklehurst et al., 1987; Miller and Jones, 1985; Weston, 1981). Chiefly this results from following the advice that it is safe to send home a patient who has been briefly unconscious or who has only a few minutes of PTA, provided that (1) a skull fracture has not been shown on x-ray, and that (2) there is a responsible person at home to whom a head injury instruction sheet can be given.

The basis for this advice is a statistical analysis of the risk factors for the development of an intracranial hematoma by Mendelow et al. (1983). This showed that the presence of skull fracture in a mildly injured patient is of much greater significance than a history of brief unconsciousness or a brief period of posttraumatic amnesia. The risk of hematoma is greater after a fall than after a high-velocity road accident, and it is two to three times greater in adults than in children. Guidelines for the management of children are being developed, and these will have to take account of the occurrence of the *pediatric concussion syndrome*. This comprises a rapid but temporary deterioration in conscious level, sometimes associated with signs of brainstem dysfunction; it is said to occur in about 15% of mildly injured children who are admitted to hospital (Snoek, Minderhoud, and Wilmink, 1984). There is, however, considerable disagreement among American pediatricians about the indications for observation in hospital after mild injuries (Dershewitz, Kaye, and Swisher, 1983).

Policies for the management of mild injuries should reflect local health care resources as well as geographical and social considerations. The much wider availability of neurosurgeons to consult in emergency rooms in the United States, as well as the tenfold greater number of CT scanners in that country, makes for a very different situation from that in Europe (Jennett, 1987), where skull x-rays are still important in triage both for scanning and for referral to regional neurosurgical units. Whether freely available CT scanners in community hospitals is necessarily beneficial without skilled neuroradiologists or neurosurgeons being ready to interpret the scans and to act on the findings remains to be established. It is of interest to Europeans to read about proposals in the United States to have more strictly regionalized centers for neurotrauma where skilled teams are available around the clock—in essence, the European pattern (American College of Surgeons, 1986; Smith 1986). Such a system requires clearly elaborated policies that are agreed upon by primary doctors and neurosurgeons, and that are expressed in the form of guidelines that all personnel can understand. There is already evidence that changing clinical policies can reduce infection rates after depressed fractures (Sande et al., 1980) and also death and disability from acute intracranial hematoma (Teasdale et al., 1982). Probably the best way to reduce avoidable mortality and morbidity from mild and moderate head injuries is to agree on protocols for the investigation and treatment of commonly occurring conditions such as these.

## REFERENCES

Prepared by the Joint Section on Trauma of the Association of Neurological Surgeons (AANS) and the Congess of Neurological Sugeons (CNS) and endoresed by the AANS Board of Directors and the CNS Executive Committee. Appendix 1 of the hospital resource document: Planning neurotrauma care. Am College Surg Bull 71 (10):22–23, 1986.

Annegers JF, Grabow JD, Kurland LT, Laws ER Jr. The incidence, causes, and secular trends of head trauma in Olstead County, Minnesota. Neurology (Minn) 30:912–919, 1980.

Brocklehurst G, Gooding M, James G. Comprehensive care of patients with head injuries. Br Med J 194:345–347, 1987.

Brookes M, MacMillan R, Cully S, Anderson E. Head injuries in Scottish accident/ emergency departments: how different are children from adults? Scott Med J 34 (in press).

Cooper KD, Tabbador K, Hauser WA, Sulman K, Feiner C, Factor PR. The epidemiology of head injury in the Bronx. Neuroepidemiology 2:70–88, 1983.

Dershewitz RA, Kaye BA, Swisher CN. Treatment of children with posttraumatic transient loss of consciousness. Pediatrics 72:602–607, 1983.

Edna T-H. Risk factors in traumatic head injury. Acta Neurochir (Wien) 69:15–21, 1983.

Edna T-H, Cappelen J. Hospital admitted head injury: a prospective study in Trondelag, Norway, 1979–80. Scand J Soc Med 12:7–14, 1984.

Fischer RP, Carlson J, Perry JF. Postconcussive hospital observation of alert patients in a primary trauma center. J Trauma 21:920–924, 1981.

Frankowski, RF. Descriptive epidemiologic studies of head injury in the United States: 1974–1984. Basel: Karger Adv Psychosom Med 16:153–172, 1986.

Frankowski RF, Annegers JF, Whitman S. The descriptive epidemiology of head trauma in the United States. In Becker DP, Povlishock JT (eds), Central Nervous System Trauma Status Report. Bethesda: NINCDS, National Institutes of Health, 1985.

Group of Neurosurgeons. Guidelines for initial management after head injury in adults. Br Med J 288:983–985, 1984.

Jagger J, Levine JI, Jane JA, Rimel RW. Epidemiologic features of head injury in a predominantly rural population. J Trauma 24:40–44, 1984.

Jennett B. Who cares for head injuries? Br Med J 3:267–270, 1975.

Jennett B. Skull x-rays after mild head injuries. Arch Emerg Med 4:133–135, 1987.

Jennett B, MacMillan R. Epidemiology of head injury. Br Med J 282:101–104, 1981.

Jennett B, Miller JD. Infection after depressed fracture of skull: implications for management of nonmissile injuries. J Neurosurg 36:333–339, 1972.

Jennett B, Teasdale G. Management of Head Injuries. Philadelphia: FA Davis, 1981.

Jennett B, Murray A, Carlin J, et al. Head injuries in three Scottish neurosurgical units. Br Med J 2:955–958, 1979.

Jones JJ, Jeffreys RV. Head injury patients admitted to general hospitals in Merseyside. Injury 14:483–488, 1982.

Kalsbeek WD, McLaurin RL, Harris BSH, et al. The national head and spinal cord injury survey: major findings. J Neurosurg [Suppl] 53(Nov):S19–S31, 1980.

Klonoff H, Thompson GB. Epidemiology of head injuries in adults. Can Med Assoc J 100:235–241, 1969.

Kraus JF, Black MA, Hessol N, et al. The incidence of acute brain injury and serious impairment in a defined population. Am J Epidemiol 119:186–201, 1984.

Mendelow AD, Teasdale G, Jennett B, et al. Risks of intracranial haematoma in head injured adults. Br Med J 287:1173–1176, 1983.

Miller JD, Jones PA. The work of a regional head injury service. Lancet 1:1141–1144, 1985.

Sande GM, Galbraith SL, McLatchie G. Infection after depressed fracture in the West of Scotland. Scott Med J 25:227–229, 1980.

Smith RW. California Association of Neurological Surgeons' emergency series committee report: Guidelines for establishment of trauma centers. J Neurosurg 65:569–571, 1986.

Snoek JW, Minderhoud JM, Wilmink JT. Delayed deterioration following mild head injury in children. Brain 107:15–36, 1984.

Strang I, MacMillan R, Jennett B. Head injuries in accident and emergency departments at Scottish hospitals. Injury 10:154–159, 1978.

Teasdale G, Galbraith S, Murray L, et al. Management of traumatic intracranial haematoma. Br Med J 285:1695–1697, 1982.

Teasdale G, Murray L. Intracranial haematomas. (personal communication)

Trauma Subcommittee of the neurosurgical society of Australasia. Neurotrauma in Australia (Report on Surveys). Aust NZ J Surg [Suppl], 1986.

Weston PAM. Admission policy for patients following head injury. Br J Surg 68:633–634, 1981.

Whitman S, Coonley-Hoganson R, Desai BT. Comparative head trauma experience in two socioeconomically different Chicago-area communities: a population study. Am J Epidemiol 119:570–80, 1984.

# II
# Experimental Models and Neuropathology

# 4

# Morphopathological Change Associated with Mild Head Injury

JOHN T. POVLISHOCK
AND THOMAS H. COBURN

There is evidence that minor and moderate head injuries are associated with structural change in various foci throughout the brain. Because such changes are likely to contribute to the ensuing neurological or behavioral abnormalities, they merit consideration. Identification of the cellular and subcellular substrates involved could shed light on the specific vulnerability, reactive capacity, and regenerative capability of various elements of the involved brain tissue. An appreciation of the brain's cellular response to minor and moderate injury would be of more than mere academic interest: Once the cellular changes and reorganization are characterized, strategies aimed at blunting, reversing, or augmenting specific traumatically induced cellular responses could be devised.

Although the need for studies in this area cannot be disputed, it seems unlikely that the technology currently available will allow direct investigation of such issues in humans sustaining minor and moderate head injury. As mild head injuries are not associated with any significant mortality, there are no routine postmortem studies that provide insight into the neuropathological (structural) sequelae of the traumatic episode. Moreover, in vivo imaging studies have not achieved the level of resolution that is needed to address the question of cellular change. For these reasons, research must be confined to experimental animals, which are subjected to minor or moderate head injury and then sacrificed in order to identify the brain's cellular response to injury and to characterize its progression and/or resolution over time.

As in the study of any disease process, animal modeling of a human condition always labors under various constraints. The typical acceleration/deceleration head injury so commonly sustained by a human in a vehicular accident is obviously difficult to replicate faithfully in animal models. Interspecies differences in neuraxis alignment, brain mass, skull thickness, and brain geometry are among the many confounding variables confronting those actively involved in the study of animal models of human head injury. Despite these rather formidable obstacles, however, advances have been made in animal modeling. At present, two specific animal models have gained widespread acceptance as providing insight into some of those features seen in head-injured humans. The angular acceleration model employed in subhuman primates and the fluid-percussion model employed primarily in cats have been shown to replicate many of the important features seen in head-injured humans, particularly those who have sustained severe head injury. Using the angular acceleration model with baboons, several investigators affiliated with the University of Pennsylvania have shown that in the case of severe head injury associated with prolonged posttraumatic coma, diffuse axonal damage constitutes a major neural cellular response which probably contributes to the genesis of coma, via the attendant disconnection of various projectional and associational fiber systems (Gennarelli et al., 1982). Because comparable axonal changes have also been described in comatose patients whose clinical course was uncomplicated by mass lesions (Adams et al., 1982), the inference can be drawn that those changes seen in subhuman primate model faithfully replicate those changes seen in head-injured humans. In this same model, minor head injury has been shown to elicit axon terminal and preterminal degeneration within the brainstem (Jane et al., 1985). Although not precisely mimicking the limited axonal damage described in isolated case reports of minor head injury (Peerless and Rewcastle, 1967; Oppenheimer, 1968), the finding of some form of axonal change in both subhuman primates and humans again suggests that the animal model replicates many of the features of the human condition.

Similar to those observations made in the baboon, experimental studies using the cat fluid-percussion model of experimental brain injury have described many of those neural changes described above in relation to head-injured humans. Again, with severe, moderate, and even minor head injury, axonal change comparable to that described for head-injured humans has been observed (Povlishock and Becker 1985; Povlishock and Kontos, 1985; Povlishock et al., 1983). Although such axonal change was confined to the brainstem and lacked the more global distribution common to human head injury, the repertoire of axonal responses so mimicked the human situation that, indeed, this fluid-percussion model in cat is also envisioned to replicate the human condition.

It is thus apparent that animal models can replicate many of the features of human head injury. In such models, as in head-injured humans, the occurrence of axonal damage throughout the neuraxis has been recognized as a consistent feature of severe, moderate, and even minor head injury, with the overall number of damaged (reactive) axons increasing with the severity of the respective injury. Therefore, considerable significance has been assigned to both occurrence and overall magnitude of the traumatically induced axonal damage. It has been assumed that with injury, the shear and tensile forces associated with the traumatic event physically tear axons, causing them to retract and expel a ball of axoplasm, resulting in the formation of a reactive axonal swelling commonly termed a *retraction ball* (Gennarelli et al., 1982; Strich, 1961). Although this concept is of interest, it is also disquieting, in that it implies that *any* injury, even the most minor, causes some immediate and irrevocable axonal damage which would preclude any therapeutic strategy aimed at blunting its occurrence or potential reactive capacity.

In the following passages, we review our experience in the cat fluid-percussion model of experimental brain injury, with emphasis on the morphopathological consequences of minor to moderate injury. Particular attention is focused upon the genesis of the axonal damage accompanying such injuries in order to test the correctness of the assumption that axons are physically torn at the moment of impact in minor to moderate injury. In this context, not only do we consider axonal damage in minor to moderate head injury, but also we explore the predilection for other forms of brain parenchymal or vascular change which may accompany and interact with the observed axonal abnormalities. We also discuss the potential for posttraumatic parenchymal rearrangement and recovery, in order to determine if the observed axonal damage signals irreversible damage or rather sets the stage for neuroplastic/regenerative changes that allow for neuronal rearrangement and possible recovery.

Through such an approach, we hope, first, to provide a possible scenario of the structural changes that occur in humans sustaining minor to moderate injuries and, second, to determine the anatomical substrates underlying both posttraumatic functional abnormality and their potential for long-term reorganization and recovery.

## AXONAL DAMAGE ACCOMPANYING MINOR TO MODERATE INJURY

We employed a cat fluid-percussion model of traumatic brain injury to assess the genesis of axonal damage with minor to moderate injury (Povlishock et al., 1979; Sullivan et al., 1976). The model essentially entails the preparation of a barbituate-anesthetized cat for placement of a 11-mm injury shaft over the midline intact dura. The hollow injury shaft is connected to a transducer which is confluent with a fluid-filled reservoir closed by a plunger mounted on O-rings. By impacting the plunger with a predetermined force, one creates a hydraulic pressure transient which impacts against the cat's intact dura, thereby eliciting a brief elastic deformation of the brain. For the purpose of inducing minor to moderate traumatic brain injuries, the pressure transient is kept between 1 and 2.4 atm and is allowed to persist for only 18–22 msec. Such brief pressure transients typically produce a typical physiological concussive response, reflected in the occurrence of transient hypertension, EEG suppression, and apnea. Posttraumatic behavioral observations were not performed because, in the interest of humane management, the animals were maintained under prolonged barbituate anesthesia; nevertheless, past experience with this model suggests that injuries in the range employed are associated with profound behavioral suppression. In previously reported studies, animals that are subjected to inhalation anesthesia which is withdrawn following injury manifest various functional abnormalities (DeSalles et al., 1987). In general, the injury produces a brief areflexia, characterized by brief reflex paralysis, and hypotonia of postural muscles and suppression of postural motor responses. While recovering from this flaccid unresponsive state, the animals pass through a transitional stuporous state during which they are relatively inattentive to external stimuli. This period of behavioral suppression never exceeds five minutes, and by 20 minutes all animals are able to walk and vocalize in response to tail shock. All animals receiving such injuries fully recover within 24 hours and display no persistent neurological or behavioral abnormalities. Additionally, postmortem examination of their brains reveals no macroscopic damage. No evidence of contusion, laceration, or intraparenchymal hemorrhage is found, and overall, the brains appear unremarkable, with the presence of occasional limited subarachnoid blood constituting the only form of macroscopic change.

To assess to genesis of axonal damage in such animals, we have, to date, employed multiple strategies employing the anterograde axoplasmic transport of various tracers to determine the potential for traumatically induced axonal damage (Povlishock and Becker, 1985; Povlishock et al., 1983). The rationale of such an approach was based upon the recognition, in the peripheral nervous system, that various axonal insults impair axoplasmic transport (Griffin et al., 1977; Martinez and Friede, 1970). Thus, it appeared reasonable to consider this possibility in the case of traumatic brain injury. To this end, various protein tracers were employed to label anterogradely the major cerebral cortical and cerebellar efferents in injured animals at various time points following injury. Some animals were studied in the early posttraumatic period (minutes to days following injury), whereas other animals were followed over a prolonged posttraumatic course (one week to three months following injury). At the end of the designated survival period, the animals were anesthetized and perfused with aldehydes, and their brains were sectioned on a vibratome. The brain sections were reacted for visualization of the anterogradely transported protein and evaluated at both the light and transmission electron microscopic levels.

Through such an approach, we recognized that both minor and moderate traumatic brain injury consistently evoked focal axonal damage within the labeled cortical and cerebellar efferents as they coursed through the brainstem, and that within 12–24 hours of the traumatic event, reactive swellings or (retraction balls) could be seen. However, contrary to the previously held belief that axons are torn with injury, no evidence for tearing could be found in any of the innumerable sections examined. Rather, it appeared that with minor to moderate injury there occurred either focal compression or stretching of axons with the generation of a focal axolemmal abnormality. Over time (i.e., one to three hours post injury), through a mechanism as yet undetermined, this focal axolemmal abnormality was associated with a focal pooling of tracers, reflecting an impairment of anterograde axoplasmic transport. This led to a local accumulation of organelles and axoplasm, with the result that the axon focally

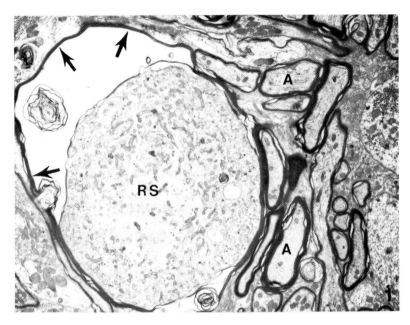

**Figure 4-1** In this electron micrograph, a reactive swelling (RS) laden with organelles and encompassed by a myelin sheath (arrows) is seen 24 hours after minor injury. Note that despite the presence of this reactive axon, the adjacent axons (A) and related brain parenchyma appear unremarkable. Magnification, ×5,000.

swelled. With continued survival, the axon displayed further focal swelling, which progressed to focal lobulation and segmentation, ultimately leading to frank separation of the proximal swollen segment from the distal swelling. By 12 hours, the proximal swelling was entirely detached from the more distal segment (Figures 4-1 and 4-2). In a majority of cases, it was covered completely by a myelin investment that involved a coalesence of the overlying myelin sheath (Figure 4-1). However, when the focal insult involved a nodal region, devoid of a myelin investment, the proximal swelling protruded into the parenchyma without any encompassing myelin (Figure 4-2). Since by 12–24 hours a swollen axoplasmic mass had formed and detached from the more distal axonal segment, it was clear that the swollen proximal axonal segment seen at this time constituted the retraction ball of classical description. Thus, the actual genesis of the reactive swelling or retraction ball involved progressive posttraumatic change rather than an immediate tearing of the axon with an extrusion of its mass. The correctness of such a hypothesis is supported indirectly by limited human data, which suggest that an individual must survive for 12 hours post injury before retraction balls can be found (Pilz, 1983), thus demonstrating that in humans also, similar evolving/progressive axonal change occurs.

The precise factors related to the genesis of such axonal damage are unknown; however, the fact that large-caliber long-tract decussating axons are

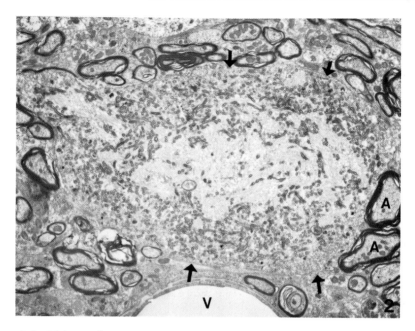

**Figure 4–2**   This reactive axon, outlined here by arrows, lacks any myelin investment. Once again, note that despite the presence of this reactive axon the surrounding brain parenchyma and vasculature (V) appear unaltered. Magnification, ×5,000.

preferentially vulnerable to injury suggests that either stretching or compression of such axons initiates the observed axonal changes. In this scenario, long-tract axons, traveling throughout the neuraxis, would most likely be stretched or compressed by the insult, with maximal stretching or compression occurring at a focal point along an axon's length. At such a focus, it is speculated that the axolemma is maximally stretched, causing alterations in its integrity and/or permeability, thereby allowing the influx of various normally extracellularly confined ions. With the influx of such ions—in particular, calcium—it is conceivable that local abnormalities in microtubular and neurofilament stability ensue, leading to focal impairment of axoplasmic transport (Lasek and Hoffman, 1976). Such impairment, over time, could lead to organelle accumulation, focal axolemmal collapse, and ultimately formation of an enlarged axonal swelling which becomes detached from the more distal axon cylinder.

Although the above scenario is speculative, it does appear quite consistent with the observations made in regard to that axonal change seen following experimental minor to moderate injury. Admittedly, much remains to be clarified regarding the causal factors underlying this axonal damage; yet the fact remains that because these events are progressive and require several hours to culminate in frank axonal detachment, there exists a posttraumatic time frame in which some therapy aimed at blunting or reversing this progression could be initiated. It is hoped that future therapeutic strategies aimed at blocking or blunting this progression of axonal change will be devised.

## LOCAL AND DISTANT PARENCHYMAL RESPONSES TO THE TRAUMATICALLY INDUCED AXONAL DAMAGE

Given that the above-described reactive axonal changes are a consistent feature of minor to moderate injury, the obvious question arises as to whether such injury involves only focal axonal injury with sparing of other focally related brain parenchymal elements, or rather evokes an avalanche of local brain parenchymal changes of which the axonal damage is but one component. This question was answered in an exhaustive series of light and electron microscopic analyses conducted in our laboratory. Somewhat to our surprise, in the hundreds of sections examined, we discovered that despite the fact that focal axonal injury was a consistent feature of the traumatic event, the focally related parenchymal and vascular tissue showed no evidence of structural abnormality (Povlishock, 1986). Typically, with minor to moderate injury, damaged axons with reactive swellings were consistently visualized in direct relation to unaltered neuronal and glial processes as well as intact microvessels (Povlishock, 1986; Povlishock and Kontos, 1985; Povlishock et al., 1983). Large organelle-laden reactive swellings were consistently seen immediately adjacent to other neuronal somatic, dendritic, and axonal profiles that displayed no ultrastructural change (Figures 4–1 and 4–2). Similarly, reactive axons coursed in direct proximity to various intraparenchymal vessels, all of which appeared unaltered. Such findings are of importance not only because they demonstrate that axons are preferentially vulnerable to shear and tensile of traumatic injury, but also because they once again prove that traumatic injury to axons does not involve direct tissue tearing. Clearly, it is impossible to conceive how an axon could be focally torn while the immediately adjacent neural and vascular elements remain intact.

Although we attach considerable significance to the fact that axonal injury can occur in isolation from other forms of local brain parenchymal change, we caution that it would be erroneous to assume that minor to moderate injuries are not associated with some form of initial and/or delayed parenchymal change. In fact, the very nature of the axonal injury would suggest otherwise: For example, when axons are damaged and ultimately separate from their target sites, this, in itself, evokes a complex and sometimes dramatic series of both immediate and delayed reactive brain parenchymal responses.

As noted, in the case of minor to moderate traumatic brain injury, the ultimate development of the formed reactive swelling is associated with the frank separation of the axon into a swollen segment in continuity with the cell body and a distal segment physically separated from the metabolically sustaining soma. Such distally separated and thereby metabolically compromised axons would be anticipated to undergo a series of changes which would include the typical Wallerian collapse of the axon cylinder followed by myelin segmentation. Additionally, with such Wallerian change, it would be expected that the axon terminals of these fibers would degenerate and trigger focal deafferentation within their respective target sites. It is of interest that when the animals that were subjected to minor or moderate injury were followed over a prolonged posttraumatic course ranging from 2 to 60 days, the previously

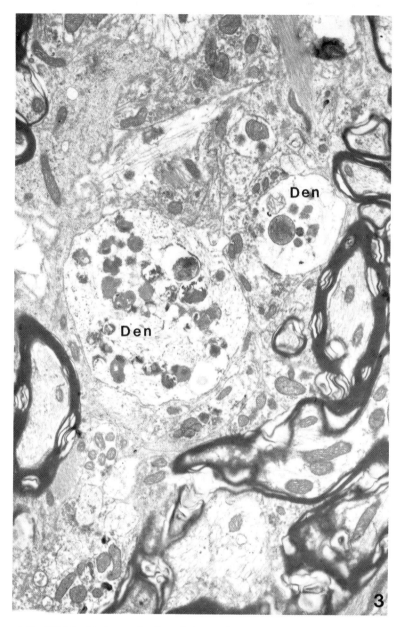

**Figure 4–3** Within 21 days of minor injury, altered dendritic profiles (Den) can be recognized within the lateral vestibular nucleus. The dendrites are enlarged and varicose, and are laden with debris. These changes suggest that the dendrites are undergoing restructuring subsequent to deafferentation. Magnification, ×15,000.

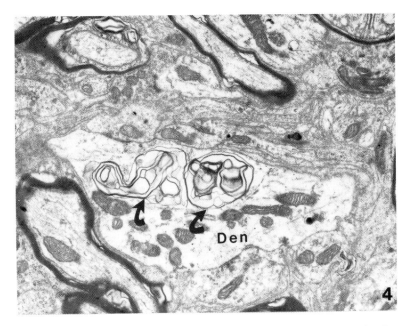

**Figure 4-4** This dendritic profile (Den) shows less dramatic change 21 days after injury and is conspicuous owing to the presence of myelin figures (curved bold arrows). Magnification, ×18,000.

described repertoire of Wallerian change was observed. In all cases, the distally separated axonal segments collapsed and underwent segmentation and fragmentation. Their axon terminals became electron-dense within days of injury and, over time, detached from their somal and dendritic targets to undergo phagocytosis by reactive glia.

In some cases, in which the initial axonal damage involved a clustering of damaged axons, these Wallerian responses were also associated within a secondary response in the target sites. Typically, in the case of minor to moderate injury, clusters of reactive swellings were observed scattered throughout the red, vestibular, reticular, and posterior thalamic nuclei, wherein the detached distal segments underwent Wallerian change with terminal loss. Most likely as a result of the clustering of such axonal injury, the axon terminal loss was dramatic, with large areas of the target neuronal somal and dendritic surface losing their synaptic input. In this situation, a complex series of changes also occurred within the deafferentated dendritic domains of the involved target sites over a 60-day period. Most commonly, dendritic profiles within these target nuclei revealed various complex inclusions, among which autophagic vacuoles appeared prominent (Figures 4-3 and 4-4). Additionally, some dendritic profiles demonstrated focal, varicose swellings which were laden with autophagic vacuoles and other forms of debris (Figure 4-3). Collectively, these dendritic changes appeared consistent with a reactive response secondary to deafferentation (Benes et al., 1977), and most likely reflected dynamic dendritic remodeling, setting the stage for possible reinnervation.

## FATE OF THE DAMAGED AXONS

In view of the previously described sequence of events, which reveals that minor to moderate traumatic brain injury consistently evokes widespread axonal damge and thereby triggers deafferentation and reorganization in distant target sites, various questions arise in regards to the neurobiological consequences of these events. Naturally, one would question the long-term fate of the traumatically induced reactive axonal swellings that are found in an otherwise unaltered brain microenvironment. Do such reactive axons ultimately degenerate, or do they mount a regenerative effort? Similarly, within the reorganizing target sites, one wonders if deafferentation persists or if various regenerating fibers and/or sprouts from intact fibers lead to the restoration of normal synaptic input. Although traditional neurobiological thought would argue that reactive axonal swellings within the central nervous system could not mount a regenerative effort and that all, if any reinnervation must arise from intact fibers, we question the validity of such assumptions. Our reluctance to accept traditional thought on this issue stems from the fact that the studies upon which such assumptions are based always utilized experimental paradigms employing relatively large focal lesions with attendant hemorrhage and gliosis to achieve axonal damage (e.g., Gibson and Stensaas, 1974; Lampert and Cressman, 1964; Ramón y Cajal, 1928). Since with minor and moderate brain injury the traumatically induced axonal swellings were identified within otherwise unaltered brain parenchyma and since they occurred without attendant vascular damage or gliosis, it appeared, from the neurobiological perspective, that we were dealing with a unique and biologically unprecedented experimental state. To investigate this issue fully, we, to date, have followed the fate of the traumatically induced reactive axonal swellings over a three-month postinjury course.

Through such an approach, it was found that some of the reactive axonal swellings persisted unchanged, whereas others degenerated and died-back, and still others mounted a sustained regenerative attempt (Povlishock and Becker, 1985; Povlishock and Kontos, 1985). In this regenerative response, the swellings displayed, in the course of the first posttraumatic week, numerous small sprouts which arose both directly from the swelling proper and from the nodal regions just proximal to the swelling (Figures 4–5 and 4–6). Over the next two to three weeks, this sprouting continued; however, now multiple growth-cone processes were observed to arise from the swelling in concert with the sprouts. Sustained sprouting and growthcone formation was associated with an overall reduction in the size of the reactive swelling proper, as it was apparent that with the outgrowth of these regenerative processes both axoplasm and organelles were redirected from the swelling proper into these newly formed processes. With continued survival, both sprouts and growthcone processes were observed to elongate and extend from the swelling through the overlying myelin sheath into the substance of the related brain parenchyma. Via semiserial section analyses some sprouts and growth cones could be observed to extend through the brain parenchyma to enter the collapsed myelin sheaths of the detached distal axonal segments which were in the early phases of Wallerian

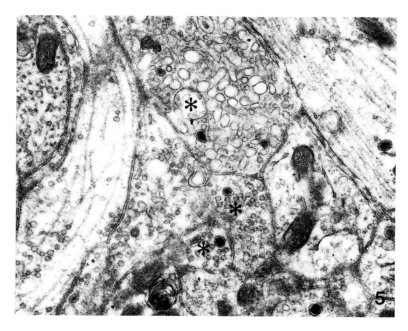

**Figure 4–5** Approximately two weeks after the traumatic episode, numerous sprouts (asterisks) can be seen originating from a damaged axon within the lateral vestibular nucleus. The sprouts contain tubular and vesicular profiles of smooth endoplasmic reticulum. Magnification, ×34,000.

degeneration (Figure 4–6). Frequently multiple sprouts and growth cones could be observed in the same collapsed axon cylinder, where they appeared to fan out and parallel its walls (Figure 4–6). Such regenerative phenomena continued over a three-month course, and, although longer periods of survival have not been considered, we would anticipate that these regenerative efforts persisted.

## SYNTHESIS AND PERSPECTIVES

In the preceding sections, we have attempted to explicate, in a very limited fashion, the structural changes occurring with minor to moderate traumatic brain injury. The data obtained using animal models clearly demonstrate that focal axonal damage is a consistent feature of minor to moderate traumatic brain injury and thus would suggest that a comparable axonal response is occurring in head-injured humans. This possibility appears all the more likely in view of the already existing isolated descriptions of axonal damage in humans sustaining minor head injury (Peerless and Rewcastle, 1967). What is most intriguing about the observed axonal response to injury is its delayed progression to frank detachment. This finding suggests that if precise subcellular mechanisms can be identified, the progressing damage may prove amenable to some posttraumatic therapeutic intervention.

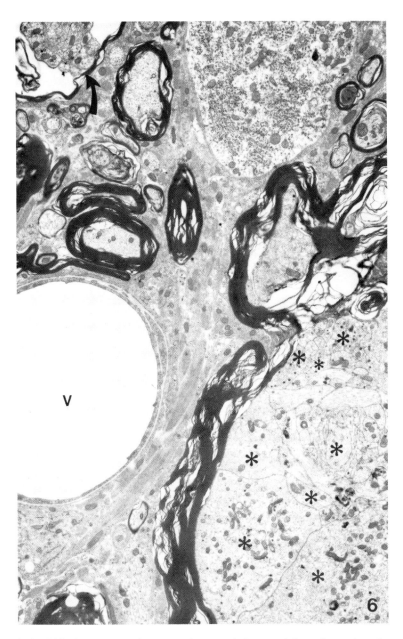

**Figure 4–6** This low-power electron micrograph is a serial section taken from the same block used for Figure 4–5. Note the numerous reactive sprouts (asterisks) that have arisen from a reactive axonal swelling. Additionally, note, in the upper-left-hand corner, those sprouts that are coursing through an empty myelin-invested (curved bold arrow) cavity. Serial section analyses confirmed that these sprouts are in continuity with those seen in the lower-right-hand corner of the figure. Once again, despite these reactive changes the related brain parenchyma and vasculature (V) appear unremarkable. Magnification, ×6,000.

One of the most remarkable observations arising from our studies is the fact that with minor to moderate trauma, axonal damage can occur in isolation from any other form of focally related brain parenchymal or intraparenchymal vascular abnormality. Upon superficial consideration, such a finding may seem of little consequence; yet, further consideration would suggest otherwise, for it is obvious that minor to moderate traumatic brain injury creates a condition which, in our estimation, is unparalleled in any other form of central nervous system insult. With other forms of CNS insult, such as cortical contusion or spinal cord trauma, axonal damage can certainly occur; however, in these conditions it is but one component of an avalanche of structural responses which include various forms of overt tissue damage, hemorrhage, and ischemic insult (Balentine, 1978a,b; Rand and Courville, 1934). Therefore, one cannot consider it to be the singular determinant of the ensuing morbidity. In minor to moderate injury, on the other hand, the isolated and focal nature of the axonal damage creates a unique situation in that one can be confident that the axonal damage alone is the major consequence of injury, and, as such, the most likely determinant of any ensuing morbidity. Although it is difficult to equate the axonal damage seen in the cat with any specific morbidity, it seems reasonable to speculate that comparable diffuse axonal damage in head-injured humans contributes to CNS pathway disconnection and thereby constitutes the morphological substrate underlying the behavioral and functional abnormalities described following relatively minor injury (Levin et al., 1987; Rimel et al., 1981, 1982).

Although there can be little doubt that the axonal damage associated with minor head injury contributes to posttraumatic morbidity, the long-term import of the axonal damage may extend far beyond its role in influencing morbidity. As the damaged axons exist in a relatively intact brain microenvironment and as they mount a sustained regenerative response, it is quite reasonable that these features of the traumatically injured axons may lead to an adaptive form of recovery. The fact that recovery has been described in humans within three months of injury (Levin et al., 1987) supports this view. The sustained sprouting and growth cone formation we have observed arising from the injured axons is, in our estimation, an unprecedented finding in the central nervous system. In that these sprouts and growth cones bear striking similarities to regenerating peripheral nerves (Friede and Bischhausen, 1980) as well as regenerating axons within the amphibian CNS (Stensaas, 1983), our conclusions regarding their regenerative capabilities appear warranted. Admittedly, we have not been able to trace these neuritic outgrowths to their target sites; nevertheless, this does not preclude the occurrence of such an event. Alternatively, even if we were to dismiss the potential for targeted regeneration from the damaged axons, the potential of sprouting (i.e., reactive synaptogenesis) from nearby intact fibers would provide another source of input to the traumatically deafferentated sites. The existence of damaged axons adjacent to intact fibers within various target nuclei would imply that even in the face of axonal injury the retention of adjacent intact fibers—most of which are of the same functional type—would provide a ready source of new sprouts (i.e., reactive synaptogenesis) for an adaptive recovery. Interestingly, as sprouting mechanisms are known to occur over a postinjury period of several months (Matthews et al., 1976a,b; Steward and Vinsant, 1983), the temporal course of the return of synaptic input would parallel the course of recovery following minor injury (Levin et al., 1987). Clearly, the temporal similarities would argue for their interrelation, and we believe that such is the case.

To address this issue more rigorously, we have conducted some preliminary studies to explore both the loss and the return of specific neurotransmitter-containing terminals following minor head injury (unpublished findings). In these experiments, we focused on the cat lateral vestibular nucleus, wherein we have observed traumatically induced axonal damage and were confident that an essentially γ-aminobutyric adic (GABA)ergic neurotransmitter population exists. Using immunocytochemical means to detect the GABAergic terminals, we attempted to confirm the above-stated assumptions. Essentially, within days of the traumatic event we observed the focal loss of GABAergic terminals, which most likely reflected the terminal degeneration previously described. Over time, however, preliminary evidence suggests restoration of the GABAergic terminals. Whether the restored GABAergic terminals arose from damaged or intact axons could not be determined; however, the fact that such a restoration occurred is notable, and supportive of the hypothesis that these factors are operant in the recovery seen following minor head injury.

Despite the apparent soundness of our argument for the recovery seen with minor injury, the obvious criticism arises that if, indeed, such mechanisms are operant, then why is recovery following moderate head injury "incomplete?" We have not explored this issue experimentally, but we believe that the answer to this criticism is readily apparent when both the nature of the injury and the postinjury regenerative effort are carefully considered. Clearly, in the case of moderate injury, focal lesions are more prevalent and are quite unlikely to undergo complete resolution; moreover—and perhaps more importantly—proportionally more axons are damaged than in the case of minor injury. In the state of moderate injury, regenerative efforts would still occur, but, owing to the magnitude of axonal damage, aberrant neurite ingrowth from "nonhomologous" fiber systems might take place; the latter would then contribute to the development of aberrant circuitry, with the end result being incomplete recovery.

In the above passages, we have emphasized the finding of damaged axons within the brain parenchyma following minor to moderate traumatic injury. Although we firmly believe in their importance for explaining both the morbidity and recovery seen with such injuries, we also would caution that morphological end points in themselves may not fully explain all of the subcellular and functional events occurring in minor to moderate injury. To date, we also have observed increased posttraumatic metabolic activity within brainstem cholinergic centers (Hayes et al., 1984) and additionally have described transient neuronal permeability alterations in other brainstem sites (Povlishock et al., 1979). However, as these changes were rather regional and proved transient, it was our impression that they were unlikely contributors to any long-term morbidity. On a similar note, in relation to the cerebral vasculature, we have noted transient functional abnormalities, despite the fact that no evidence for direct structural vascular disruption was consistently found. In animals equipped with cranial windows for the direct visualization and measurement of the underlying pial vasculature, minor or moderate injury was recognized to elicit some form of vascular functional abnormality. In general, minor to moderate injury was associated with pial arteriolar dilation which persisted beyond the duration of the posttraumatic hypertensive episode and also was quantitatively related to the magnitude of the traumatic event (DeWitt et al., 1986; Wei et al., 1980). Small arterioles generally dilated to a greater extent than large arterioles, and such dilatory responses tended to subside readily within several hours following injury. Abnormal vascular responsivity accompanied the arteriolar dilation. The normal arteriolar vasoconstrictor response to hypocapnia was reduced and an impairment in autoregulation was also recognized (Lewelt et al., 1980, 1982; Wei et al., 1980). Interestingly, vasodilator agents, such as acetylcholine, that act via the secondary release of an endothelium-derived relaxant factor manifested altered responsivity. In some instances, the arterioles failed to dilate in the presence of acetylcholine, whereas others vasoconstricted slightly (Kontos and Povlishock, 1986). As was the case for the observed pial arteriolar dilation, all the above-described changes in responsivity tended to normalize within several hours. Because these vascular abnormalities were rapidly reversible and were not associated with a reduction in cerebral blood flow, they would not appear to influence the morbidity that accompanies minor or moderate injury. Perhaps only with a secondary insult would the existence of altered vascular responsivity suggest the potential of adverse impact. However, because minor and moderate traumatic brain injuries are not generally associated with secondary insults, this consideration may be academic.

In summary, in this review we have attempted to provide compelling evidence from both animals and humans that axonal injury is the most consistent feature of minor to moderate injury. Additionally, given the fact that such axonal injury occurs without attendant change in the related brain parenchyma and vasculature, we have attempted to explain how the retention of such an intact brain microenvironment might facilitate regeneration and recovery. We would argue that from a neurobiological perspective, minor to moderate injury evokes a parenchymal response that cannot be appreciated in terms of traditional thought. Further studies appear warranted, not only to provide new information on head injury but also reshape current thinking on CNS regeneration.

## ACKNOWLEDGMENTS

Most of the experimental work reported in this chapter was supported by NIH Grant NS 20193.

## REFERENCES

Adams JH, Graham DI, Murray LS, Scott G. Diffuse axonal injury due to nonmissile head injury in humans. Ann Neurol 12:557–563, 1982.

Balentine JD. Pathology of experimental spinal cord trauma. I. The necrotic lesion as a function of vascular injury. Lab Invest 39:236–253, 1978a.

Balentine JD. Pathology of experimental spinal cord trauma. II. Ultrastructure of axons and myelin. Lab Invest 39:254–266, 1978b.

Benes FM, Parks TN, Rubel EW. Rapid dendritic atrophy following deafferentation: an EM morphometric analysis. Brain Res 122:1–13, 1977.

DeSalles AAF, Newlon MS, Katayama Y, Dixon CE, Becker DP, Stonnington HH, Hayes RL. Transient suppression of event-related evoked potentials produced by mild head injury in the cat. J Neurosurg 66:102–108, 1987.

Dewitt DS, Jenkins LW, Wei EP, Lutz H, Becker DP, Kontos HA. Effects of fluid-percussion on regional cerebral blood flow and pial vessel diameter. J Neurosurg 64:787–794, 1986.

Friede RL, Bischhausen, R. The fine structure of stumps of transected nerve fibers in subserial sections. J Neurol Sci 44:181–188, 1980.

Gennarelli TA, Thibault LE, Adams JH, Graham DI, Tompson CJ, Marcincin RP. Diffuse axonal injury and traumatic coma in the primate. Ann Neurol 12:564–575, 1982.

Gibson BC, Stensaas LJ. Early axonal changes following lesions of the dorsal columns in rats. Cell Tissue Res 149:1–17, 1974.

Griffin JW, Price DL, Engel WK, Drachman DB. The pathogenesis of reactive axonal swellings: role of axonal transport. J Neuropathol Exp Neurol 36:214–226, 1977.

Hayes RL, Pechura CM, Katayama Y, Povlishock JT, Giebel ML, Becker DP. Activation of pontine cholinergic sites implicated in unconsciousness following cerebral concussion in the cat. Science 233:301–303, 1984.

Jane JA, Steward O, Gennarelli TA. Axonal degeneration induced by experimental non-invasive minor head injury. J Neurosurg 62:96–100, 1985.

Kontos HA, Povlishock JT. Oxygen radicals in brain injury. J Cent Nerv Syst Trauma 3:257–263, 1986.

Lampert PW, Cressman M. Axonal regeneration in the dorsal columns of the spinal cord of adult rats. Lab Invest 13:825–839, 1964.

Lasek RF Hoffman PN. The neuronal cytoskeleton, axonal transport and axonal growth. In Goldman R, Pollard T, Rosenbaum M (eds), Microtubules and Related Proteins. Cold Spring Harbor, NY: Cold Spring Harbor Laboratories, 1976, pp 1021–1049.

Levin HS, Mattis S, Ruff RM, Eisenberg HM, Marshall LT, Tabaddor K, High WM, Frankowski RF. Neurobehavioral outcome following minor head injury: a three center study. J Neurosurg 66:234–243, 1987.

Lewelt W, Jenkins LW, Miller JD. Autoregulation of cerebral blood flow after experimental fluid percussion injury of the brain. J Neurosurg 53:500–511, 1980.

Lewelt W, Jenkins LW, Miller JD. Effects of experimental fluid percussion injury of the brain on cerebrovascular reactivity to hypoxia and to hypercapnia. J Neurosurg 56:332–338, 1982.

Martinez AJ, Friede RL. Accumulation of axoplasmic organelles in swollen nerve fibers. Brain Res 19:185–198, 1970.

Matthews DA, Cotman C, Lynch G. An electron microscopic study of lesion-induced synaptogenesis in the dentate gyrus of the adult rat. I. Magnitude and time course of degeneration. Brain Res 115:1–21, 1976a.

Matthews DA, Cotman C, Lynch G. An electron microscopic study of lesion-induced synaptogenesis in the dentate gyrus of the adult rat. II Reappearance of morphologically normal synaptic contacts. Brain Res 115:23–41, 1976b.

Oppenheimer DR. Microscopic lesions in the brain following head injury. J Neurol Neurosurg Psychiatry 31:299–306, 1968.

Peerless SJ, Rewcastle NW. Shear injuries of the brain. Can Med Assoc J 96:577–582, 1967.

Pilz P. Axonal injury in head injury. Acta Neurochir (Wien) [Suppl] 32:119–124, 1983.

Povlishock JT. Traumatically induced axonal damage without concomitant change in focally related neuronal somata and dendrites. Acta Neuropathol (Berl) 70:53–59, 1986.

Povlishock JT, Becker DP. Fate of reactive axonal swellings induced by head injury. Lab Invest 52:540–552, 1985.

Povlishock JT, Kontos HA. Continuing axonal and vascular change following experimental brain trauma. J Cent Nerv Syst Trauma 2:285–298, 1985.

Povlishock JT, Becker DP, Miller JD, Jenkins LW, Dietrich WD. The morphopathologic substrates of concussion? Acta Neuropathol (Berl) 47:1–12, 1979.

Povlishock JT, Becker DP, Cheng CLY, Vaughan GW. Axonal change in minor head injury. J Neuropathol Exp Neurol 42:225–242, 1983.

Ramón Y Cajal S. Degeneration and Regeneration of the Nervous System. London: Oxford University Press, 1928.

Rand CW, Courville CB. Histologic changes in the brain in cases of fatal injury to the head. Arch Neurol Psychiatry 31:527–542, 1934.

Rimel RW, Giordani B, Barth JT, Boll TJ, Jane JA. Disability caused by minor head injury. Neurosurgery 9:221–228, 1981.

Rimel RW, Giordani B, Barth JT, Jane JA. Moderate head injury: completing the clinical spectrum of brain trauma. Neurosurgery 11:344–351, 1982.

Stensaas LJ. Regeneration in the spinal cord of the newt notophthalmus *(Triturus) pyrrhogaster. In* Kao CC, Bunge RP, Reier PJ (eds), Spinal Cord Reconstruction. New York: Raven Press, 1983, pp 121–143.

Steward O, Vinsant SL. The process of reinnervation in the dentate gyrus of the adult rat: a quantitative electron microscopic analysis of terminal proliferation and synaptogenesis. J Comp Neurol 214:370–386, 1983.

Strich SJ. Shearing of nerve fibers as a cause of brain damage due to head injury. Lancet 2:443–448, 1961.

Sullivan HG, Martinez AJ, Becker DP, Miller JD, Griffith R, Wist AO. Fluid-percussion model of mechanical brain injury in the cat. J Neurosurg 45:520–534, 1976.

Wei EP, Dietrich WD, Povlishock JT, Navari RM, Kontos HA. Functional morphologic and metabolic abnormalities of the cerebral microcirculation after concussive brain injury in cats. Circ Res 46:37–47, 1980.

# 5

# Neurochemical Mechanisms of Mild and Moderate Head Injury: Implications for Treatment

RONALD L. HAYES,
BRUCE G. LYETH,
AND LARRY W. JENKINS

Over the past several years, research in our laboratories has focused on cholinergic mechanisms of brain injury. Much of our earlier investigations examined traumatically induced changes in functional activity within endogenous neural systems potentially regulating states of consciousness. As outlined below, these initial studies represented the first systematic exploration of possible neural mechanisms mediating transient unconsciousness produced by mild to moderate levels of concussive head injury. However, these observations provided little insight into mechanisms mediating the more enduring neurological deficits which may persist long after disturbances of consciousness produced even by mild head injury (Binder, 1986; Carlsson et al., 1987; Leininger, 1987; Levin et al., 1987; Rimel et al., 1981, 1982).

More recently, data from our laboratory have suggested that cholinergic mechanisms may also mediate some of the more enduring neurological deficits following brain injury. Cholinergic mechanisms mediating transient unconsciousness may be quite different from those mediating long-term deficits (Figure 5–1). However, an understanding of multiple changes in cholinergic function produced by mechanical brain injury could have profound implications for the treatment of human head injury. Indeed, the principal clinical implication of the data presented here is that appropriate anticholinergic therapy could reduce the duration of transient unconsciousness as well as attenuate the magnitude of longer-term deficits following mild to moderate human head injury.

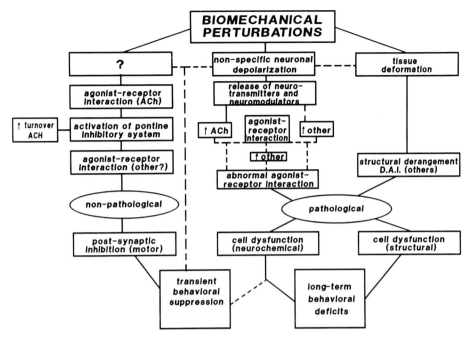

**Figure 5-1**   A schematic representation of various processes that could contribute to transient behavioral suppression (i.e., unconsciousness) or long-term behavioral deficits following mild to moderate mechanical brain injury. The principal feature of the schematic is that transient unconsciousness may be produced by a nonpathological activation of an endogenous, cholinergic inhibitory system. In contrast, long-term behavioral deficits may result from pathological changes resulting in neurochemically mediated perturbations in intracellular and extracellular information flow pathways. These neurochemical perturbations may be mediated by the binding of acetylcholine (ACh) or other endogenous excitatory neurotransmitters or neuropeptides to their respective receptors. Long-term behavioral deficits may also result from structural derangements such as diffuse axonal injury (D.A.I.). See text for details.

## PRODUCTION OF EXPERIMENTAL BRAIN INJURY: DESCRIPTION AND CLINICAL RELEVANCE

Before presenting data from our laboratories, we wish to give some detailed consideration to issues central to the experimental production of brain injury. Functional and structural disturbances of the brain produced by sudden impact to the skull represent a fundamental problem in the neurosurgical treatment of head trauma. The development of appropriate animal models has made possible much progress in describing the neurophysiological correlates of pathologies affecting the human central nervous system, including stroke, epilepsy, sleep disorders, and chronic pain. Thus, animal models are also prerequisites for the development of rational modes of prevention, diagnosis, and treatment of head injury. Adequate animal models should allow studies of both biomechanical and physiological variables relevant to mechanical injury to neural tissue.

When mechanical loads are applied to a structure such as the brain, the forces acting on that structure may cause deformation. This deformation is felt to be the principal damaging factor (see Hayes et al., 1987c; Hayes and Ellison [in press] for a more detailed treatment of these issues). The biomechanical determinants of damage related to deformation may be discussed in terms of velocity, acceleration, and the magnitude of displacement of neural tissue. These variables, in turn, depend upon the onset and duration of the mechanical load and the material properties of the tissue. Thus, a desirable model of head injury should make possible quantifiable changes in the parameters influencing brain deformation. In some models simulating mechanical head injury, the brain has been loaded by an extracranial impact to the intact skull or by forcing the head to change its motion. However, when methods such as these are used, it is difficult to analyze, quantify, and control the forces producing brain deformation, and, with notable exceptions (see Thibault and Gennarelli, 1985), attempts to measure deformation have often resulted in only rough qualitative estimates of brain displacement.

An alternative strategy is to introduce fixed volumes of fluid intracranially in order to produce brain deformation. A number of techniques have been used since Duret's experiments in 1878 (see Hayes and Ellison, in press). More recently, Lindgren and Rinder (1969) developed a head trauma model in the rabbit which introduces a volume of fluid intracranially. One of the advantages of the Lindgren and Rinder fluid percussion model is that the variables influencing damage to neural tissue by deformation can be more precisely identified and controlled. For example, although the velocity, acceleration, and magnitude of deformation of brain tissue cannot easily be measured directly, these variables should be invariantly related to the velocity, acceleration, and magnitude of fluid volume loading in a relatively closed system such as the craniospinal cavity. In contrast to neural tissue, these variables can be accurately assessed for the fluid medium used to produce deformation (e.g., Stalhammar et al., 1987).

In all studies conducted in our laboratories, experimental brain injury is produced with a fluid percussion device (see Sullivan et al., 1976) similar to the one developed by Lindgren and Rinder (1969). Briefly, it consists of a Plexiglas cylindrical reservoir, 60 cm long and 4.5 cm in diameter, bounded at one end by a Plexiglas cork-covered piston mounted on O-rings (Figure 5–2). The opposite end of the reservoir is fitted with a 2-cm-long metal housing on which a transducer is mounted. Fastened to the end of this is a tube that ends with a male Leur-Loc fitting. This is connected to a female Leur-Loc fitting that has been chronically implanted over the exposed dura overlying the parietal cortex. The entire system is filled with 37°C isotonic saline. The injury is induced by a metal pendulum which strikes the piston of the injury device from a predetermined height. The resulting pressure pulse is measured extracranially by the transducer at the time of injury. The device injects varying volumes of saline into the closed cranial cavity, thereby producing brief displacement and deformation of neural tissue. Increased magnitudes of tissue deformation are

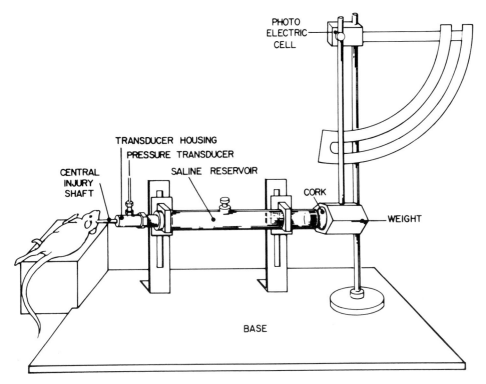

**Figure 5–2**  Diagram of the fluid-percussion model of brain injury in the rat. A 4-mm central craniectomy is connected to one end of a Plexiglas cylinder filled with physiological saline. At the other end in the cylinder is a Plexiglas cork mounted on O-rings. Injury is produced by striking the cork with a 4.8-kg pendulum dropped from a specific height. The pressure transient is recorded on a storage oscilloscope with an extracranial transducer. (Reproduced from Dixon et al., 1987, by permission)

associated with increased magnitudes of brain injury. The magnitude of the injury is regulated by varying the height of the pendulum. This also results in corresponding variations of extracranial pressure pulses expressed in atmospheres (atm). Extracranial pressure pulses produced by fluid percussion injury have been found to be closely associated with intracranial pressure changes (Lindgren and Rinder, 1966, 1969; Stalhammar et al., 1987). For additional details on surgical preparation, see Dixon et al., 1987; Lyeth et al., 1988a,b.

The fluid percussion technique has been widely used by a number of laboratories and produces many features of brain injury resembling pathophysiological responses seen in human head injury. These include (1) production of brief pressure transients, similar to those recorded in human cadaver skulls during sudden impact (Lindgren and Rinder, 1966); and (2) suppression of behavioral responses and neurological signs (Dixon et al., 1987; Hayes et al., 1984; 1988; Katayama et al., 1988a,b), resembling traumatic unconsciousness in humans (Teasdale, 1976). Similar even to mild and moderate head injury in humans (Binder et al., 1986; Levin et al., 1987; Rimel et al., 1981, 1982), fluid percussion injury also produces deficits in (3) motor function (Dixon et al., 1987), (4) attention (DeSalles et al., 1987) and (5) memory (Lyeth et al., 1987), which persist after resolution of disturbed states of consciousness. Injury by this method also (6) reduces or abolishes cerebrovascular responsiveness to changes in $P_{CO_2}$ (Lewelt et al., 1982; Saunders et al., 1979; Wei, 1980), and (7) causes loss of pressure autoregulation (Lewelt et al., 1980) similar to clinical reports of loss of $P_{CO_2}$ responsivity (Fieschi et al., 1974; Gennarelli et al., 1979; Overgaard and Tweed, 1974) and, to a greater extent, pressure autoregulation (Fieschi et al., 1974; Overgaard and Tweed, 1974) following human head injury. (8) These experimentally produced cerebrovascular perturbations are not accompanied by ischemia at the moderate levels of injury used in these experiments (DeWitt et al., 1986; Jenkins et al., 1986; Lewelt et al., 1980, 1982). Similarly, ischemia does not seem to be a primary feature of mechanical injury to the human brain in the absence of secondary insults (Deutsch and Eisenberg, 1987; Obrist et al., 1984).

9. As is the case in humans (e.g., Marshall et al., 1979; Miller et al., 1981), fluid percussion injury produces late-developing increases in intracranial pressure (Rosner and Becker, 1982).

10. Brain swelling, a prominent feature of human head injury (Becker et al., 1977; Marshall et al., 1979), also develops after fluid percussion injury (Becker, 1986).

11. This injury model also produces decreased rates of energy metabolism (Hayes et al., 1984; in press), similar to decreased rates reported following human head injury (Obrist et al., 1984).

12. Similar to human head injury (Clifton et al., 1981), fluid percussion injury also increases circulating catecholamines (Rosner et al., 1984) and results in immunosuppression (Schall-Vess et al., submitted).

13. As is the case with moderate head injury in humans (Becker, 1986; Gennarelli et al., 1986), fluid percussion injury is not usually associated with mass lesions (Dixon et al., 1987; Povlishock, 1985; Sullivan et al., 1976).

14. Diffuse axonal injury is a feature of both human head injury (Becker, 1986; Gennarelli et al., 1986) and fluid percussion injury in the cat (Povlishock, 1985, 1986; Povlishock et al., 1983).

15. Cell death is not prominent following low levels of human head injury Oppenheimer, 1968) or fluid percussion injury (Jenkins et al., 1986, 1987; Lyeth et al., 1987).

16. As may be the case for human head injury (Langfitt and Gennarelli, 1982; Miller et al., 1978), fluid percussion injury results in an enhanced pathological response to secondary ischemic insult (Jenkins et al., 1986, 1987).


## MECHANISMS MEDIATING TRANSIENT BEHAVIORAL SUPPRESSION

### Experimental Data

Prior to our research, no investigators had rigorously examined changes in neural processes associated with temporary unconsciousness following brain injury. Most researchers assumed that unconsciousness must result from an injury-produced depression of activity within the reticular activating system (e.g., Foltz and Schmidt, 1956; French, 1952; Hass, 1980; Ommaya, 1982). Sufficient levels of neural activity in this system are thought to be necessary to maintain the organism in an aroused, alert state (Moruzzi and Magoun, 1949). Although destruction of parts or all of the reticular activating system may contribute to prolonged coma following severe brain injury, we believe that, rather than depression of an activating system, activation of an inhibitory system may be a primary neurophysiological process mediating transient unconsciousness following brain injury.

Our laboratories have provided several lines of evidence consistent with the hypothesis that activation of a muscarinic, cholinergic neural system located in the rostral pons contributes to components of behavioral suppression associated with transient unconsciousness following concussive brain injury (for review, see Hayes et al., 1986). Data in support of this hypothesis include studies, summarized below, indicating that:

1. Destruction of the reticular activating system is not sufficient to produce EEG changes observed during periods of the flaccid, comatose state following low levels of concussion in the cat (Hayes et al., 1988).
2. Functional changes in regions bounded by collicular and midpontine transections contribute to at least motor components of the behavioral suppression associated with concussion in the cat (Hayes et al., 1987b; Katayama et al., 1985a, 1988).
3. Local rates of glucose utilization increase in restricted areas bounded by these same collicular and midpontine transections following concussive injury to the cat (Hayes et al., 1983, 1984; see also Hayes et al., in press); microinjections of carbachol into these same hypermetabolic regions produce changes in EEG (Katayama et al., 1984a, 1986, submitted) and in event-related potentials (Katayama et al., 1985c; see also DeSalles et al., 1987) as well as behavioral suppression (Hayes et al., 1984, 1988; Katayama et al., 1984a, 1986, submitted), resembling changes following concussion.
4. Systemic administrations or microinjections of the muscarinic antagonist, atropine, but not the nicotinic antagonist, mecamylamine, can antagonize the behavioral suppression produced by carbachol microinjections in the cat (Hayes et al., 1984; Katayama et al., 1984a, 1986, submitted).
5. The turnover rate of acetylcholine in the pons is transiently increased after low-level concussion in the rat (Hayes et al., 1987c; Robinson et al., 1986b; Saija et al., 1988).
6. Pretreatment or posttreatment with the muscarinic antagonist, scopolamine, but not mecamylamine, can attenuate the transient behavioral suppression following concussive injury to the rat (Hayes et al., 1985, 1986b; Lyeth et al., 1988a).

As we emphasize elsewhere in this chapter, these final data are consistent with clinical reports that anticholinergics can reduce disturbances in consciousness following brain injury (e.g., Heppner and Diemath, 1958; Ward, 1950).

Although lesions of the reticular activating system (RAS) have been reported to result in a comatose state, some data indicate that RAS disruption may not be necessary to produce a flaccid comatose state following head injury. For example, lesions of the RAS typically result in marked increases in slow wave (5–11 Hz) activity. In experiments conducted in our laboratories (Hayes et al., in press), cats in which rostral projections of the RAS were interrupted by transections of the rostral midbrain tegmentum *(cerveau isolé)* also showed a predominance of slow-wave activity. However, cats subjected to low levels of concussive injury never show abnormal slow waves or a predominance of low-frequency activity associated with the prolonged flexion reflex suppression and postural hypotonia (i.e., coma) produced by the injury. In fact, low levels of concussion resulted in a transient increase in high-frequency (11–23 Hz) activity following fluid percussion. Thus, at least transient, reversible comatose states are probably not associated with functional changes in the brainstem similar to the effects produced by lesions of the RAS.

Additional data from our laboratories, using systematic transections at varying levels of the neuraxis, indicate that changes in functional activity within restricted areas of the brainstem differentially contribute to components of sensory and motor suppression following experimental concussion (Hayes et al., 1987b; Katayama et al., 1985a,b). These experiments used electrophysiological measures of spinal cord sensory input, assessed by recording primary afferent depolarization (PAD); and of motor output, assessed by recording monosynaptic and polysynaptic ventral root potentials (VRPs). These electrophysiological indices of spinal cord sensorimotor integration were used because suppression of spinally mediated reflexes (e.g., flexion to noxious stimuli) is a prominent feature of a flaccid comatose state.

Studies in untransected cats showed that low levels of fluid percussion injury suppressed PAD and VRPs over the approximate time periods during which flaccid coma had been observed in separate neurological studies. Concussive injury to cats with prior spinal cord transections failed to produce the suppression of PAD and VRPs typically seen in intact animals subjected to low levels of concussion. These data indicate that disruptions of spinal cord functions following concussion are not attributable to the direct effects of mechanical forces acting on the spinal cord itself. Rather, spinal reflex suppression is attributable to changes in CNS function at supraspinal sites. Injured animals with transections at the midpontine level in which neural pathways between the pontomedullary reticular formation and spinal cord were preserved, showed significantly less suppression of monosynaptic and polysynaptic VRPs than was observed in intact cats. However, PAD in these injured, midpontine-transected cats was suppressed, similar to intact cats following concussion. Thus, whereas areas between the midpontine and spinal transections are critical for production of PAD suppression following concussion, areas rostral to the midpontine level appear critical for the motor suppression. In cats with more rostral transections at collicular levels, concussion produced VRP suppression, similar to that seen in intact animals. Therefore, the predominance of descending inhibitory influences on spinal cord somatomotor functions following injury appears to originate from areas bounded rostrally by sites of collicular transections and caudally by sites of midpontine transections.

Other studies conducted in our laboratories suggested that increased functional activity of cholinergic systems within areas bounded by the collicular and midpontine transections contributed to features of behavioral suppression following concussion (Hayes et al., 1983, 1984, in press). For at least two hours following low levels of concussion, there were increased rates of glucose utilization in regions within the dorsomedial pontine tegmentum. These increased rates of glucose utilization presumably reflected increased functional activity within these regions. Pharmacological activation of these same hypermetabolic zones produces electrophysiological changes similar to those seen following concussion. For example, carbachol microinjection into these zones in awake cats produces desynchronization of parietal EEG (Katayama et al., 1984a, 1986, submitted). This suggests that, similar to data for concussion, the resultant stuporous and comatose states are not induced by generalized depression of forebrain activities, such as that produced by disruption of the RAS. Other data showed that cholinergic activation of these same zones produced reversible suppression of event-related evoked potentials (Katayama et al., 1985c). These potentials have been attributed to endogenous neural processes related to selective attention and/or orienting responses. Similar suppression of these potentials is produced by fluid percussion injury (DeSalles et al., 1987). Thus, it is possible that cholinergic activation of this region following concussion could contribute to transient deficits in higher-order brain functions.

Additional studies showed that pharmacological activation of these hypermetabolic regions by bilateral microinjections of a cholinergic agonist, carbachol, produced behavioral (i.e., motor) suppression, resembling that following low levels of concussion (Hayes et al., 1984; Katayama et al., 1984a, 1986, submitted). Identical microinjections in surrounding zones showed significantly less behavioral suppression. Tetracaine failed to produce behavioral suppression when microinjected into regions corresponding to the hypermetabolic foci at doses shown to produce reversible inactivation of other neural systems. Other studies showed that systematically administered or microinjected atropine, a muscarinic antagonist, reversed the behavioral effects of carbachol. Equimolar doses of mecamylamine, a nicotinic antagonist, failed to reverse the behavioral effects of carbachol.

Other studies examined the effect of fluid percussion head injury on the activity of cholinergic neurons in specific brain areas of the rat 12 minutes, 4 hours, and 24 hours following injury (Hayes et al., 1987c; Robinson et al., 1986b; Saija et al., 1988). Acetylcholine (ACh) turnover, used as an index of cholinergic neuronal activity, was determined by use of a gas chromatographic-mass spectrometric technique. The most striking changes in cholinergic activity were observed in the dorsal pontine tegmentum, where concussive head injury produced an increase in ACh turnover 12 minutes and 4 hours following injury. This area included regions that our previous research, described above, associated with behavioral changes observed following concussive injury. ACh turnover in the thalamus, a region to which pontine cholinergic neurons projects, also tended to increase four hours following injury. On the other hand, ACh turnover decreased in amygdala four hours following injury. Although there were no significant changes in hippocampal ACh turnover following injury, ACh content did increase in that brain region 12 minutes following injury. There were no significant effects of injury on cholinergic neurons in the hypothalamus or cingulate/frontal cortex. These data provided additional evidence that activation of cholinergic neurons in the pontine region may contribute to components of behavioral suppression associated with reversible traumatic unconsciousness.

If activation of muscarinic cholinergic systems contribute to coma, pharmacological blockage of cholinergic systems would be expected to attenuate coma. Data from our laboratories indicate that administration of a muscarinic cholinergic antagonist can attenuate transient behavioral suppression following a moderate level of concussion (Hayes et al., 1985, 1986; Lyeth et al., 1988a). Increasing doses (0.1, 1.0, 10.0 mg/kg) of scopolamine were systemically (i.p.) administered to rats subjected to moderate fluid percussion brain injury. Scopolamine treatment (1.0 mg/kg, i.p.) 15 minutes prior to trauma significantly reduced mortality and the duration of transient behavioral suppression assessed by a variety of measures. These measures include assessments of pinna, corneal, flexion, and righting reflexes as well as spontaneous locomotion and organized escape behavior. No differences were observed between saline- and scopolamine-treated animals in either the incidence or duration of transient apnea associated with injury. Preinjury treatment with methylscopolamine (1.04 mg/kg) or mecamylamine (1.0 mg/kg) had no effect on transient behavioral suppression, indicating that scopolamine's behavioral effects were mediated by muscarinic receptors within the central nervous system. Except for increased heart rate, preinjury treatment with scopolamine (1.0 mg/kg) did not significantly alter systemic physiological responses to injury, further suggesting that scopolamine's beneficial effects were related to changes in neural function. Rats treated with scopolamine (1.0 mg/kg, i.p.) 30 seconds after injury also tended to have shorter durations of reflex and response suppression.

## Discussion

The lines of evidence reviewed above and elsewhere (Hayes et al., 1986) indicate that activation of an inhibitory cholinergic neural system located in the rostral pons contributes to components of behavioral suppression accompanying transient unconsciousness produced by experimental concussive brain injury. This hypothesis makes no statement regarding any pathological or injurious process. Temporary traumatic unconsiousness, although precipitated by a blow to the head, is posited to result from changes in activity within endogenous neural systems. These changes in activity are not pathological since they probably do not exceed the magnitudes of neural activity encountered in normally functioning neurons (Hayes et al., 1987c; Robinson et al., 1986b; Saija et al., 1988). Although these nonpathological processes probably do not mediate the long-term deficits observed in the studies reported here, we believe the discussion of active inhibitory mechanisms included below can enhance the understanding of multiple neural processes that may differentially influence acute and chronic responses to closed head injury.

First, however, we wish to emphasize the possible relevance of this hypothesis to mechanisms of traumatic unconsciousness following human head injury. The fluid percussion model of injury best approximates mild to moderate levels of human head injury associated with relatively brief periods of unconsciousness. Thus, the laboratory data suggest that active inhibitory mechanisms most likely contribute to reversible unconsciousness following less severe levels of human head injury and that timely initiation of anticholinergic therapy could reduce the duration of this period of unconsciousness or "posttraumatic amnesia." Mechanisms of clinically observed flaccid coma following severe injury are also poorly understood, except for cases in which lesions of the pontomedullary reticular formation are implicated. Among patients with severe head injury treated at our institution, 8% exhibited flaccidity on admission and 76% of these patients died (Butterworth et al., 1981). Despite this high mortality rate, this is apparently a group of flaccid patients who make a good recovery (Butterworth et al., 1981; Levine et al., 1979). Thus, a flaccid comatose state does not always indicate an extremely severe insult to the brain. Therefore, it is possible that reversible physiological changes, including activation of a cholinergic inhibitory system, may mediate reversible flaccid coma following even more severe levels of injury. Consistent with this hypothesis, anticholinergic therapy has been reported to attenuate disturbances of consciousness following mild to moderate (e.g., Heppner and Diemath, 1958) as well as severe levels of head injury (e.g., Heppner and Diemath, 1958; Ward, 1950).

Other researchers have suggested that coma may be attributable to increases in neural activity. More than three decades ago, Araki and his colleagues (1949; see also Katayama et al., 1986) demonstrated several lines of evidence indicating that abnormal neural excitation within the mesencephalic or the pontomesencephalic region induced either by mechanical, electrical, or chemical stimulation results in coma. They reported their experiments under the term "coma-puncture." Stockard et al. (1975) recently suggested, on the basis of their experiences with a large series of posttraumatic coma, that in some cases coma is a more active process than was formerly supposed, and involves overaction of inhibitory centers or some other imbalance in the brain stem activating system.

Although a departure from earlier explanations (e.g., Hass, 1980; Ommaya, 1982), the possibility that transient unconsciousness may result from activation of specific inhibitory systems is also consistent with our understanding of more general neural processes regulating the organism's responses to external stimuli. Recent observations have firmly established the concept that active inhibitory mechanisms located in the brain stem can modulate sensory input and/or motor output in response to changing environmental events or vegetative states. For example, prior exposure to stressful (e.g., painful stimuli) or nonstressful (e.g., novel stimuli) situations can activate endogenous cholinergic neural systems which reduce noxious sensory input (Hayes and Katayama, 1986; Watkins and Mayer, 1982). Endogenous inhibitory mechanisms capable of immobilizing animals during dream sleep have also been described (e.g., Morrison and Reiner, 1985). The neuroanatomical substrate for rapid eye movement (REM) or "dream" sleep motor inhibition (Hendricks et al., 1982) resembles that for active motor inhibition accompanying concussive uncon- sciousness (Hayes et al., 1984; Katayama et al., 1984a, 1986). Activation of the cholinergic sites producing a comatose state in cats also results in elevated intracranial pressures, similar to those seen during REM sleep (Katayama et al., 1984b). EEG patterns resembling those of sleep have also been observed in comatose head-injured patients (Chatrian et al., 1963). Activity of a central cholinergic inhibitory system may also mediate tonic immobility in chickens (Klemm, 1969, 1971; Thompson et al., 1974). Activation of neural systems, as indicated by a relative sparing of decreases in brain glucose metabolism in selected brain regions, may also accompany general anesthesia produced by pentobarbital, ether, and chloral hydrate (Herkenhan, 1981) as well as during hibernation (Kilduff et al., 1983). Thus, there is a significant possibility that an active inhibitory mechanism or mechanisms mediate(s) immobility in a vari- ety of contexts.

The larger task confronting researchers investigating these phenomena will be to describe systematically the environmental situations producing motor suppression, their associated neural mechanism(s), and the relationship of these modulatory motor mechanisms to mechanisms modulating sensory input (e.g., Katayama et al., 1984a). During the conduct of these studies, it will be important to remember that activity in these inhibitory systems may con- tribute to other changes in addition to sensory and motor modulation. As pointed out above, cholinergic activation of sites producing a comatose state in cats also results in elevated intracranial pressures, possibly associated with increased cerebral metabolism and reduced cervical sympathetic vasoconstric- tion tone (Katayama et al., 1984b). These sites were located near a brain area that has been reported to produce changes in forebrain blood flow (De la Torre, 1977; Katayama et al., 1981; Raichle et al., 1976) and cerebrovascular perme- ability (Raichle et al., 1976), following cholinergic or electrical stimulation (see also Preskorn et al., 1980, 1981). Understanding the nature of associations between immobilization and more global changes in the regulation of cerebral metabolism and cerebrovascular responsivity could provide insights into the functional roles of naturally occurring or traumatically induced immobilization.

One may ask, what initial events are triggered by a blow to the head that result ultimately in activation of an endogenous system capable of rendering the animal completely unresponsive even to the most intense stimulation? As implied by the schematic in Figure 5–1, nonspecific central nervous system excitation may activate this inhibitory system. Tissue deformation alone could produce neural depolarization (e.g., Julian and Goldman, 1962; Krivanek, 1981; Takahashi et al., 1981) and the resultant excitation. If this were true, concussive unconsciousness might share at least some common mechanisms with postictal depression. Rats receiving electroconvulsive shock show behav- ioral suppression, decreased blood pressure, and respiratory depression (Belenky and Holaday, 1979; Urca et al., 1981), all of which are produced by concussive injury to the rat (Dixon et al., 1987). Studies investigating possible similarities between postictal and concussive behavioral depression are cur- rently in progress in our laboratories.

Obviously, this line of inquiry ultimately raises teleological questions. Why would an "immobilization system" evolve? Such a system might have some survival value for the organism. Because apnea is a reliable feature of concussive injury (e.g., Dixon et al., 1987; Hayes et al., 1988), immobilization of the animal would reduce competition of skeletal muscles with the more vulnerable brain for a reduced oxygen substrate. Mechanical brain injury can also compromise the brain's ability to regulate blood flow in response to changes in $P\text{CO}_2$ (Fieschi et al., 1974; Gennarelli et al., 1979; Lewelt et al., 1982; Overgaard and Tweed, 1974; Saunders et al., 1979; Wei et al., 1980) or systemic blood pressure (Fieschi et al., 1974; Lewelt et al., 1980; Overgaard and Tweed, 1974). Reduced behavioral activity may attenuate regional differences in brain energy demands, a desirable situation when mechanisms mediating coupling of cerebral blood flow to local metabolic demand may be disturbed. As pointed out earlier, brain injury may also produce an initial nonspecific increase in neural activity. Thus, the pontine inhibitory system may be a component of a negative feedback system which would attempt to dampen massive increases in neural activity accompanying concussion. This negative feedback hypothesis is a teleological corollary of the above assertion that active inhibition is invoked by the initial surge in brain activity following injury. Finally, it is possible that the temporary abolition of all movement could be ethologically adaptive when impaired brain functions from a blow to the head prevent the organization of appropriate responses. Studies have widely documented "no movement" strategies (freezing responses) in a variety of species, including rodents, when placed in stressful or threatening situations (Bolles, 1970; Gallup and Maser, 1977; Meyer-Holzapfel, 1968). For many animals, movement is a stimulus for continued predation (e.g., Herzog and Burghardt, 1974). Data on a number of species collected both in the laboratory and field suggest that immobility can minimize stimulation for further attack (e.g., Gallup and Maser, 1977; Sargeant and Eberhardt, 1975).

## MECHANISMS MEDIATING LONGER-TERM BEHAVIORAL DEFICITS

### Experimental Data

As discussed above, our studies had led us to the important observation that treatment with anticholinergics could reduce acute traumatic unconsciousness, at least in rodents. However, there was no a priori reason to believe that a reduced period of unconsciousness would benefit the animal. It seemed equally plausible that by interrupting possibly compensatory processes accompanying unconsciousness, anticholinergics could exacerbate long-term deficits. Therefore, we designed studies to determine if reduction in transient behavioral suppression with scopolamine treatment would also be associated with changes in long-term deficits resulting from brain injury. The specific aims of these studies were to determine (1) whether scopolamine administered prior to concussive brain injury could attenuate components of the long-term behavioral deficits following such injury, and, if so, (2) the optimum dose of scopolamine producing changes in long-term deficits; (3) whether scopolamine

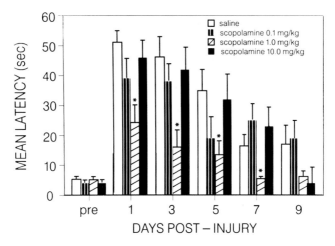

**Figure 5–3**   The effects of scopolamine treatment on beam-walking performance after moderate fluid percussion head injury in rats. Drugs were administered intraperitoneally (i.p.) 15 minutes prior to injury. The data represent mean latencies to traverse the beam ($\pm$ SEM, $n = 10$ animals per group; $*p < .05$ versus saline-treated animals). Note that pretreatment with 1.0 mg/kg of scopolamine significantly reduced this long-term deficit. Rats treated with 1.0 mg/kg of scopolamine were able to traverse the beam much more quickly than saline-treated rats. Similar effects were seen when scopolamine was administered immediately after injury. See text for details.

administered after fluid percussion injury could attenuate components of the long-term behavioral deficits; and (4) whether a dose of scopolamine that produced maximum attenuation of long-term head injury deficits could attenuate long-term motor deficits produced by compressive spinal cord injury. These studies are reported in more detail elsewhere (Lyeth et al., 1985, 1986, 1988b).

Scopolamine (0.1, 1.0, or 10.0 mg/kg) or saline was systemically (i.p.) administered to rats 15 minutes prior to concussive fluid percussion brain injury. Motor deficits were assessed by evaluating rats' abilities to balance on a narrow wooden beam or to traverse a beam to escape aversive noise and light by entering a darkened goal box. Animals pretreated with the 1.0-mg/kg dose exhibited significantly ($p < .05$) fewer motor deficits (e.g., Figure 5–3) and less body weight loss and recovered to baseline performance sooner than saline-treated rats. Mortality and associated convulsions were significantly lower in rats pretreated with the 1.0-mg/kg dose of scopolamine. A 1.0-mg/kg dose of scopolamine administered (i.p.) 30 seconds after injury also significantly reduced behavioral deficits. No differences were observed between saline- and scopolamine-treated animals in either the incidence or the duration of transient apnea following injury. A 1.0-mg/kg dose of scopolamine administered (i.p.) 15 minutes prior to epidural clip compression of the spinal cord had no effect on the severity of motor function deficits assessed by an inclined plane test.

## Discussion

The data from these studies indicate that, as with reversible traumatic unconsciousness, at least some of the long-term behavioral deficits following mild
and moderate levels of brain injury may be attributable to binding of acetylcholine to its muscarinic receptor. As suggested by data reported elsewhere
(Lyeth et al., 1988a), these receptors are probably located on neurons within
the central nervous system. Scopolamine's effects on the neurological consequences of brain injury do not seem to be mediated by its binding to peripheral
nervous system receptors or by scopolamine-mediated changes in cerebrovascular or systemic responses to injury. However, as Figure 5-1 schematically
represents, this binding may invoke quite different but concurrently occurring
processes that separately mediate transient behavioral suppression and long-
term behavioral deficits.

Several observations suggest that increased activity in the discrete cholinergic inhibitory system producing temporary behavioral suppression may not
mediate long-term deficits. First, it seems unlikely that the same mechanism
would mediate behavioral changes characterized by such widely differing time
courses (minutes versus days in the rat). Second, pharmacological activation
of the cholinergic pontine inhibitory area producing unconsciousness does not
seem to result in enduring deficits (Hayes et al., 1984; Katayama et al., 1984a,
1985c). Third, increases in turnover of acetylcholine in the rostral pons do not
persist even for 24 hours after concussive injury to the rat (Hayes et al., 1987c;
Robinson et al., 1986b; Saija et al., 1988)—a time at which many deficits are
still present. Moreover, we are currently conducting experiments in our laboratories in an attempt to dissociate mechanisms mediating transient unconsciousness and long-term deficits. These efforts include studies examining the
possibility of differential effects of neuropharmacological alterations on unconsciousness and long-term deficits. For example, we have recently shown that
pretreatment with phencyclidine can reduce certain long-term behavioral deficits following concussive injury in the rat without affecting the duration of
transient unconsciousness (Hayes et al., 1987a). Finally, and perhaps most
importantly, recent clinical data from our institution also suggest that minor
head injury produces similar degrees of residual cognitive deficits independently of whether or not patients also experienced loss of consciousness (Leininger, 1987). A recent study also indicates that head injuries with impaired
consciousness, no matter how brief, can produce permanent sequelae (Carlsson
et al., 1987; but see Levin et al., 1987). These clinical data at least further suggest the possibility that independent mechanisms could mediate acute traumatic unconsciousness and enduring neurological deficits.

Our current hypothesis is that long-term behavioral deficits result from
widespread excitation of neurons produced by excessive release of acetylcholine (and possibly other excitatory neurotransmitters) following concussion
(Hayes et al., 1987a). Formally stated, our hypothesis is that concussive brain
injury results in increased levels of free acetylcholine which bind to (muscarinic) cholinergic receptors, thereby increasing excitatory influences on neural
tissue already subjected to mechanical stresses. This abnormal excitation can

alter cellular information flow pathways, resulting in transient, long-term and/ or irreversible changes in cell function. However, neurochemical disturbances resulting from abnormal excitation may not be associated with structural alterations—at least, alterations detectable at the light microscopic level. Aside from diffuse axonal injury (Povlishock, 1985, 1986; Povlishock et al., 1983), no light microscopic structural changes have been detected in mild to moderate fluid percussion injury (L. Jenkins, preliminary observation; Jenkins et al., 1986, 1987; Lyeth et al., 1987). However, some subtle ultrastructural changes have been observed (Povlishock et al., 1979). Although human autopsy following mild and moderate brain injury is rare, case reports (e.g., Oppenheimer, 1968) are consistent with the morphopathological features described in the laboratory. We do, of course, recognize that structural alterations such as diffuse axonal injury could contribute to long-term deficits (Figure 5–1).

This excitotoxic hypothesis is derived from the original observations of Olney and co-workers (Olney, 1978, 1983; Olney et al., 1974, 1975, 1979), who discovered a series of glutamate/aspartate analogues. The order of potencies for toxic activities of these compounds (kainic acid, $N$-methyl-D-aspartate [NMDA], homocysteic acid, glutamate) corresponded with their potencies for excitation. Small quantities of these "excitatory amino acids" could cause postsynaptic swelling of dendrites and somal changes as well as cell death. More recently, investigators have examined the possibility that excitotoxic mechanisms contribute to certain brain diseases and the associated pathophysiology of selective vulnerability. As reviewed by Collins (1986), seizures, hypoxia/ischemia, and hypoglycemia may cause the release of excitatory amino acids which could function as endogenous excitotoxins. By selectively binding to receptors that are specialized for excitatory neurotransmission, these excitotoxins, upon release, could, in some circumstances, precipitate burst discharges, large fluxes of ions and water, and, ultimately, cell death. Other recent research on the biochemistry of memory has suggested that high levels of excitation can produce adaptive long-term functional changes and dendritic structural alterations not associated with cell death or dysfunction (Lynch and Baudry, 1984). Thus, it is possible that brain injury could invoke processes similar to those postulated for memory. However, unlike excitation mediating memory, injury produced excitation would not be restricted to specific neural circuits and would be of sufficiently greater magnitude to mediate maladaptive functional changes not associated with cell death.

There are data suggesting that acetylcholine can have excitotoxic effects in some situations. Seizures and postsynaptic neuronal necrosis result from cholinergic activation by a variety of means including administration of acetylcholine, cholinomimetics, and cholinesterase inhibitors as well as stimulation of cholinergic tracts (e.g., Olney et al., 1983a,b; Sloviter, 1983; Turski et al., 1983). The neurotoxic effects of some organophosphates may be attributable to their ability to inhibit cholinesterase (e.g., Robinson et al., 1986a; Samson et al., 1985). Cholinergic excitotoxic effects are not restricted to the nervous system, since myopathy results from sustained action of cholinergic agonists (Leonard and Salpeter, 1979).

There are at least three lines of evidence suggesting a possible excitotoxic role for acetylcholine following mechanical brain injury. First, there are data at least indirectly suggesting that mechanical brain injury can produce widespread neural excitation and depolarization, a prerequisite for liberation of large amounts of acetylcholine and other excitatory agents. Studies in our laboratory have documented that the first one to five minutes after concussive injury are often associated with increased cerebral blood flow (DeWitt et al., 1986), muscle hypertonia, and desynchronous EEG (Hayes et al., 1988), all of which are compatible with a nonspecific increase in brain activity. Other investigators have reported that concussive injury produces increased oxidation of mitochondrial cytochromes, suggesting an increase in brain energy demand (Duckrow et al., 1981). We, as well as others, have also provided preliminary data that experimental concussion produces transient increases in extracellular potassium presumably related to neuronal depolarization (DeSalles et al., 1986; Takahashi et al., 1981).

Second, other research has indicated that brain injury can liberate significant amounts of unbound acetylcholine which may persist for several days. Laboratory studies have reported that mechanical brain injury results in increased levels of acetylcholine both in cerebrospinal fluid (Bornstein, 1946; Metz, 1971; Ruge, 1954; Sachs, 1957) and in brain (Robinson et al., 1986b; Saija et al., 1988). Increased levels of acetylcholine have also been observed in blood (Grashchenkov et al., 1966) and in cerebrospinal fluid of head-injured humans (Cone et al., 1948; Haber and Grossman, 1980; Tower and McEachern, 1949a,b).

A third line of evidence suggests that increased levels of acetylcholine are, in fact, injurious. Both laboratory (Sachs, 1957) and clinical (Grashchenkov et al., 1966; Haber and Grossman, 1980; Sachs, 1957; Tower and McEachern, 1949a) studies indicate that higher levels of acetylcholine in cerebrospinal fluid are associated with higher magnitudes of injury and/or poor clinical outcome. More importantly, in addition to the data presented here, other laboratory data indicate that administration of anticholinergics can improve outcome after experimental brain injury (Bornstein, 1946; Ruge, 1954). These laboratory findings parallel a series of clinical reports, totalling over 2,000 patients, indicating that treatment with anticholinergics might improve outcome following human head injury (Heppner and Diemath, 1958; Jenkner and Lechner, 1954, 1955a,b; Sachs, 1957; Ward, 1950, 1966). However, it is important to remember that these early clinical data were not derived from prospective, randomized clinical trials required for a rigorous evaluation of drug effects. Equally important from a scientific as well as a clinical perspective, these studies frequently lacked systematic outcome assessments and careful distinctions between acute deficits associated with disturbances of consciousness and neuropsychological problems that persist after normal consciousness returns.

The potential usefulness of anticholinergics to treat human head injury may seem incompatible with the observations of Luria and colleagues, who reported that increasing brain cholinergic tone could improve the clinical status of brain-injured patients (Luria et al., 1969). However, we believe our data are not necessarily discrepant with those of Luria. First, many of Luria's patients suffered missile injuries and/or head injuries of unspecified magni-

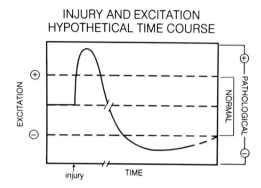

**Figure 5-4** A schematic representation of the effects of mechanical brain injury on levels of excitation within the central nervous system. Injury may initially result in an increase in excitation that could exceed normal physiological limits. Pathological increases in excitation could result in abnormal, excitatory agonist–receptor interactions producing neural injury. During this initial time period, blockade of receptors for excitatory neurotransmitters could reduce injury and improve outcome. In contrast, after neural injury has occurred, a chronic state of hypoexcitability and reduced neural function may persist. During this later time period, agents supplementing neurotransmission may be useful. See text for details.

tudes. There is no reason to believe that anticholinergic therapy would work on every type and/or magnitude of central nervous system injury. Although we have presented data that scopolamine may be useful in the treatment of mild and moderate head injury, we also have reported that scopolamine was ineffective in a rodent model of spinal cord injury. Second, as illustrated in Figure 5-4, the brain's response to mechanical injury may be a dynamic one. The appropriate neuropharmacological approach to therapy could importantly depend on the time after injury at which the drug is administered. Injury may produce a transient increase in levels of acetylcholine or other excitatory agents. Administration of receptor antagonists during this period could provide therapeutic benefits. This possibly damaging "storm" of excitation may be followed by a more enduring chronic phase associated with long-term neuronal injury and reduced neurotransmitter function. During this chronic phase, supplementing neurotransmission may be beneficial, as seems to have been the case with Luria's observations. Obviously, defining the time courses of these very different therapeutic windows represents a critical area for laboratory and clinical studies of the neuropharmacology of brain injury.

## FUTURE RESEARCH

This chapter has focused on the role of acetylcholine and, tangentially, excitatory amino acids. As reviewed by Feeney and Sutton (1987), a number of other pharmacological events may accompany head injury. We certainly do not wish to imply that future research on, for example, GABAergic or catecholaminergic responses to brain injury will not provide important data. The two hypotheses presented here attempt to account for both reversible unconsciousness and long-term behavioral deficits. Future research on the discrete cholinergic systems mediating traumatic unconsciousness should focus on the descending and ascending neural circuits and other neurotransmitters mediating suppression of motor functions and higher order activities, respectively. Additional studies are also needed to confirm that separate processes do, in fact, contribute to unconsciousness and more persistent deficits.

If the excitotoxic hypothesis is correct, many of the features of mechanical brain injury should resemble those of excitotoxicity. For example, injury should be especially prominent in regions containing large numbers of receptors for excitatory amino acids and/or other excitatory neurotransmitters. Thus, studies of receptor binding could prove sensitive indices of regional perturbations produced by mechanical injury. Appropriate receptor antagonists, including antagonists of excitatory amino acids, should attenuate at least some pathophysiological consequences of injury. Preliminary data from our laboratory indicate that blockade of the NMDA receptor can reduce long-term behavioral deficits following concussive injury to the rat (Hayes et al., 1987a).

It will be particularly important for future studies to systematically compare the histopathological consequences of mechanical brain injury and excitotoxins. Although cell death is a classic consequence of excitotoxic processes, cell death may not result from diffuse mechanical brain injury not associated with other insults (e.g., Lyeth et al., 1987). However, because important differences have been described for the histopathological consequence of seizures, hypoxia/ischemia, and hypoglycemia, mechanical brain injury may also possess unique histopathological properties still consistent with excitotoxic mechanisms. One might at least expect significant alterations in dendrosomatic morphology resembling those reported in studies of excitotoxicity (Collins, 1986) or memory (Lynch and Baudry, 1984).

Studies of excitotoxic phenomena could also provide insights into intracellular changes producing cellular dysfunction following mechanical brain injury. If so, increases in intracellular levels of free calcium implicated in functional changes associated with excitotoxicity (Collins, 1986) or memory storage (Lynch and Baudry, 1984) could also mediate long-term functional deficits produced by mechanical injury. Calcium entry mediates damage to skeletal muscle produced by cholinergic agonists (Leonard and Salpeter, 1979). However, as Choi (1987) has pointed out in the case of glutamate neurotoxicity, toxic consequences of exposure to excitatory neurotransmitters can be separated into two components, one dependent on extracellular Na and Cl and the second dependent on extracellular Ca. Similar patterns of ionic dependence may be present in mechanical brain injury.

Finally, we belive that the possibility that receptor-mediate events contribute to the pathophysiology of mechanical brain injury has far-reaching clinical implications. Such data suggest that development of successful therapies for brain injury should emphasize agents that bind to specific neural receptors. In contrast, efforts to manipulate endogenous levels of ions, neuropeptides, neurotransmitters, and other potentially injurious substances (e.g., free radicals; see Kontos and Povlishock, 1986) frequently involve administrations of incompletely understood agents with side effects that could compromise their clinical usefulness. Receptor interactions, however, are well studied neuropharmacological processes. Improved understanding of these processes in the mechanically injured brain could provide tangible benefits for head-injured patients. In view of the data reviewed here, we have implemented a trial at our institution to evaluate the effects of anticholinergics on mild and moderate human head injury.

## SUMMARY

In this chapter, we review data suggesting that mild to moderate (and possibly severe) levels of human head injury may be successfully treated with currently available anticholinergic drugs. The data are derived from a number of laboratory and clinical studies indicating that cholinergic agonist–receptor interactions could mediate both reversible unconsciousness and long-term behavioral deficits following mild and moderate levels of concussive injury. However, these agonist–receptor interactions may involve quite different but concurrently occurring processes that separately mediate reversible unconsciousness and long-term behavioral deficits.

Activation of a muscarinic cholinergic neural system located in the rostral pons may contribute to components of behavioral suppression accompanying transient unconsciousness following concussion. Thus, we hypothesize that temporary traumatic unconsciousness results from increases in activity within endogenous, inhibitory neural systems. This increased activity is not pathological since it does not exceed magnitudes of neural activity encountered in normally functioning neurons. In contrast, long-term behavioral deficits may result from widespread, pathological excitation of neurons produced by excessive release of acetylcholine (and possibly other excitatory neurotransmitters) following concussion. This abnormal excitation could alter cellular information flow pathways resulting in transient, long-term and/or irreversible changes in cell functions. Neurochemical disturbances resulting from abnormal excitation may not be associated with structural alterations detectable at the light microscopic level.

## REFERENCES

Araki C, Taketomo T, Toda T. Coma-puncture: exact experimental proof of the presence of the center of unconsciousness in the brain stem. Acta Sch Med Univ Kyoto 27:205–214, 1949.
Becker DP, Miller JD, Ward JD, Greenberg RP, Young HF, Sakalas R. The outcome from severe brain injury with early diagnosis and intensive management. J Neurosurg 47:491, 1977.
Becker DP. The temporal genesis of primary and secondary brain damage in experi-

mental and clinical head injury. *In* Baethmann A, Go KG, Unterberg A (eds), Mechanisms of Secondary Brain Damage. New York: Plenum, 1986, pp 47–64.

Belenky GL, Holaday JW. The opiate antagonist naloxone modifies the effects of electroconvulsive shock (ECS) on respiration, blood pressure and heart rate. Brain Res 197:414–417, 1979.

Binder LM. Persisting symptoms after mild head injury: a review of the post-concussion syndrome. J Clin Exp Neuropsychol 8(4):323–346, 1986.

Bolles RC. Species-specific defense reactions and avoidance learning. Psychol Rev 77:32–48, 1970.

Bornstein MB. Presence and action of acetylcholine in experimental brain trauma. J Neurophysiol 9:349–366, 1946.

Butterworth JF IV, Selhorst JB, Greenberg RP, Miller JD, Gudeman SK. Flaccidity after head injury: diagnosis, management and outcome. Neurosurgery 9:242–248, 1981.

Carlsson GS, Svärdsudd K, Welin L. Long-term effects of head injuries sustained during life in three male populations. J Neurosurg 67:197–205, 1987.

Chatrian GE, White LE, Daly D. Electroencephalographic patterns resembling those of sleep in certain comatose states after injuries to the head. Electroencephalogr Clin Neurophysiol 15:272–280, 1963.

Choi DW. Ionic dependence of glutamate neurotoxicity. J Neurosci 7:369–379, 1987.

Clifton GL, Ziegler MG, Grossman RG. Circulating catecholamines and sympathetic activity after head injury. Neurosurgery 8:10–14, 1981.

Collins RC. Selective vulnerability of brain: new insights from the excitatory synapse. Metab Brain Dis 1:231–240, 1986.

Cone WV, Tower DB, McEachern D. Acetylcholine and neuronal activity in epilepsy. Trans Am Neurol Assoc 73:59–63, 1948.

De la Torre JC. Local cerebral blood flow following stimulation of locus coeruleus in monkeys and rats. *In* Owman C, Edvinsson L (eds), Neurogenic Control of Brain Circulation. Oxford: Pergamon, 1977, pp 443–454.

DeSalles AAF, Jenkins LW, Anderson RL, Opoku-Edusei T, Marmarou A, Hayes RL. Extracellular potassium activity following concussion. A microelectrode study in the cat. Soc Neurosci Abstr 12:967, 1986.

DeSalles AAF, Katayama Y, Newlon PG, Dixon CE, Becker DP, Stonnington HH, Hayes RL. Transient suppression of event-related evoked potentials in the cat produced by mild head injury. J Neurosurg 66:102–108, 1987.

Deutsch G, Eisenberg HM. Frontal blood flow changes in recovery from coma. J Cereb Blood Flow Metab 7:29–34, 1987.

DeWitt DS, Jenkins LW, Wei EP, Kontos HA, Becker DP. The effects of fluid percussion brain injury on regional and total cerebral blood flow and pial vessel diameter: a combined pial window and microsphere study. J Neurosurg 64:787–794, 1986.

Dixon CE, Lyeth BG, Povlishock JT, Findling RL, Hamm RJ, Marmarou A, Young HF, Hayes, RL. A fluid percussion model of experimental brain injury in the rat. J Neurosurg 67:110–119, 1987.

Duckrow RB, LaManna JC, Rosenthal M, Levasseur JE, Patterson JL. Oxidative metabolic activity of cerebral cortex after fluid percussion head injury in the cat. J Neurosurg 54:607–614, 1981.

Duret H. Etudes experimentales et clinique sur les traumatismes cerebraux. Thèse de Paris, 1878.

Feeney DM, Sutton RL. Pharmacotherapy for recovery of function after brain injury. CRC Crit Rev Neurobiol 3:135–197, 1987.

Fieschi C, Battistini N, Beduschi A, Boselli L, Rossanda M. Regional cerebral blood flow and intraventricular pressure in acute head injuries. J Neurol Neurosurg Psychiatry 37:1378–1388, 1974.

Foltz EL, Schmidt RP. The role of the reticular formation in the coma of head injury. J Neurosurg 13:145–154, 1956.

French JD. Brain lesions associated with prolonged unconsciousness. Arch Neurol Psychiatry 68:727–740, 1952.

Gallup GG Jr, Maser JD. Tonic immobility: evolutionary underpinnings of human catalepsy and catatonia. *In* Maser JD, Sellymann MEP (eds), Psychopathology: Experimental Models. San Francisco: Freeman, 1977, pp 334–357.

Gennarelli TA, Obrist WD, Langfitt TW, Segawa H. Vascular and metabolic reactivity to changes in $P_{CO_2}$ in head injured patients. *In* Papp AJ, Bourke RS, Nelson LR, Kimelberg HK (eds), Neural Trauma. New York: Raven Press, 1979.

Gennarelli TA, Adams JH, Graham DI. Diffuse axonal injury—a new conceptual approach to an old problem. *In* Baethmann A, Go KG, Unterberg A (eds), Mechanisms of Secondary Brain Damage. New York: Plenum, 1986, pp 15–28.

Grashchenkov NI, Boeva EM, Irger JM, Kassil GN, Kamenetskaya BI, Fishman MN. Clinical and pathophysiological analysis of acute closed craniocerebral injury. *In* DeVett AC (ed), Proceedings of the Third International Congress of Neurological Surgery. Excerpta Medica Foundation, Amsterdam, 1966, pp 119–125.

Haber B, Grossman RG. Acetylcholine metabolism in intracranial and lumbar cerebrospinal fluid and in blood. *In* Wood JH (ed), Neurobiology and Cerebrospinal Fluid. New York: Plenum, 1980, pp 345–350.

Hass W. Regional studies of glucose metabolism in coma. *In* Passonneau J, Hawkins R, Lust W, Welsh F (eds), Cerebral Metabolism and Neural Function. Baltimore: Williams & Wilkins, 1980, pp. 382–386.

Hayes RL, Ellison MD. Animal models of concussive head injury. *In* Becker DB (ed), Head Injury, Philadelphia: WB Saunders, In Press.

Hayes RL, Katayama Y. Range of environmental stimuli producing nociceptive suppression: implications for neural mechanisms. Ann NY Acad Sci 467:1–13, 1986.

Hayes RL, Lewelt W, Yeatts ML, Jenkins LW, Katayama Y, Newlon PG, Pechura CM, Povlishock JT, Becker DP, Miller JD. Metabolic, behavioral and electrophysiological correlates of experimental brain injury in the cat. J Cereb Blood Flow Metab 3(Suppl 1):39–40, 1983.

Hayes RL, Pechura CM, Katayama Y, Povlishock JT, Giebel ML, Becker DP. Activation of pontine cholinergic sites implicated in unconsciousness following cerebral concussion in the cat. Science 233:301–303, 1984.

Hayes RL, Lyeth BG, Dixon CE, Becker DP. Cholinergic antagonist reduces neurological deficits following cerebral concussion in the cat. J Cereb Blood Flow Metab 5(1):395–396, 1985.

Hayes RL, Stonnington HH, Lyeth BG, Dixon CE, Yamamoto T. Metabolic and neurophysiologic sequellae of brain injury: a cholinergic hypothesis. J Cent Nerv Syst Trauma 3(2):163–173, 1986.

Hayes RL, Chapouris R, Lyeth BG, Jenkins L, Robinson SE, Young HF, Marmarou A. Pretreatment with phencyclidine (PCP) attenuates long-term behavioral deficits following concussive brain injury in the rat. Soc Neurosci Abst, 13:1254, 1987a.

Hayes RL, Katayama Y, Stonnington HH. Effects of experimental concussion on spinal cord integration of sensory input: relationship to acute traumatic unconsciousness. *In* Pubols LM, Sessle B (eds), Effects of Injury on Trigeminal and Spinal Somatosensory Systems. New York: Alan R Liss, 1987b, pp 411–418.

Hayes RL, Lyeth BG, Robinson SE, Young HF. Regional changes in brain acetylcholine (ACh): relationship to scopolamine effects on behavioral deficits following experimental brain injury. J Cereb Blood Flow Metab 7(Suppl 1):S635, 1987c.

Hayes RL, Katayama Y, Young HF, Dunbar JG. Coma associated with flaccidity produced by fluid percussion concussion in the cat. Part 1: Is it due to depression of activity within the brainstem reticular formation? Brain Injury, 2:31–49, 1988.

Hayes RL, Katayama Y, Jenkins LW, Lyeth BG, Clifton GL, Gunter J, Povlishock JT, Young HF. Regional rates of glucose utilization in the cat following concussive head injury. J. Neurotrauma (in press).

Hendricks JC, Morrison AR, Mann GL. Different behaviors during paradoxical sleep without atonia depend on pontine lesion site. Brain Res 239:81–105, 1982.

Heppner F, Diemath HE. Clinical experience with anticholinergic therapy of covered craniocerebral injuries. Monatsschr Unfallheilk Versicherungsmed 61:257–265, 1958.

Herkenhan M. Anesthetics and the habenulo-interpeduncular system: selective sparing of metabolic activity. Brain Res 210:461–466, 1981.

Herzog HA, Burghardt GM. Prey movement and predatory behavior of juvenile western yellow-bellied racers, *Coluber constrictor mormon.* Herpetologica 30:285–289, 1974.

Jenkins LW, Marmarou A, Lewelt W, Becker DP. Increased vulnerability of the traumatized brain to early ischemia. *In* Baethmann A, Go KG and Unterberg A (eds), Mechanisms of Secondary Brain Damage. New York: Plenum, 1986, pp 273–282.

Jenkins LW, Lewelt W, Moszynski K, Lyeth BG, Hayes RL, DeWitt DS, Robinson SE, Allen A, Opoku J, Marmarou A, Young HF. Increased vulnerability of the mildly traumatized rat brain to cerebral ischemia: the use of a controlled second insult as a research tool. Soc Neurosci Abstr 13:1253, 1987.

Jenkner FL, Lechner H. About the influence of scopolamine on the EEG in closed head injury. Fortschr Neurol Psychiatr 22:270–276, 1954.

Jenkner FL, Lechner H. The effect of diparcol on the electroencephalogram in the normal subject and in those with cerebral trauma. Electroencephalogr Clin Neurophysiol 7:303–305, 1955a.

Jenkner FL, Lechner H. Anticholinergic therapy in closed craniocerebral trauma. Langenbecks Arch U Dtsch Z Chir 280:354–361, 1955b.

Julian FJ, Goldman DE. The effects of mechanical stimulation on some electrical properties of axons. J Gen Physiol 46:297–313, 1962.

Katayama Y, Ueno Y, Tsukiyama T, Tsubokawa T. Long-lasting suppression of firing of cortical neurons and decrease in cortical blood flow following train pulse stimulation of the locus coeruleus in the cat. Brain Res 216:173–179, 1981.

Katayama Y, DeWitt DS, Becker DP, Hayes RL. Behavioral evidence for a cholinoceptive pontine inhibitory area: descending control of spinal motor output and sensory input. Brain Res 296:241–262, 1984a.

Katayama Y, Nakamura T, Becker DP, Hayes RL. Intracranial pressure variations associated with activation of the cholinoceptive pontine inhibitory area in the unaesthetized drug-free cat. J Neurosurg 61(4):713–724, 1984b.

Katayama Y, Watkins LR, Becker DP, Hayes RL. Non-opiate analgesia induced by carbachol microinjection into the pontine parabrachial region of the cat. Brain Res 296:263–283, 1984c.

Katayama Y, Becker DP, Hayes RL. Depression of afferent-induced primary afferent depolarization at the lumbar spinal cord following concussive head injury. Brain Res 335(2):392–395, 1985a.

Katayama Y, Glisson JD, Becker DP, Hayes RL. Concussive head injury produces suppression of sensory transmission within the spinal cord. J Neurosurg 63:97–105, 1985b.

Katayama Y, Reuther S, Dixon CE, Becker DP, Hayes, RL. Dissociation of endogenous components of auditory evoked potentials following carbachol microinjections into the cholinoceptive pontine inhibitory area. Brain Res 334:366–371, 1985c.

Katayama Y, Tsubokawa T, Abekura M, Hayes RL, Becker DP. Coma induced by cholinergic activation of a restricted region in the pontine reticular formation—a model of reversible forms of coma. Neurol Med Chir (Tokyo) 26:1–10, 1986.

Katayama Y, Young HF, Dunbar JG, Hayes RL. Coma associated with flaccidity produced by fluid percussion concussion in the cat. Part 2: Contribution of activity in the pontine inhibitory system. Brain Injury, 2:51–66, 1988.

Katayama Y, Abekura M, Young HF, Hayes RL. Cholinergic activation of a restricted region in the rostral pons of the cat produces a flaccid comatose state. Pharmacol Biochem Behav, submitted.

Kilduff TS, Sharp FR, Heller HC. Relative 2-deoxyglucose uptake of the paratrigeminal nucleus increases during hibernation. Brain Res 262:117–123, 1983.

Klemm WR. Mechanisms of the immobility reflex ("animal hypnosis"). II. EEG and multiple unit correlates in the brain stem. Commun Behav Biol 3:43–52, 1969.

Klemm WR. Neurophysiologic studies of the immobility reflex ("animal hypnosis"). In Ehrenpreis S, Solnitzky OC (eds), Neuroscience Research, Vol 4. New York: Academic Press, 1971, pp 165–212.

Kontos HA, Povlishock JT. Oxygen radicals in brain injury. J Cent Nerv Syst Trauma 3:257–263, 1986.

Krivanek J. Some metabolic changes accompanying Leao's spreading cortical depression in the rat. J Neurochem 6:182–189, 1981.

Langfitt TW, Gennarelli TA. Can the outcome from head injury be improved? J Neurosurg 56:19–24, 1982.

Leininger BE. Comparison of Two Minor Head Injury Groups: Importance of Loss of Consciousness in the Production of Cognitive Deficits. Unpublished Master's thesis, Department of Psychology, Virginia Commonwealth University, 1987.

Leonard JP, Salpeter MM. Agonist induced myopathy at the neuromuscular junction is mediated by calcium. J Cell Biol 82:811–819, 1979.

Levin HS, Mattis S, Ruff RM, Eisenberg HM, Marshall LF, Tabaddor K, High WM, Frankowski, RA. Neurobehavioral outcome following minor head injury: a three-center study. J Neurosurg 66:234–243, 1987.

Levin JE, Becker D, Chun T. Reversal of incipient brain death from head injury apnea at the scene of accidents. N Engl J Med 301:109, 1979.

Lewelt W, Jenkins LW, Miller JD. Autoregulation of cerebral blood flow after experimental fluid percussion injury of the brain. J Neurosurg 53:500–511, 1980.

Lewelt W, Jenkins LW, Miller JD. Effects of experimental fluid-percussion injury of the brain on cerebrovascular reactivity to hypoxia and to hypercapnia. J Neurosurg 56:332–338, 1982.

Lindgren S, Rinder L. Experimental studies on head injury. II. Pressure propagation in "percussion-concussion." Biophysik 3:174–180, 1966.

Lindgren S, Rinder L. Production and distribution of intracranial and intraspinal pressure changes at sudden extradural fluid volume input in rabbits. Acta Physiol Scand 76:340–351, 1969.

Luria AR, Naydin VL, Tsvetkova LS, Vinarskaya EN. Restoration of higher cortical function following local brain damage. In Vinken PJ, Bruyn GW (eds), Handbook of Clinical Neurology, Vol 3: Disorders of Higher Nervous Activity. Amsterdam: North-Holland, 1969, pp 368–433.

Lyeth BG, Dixon CE, Hamm RJ, Yamamoto T, Giebel ML, Stonnington HH, Becker DP, Hayes RL. Neurological deficits following experimental cerebral concussion in the rat attenuated by scopolamine pretreatment. Soc Neurosci Abstr 11:432, 1985.

Lyeth BG, Dixon CE, Giebel ML, Robinson SE, Hamm RJ, Stonnington HH, Young

HF, Hayes RL. The effects of scopolamine pre-and post-treatment on the responses to concussive brain injury in the rat. Soc Neurosci Abstr 12:967, 1986.

Lyeth BG, Jenkins LW, Hamm RJ, Robinson SE, Dixon CE, Giebel ML, Allen A, Schaeffer M, Oleniak L, Opoku J, Chapouris RG, Marmarou A, Young HF, Hayes RL. Enduring short-term memory deficits in the absence of hippocampal cell death following moderate head injury in the rat. Soc Neurosci Abstr, 13:1253, 1987.

Lyeth BG, Dixon CE, Hamm RJ, Jenkins LW, Young HF, Stonnington HH, Hayes RL. Effects of anticholinergic treatment on transient behavioral suppression and physiological responses following concussive brain injury to the rat. Brain Research 448:88–97, 1988a.

Lyeth BG, Dixon CE, Jenkins LW, Hamm RJ, Alberico A, Stonnington HH, Young HF, Hayes RL. Effects of scopolamine treatment on long-term behavioral deficits following concussive brain injury in the rat. Brain Research 452:39–48, 1988b.

Lynch G, Baudry M. The biochemistry of memory: a new and specific hypothesis. Science 224:1057–1063, 1984.

Marshall LF, Smith RW, Shapiro HM. The outcome with aggressive treatment in severe head injuries. 1. The significance of intracranial pressure monitoring. J Neurosurg 50:20–25, 1979.

Metz B. Acetylcholine and experimental brain injury. J Neurosurg 35:523–528, 1971.

Meyer-Holzapfel M. Abnormal behavior in zoo animals. In Fox MW (ed), Abnormal Behavior in Animals. Philadelphia: WB Saunders, 1968, p 477.

Miller JD, Sweet RC, Narayan R, Becker DP. Early insults to the injured brain. JAMA 240:439–442, 1978.

Miller JD, Butterworth JF, Gudeman SK, Falkner JE, Choi SC, Selhorst J, Harbison J, Lutz HA, Young HF, Becker DP. Further experience in the management of severe head injury. J Neurosurg 54:289–299, 1981.

Morrison AR, Reiner PB. A dissection of paradoxical sleep. In McGinty DJ, Drucker-Colin R, Morrison A, Parmeggiani PL (eds), Brain Mechanisms of Sleep. New York: Raven Press, 1985, pp 97–110.

Moruzzi G, Magoun HW. Brain stem reticular formation and activation of the EEG. Electroencephalogr Clin Neurophysiol 1:455–473, 1949.

Obrist WD, Langfitt TW, Jaggi JL, Cruz J, Gennarelli TA. Cerebral blood flow and metabolism in comatose patients with acute head injury. J Neurosurg 6:241–253, 1984.

Olney JW. Neurotoxicity of excitatory amino acids. In McGeer E, Olney JW, McGeer P (eds), Kainic Acid as a Tool in Neurobiology. New York: Raven Press, 1978, pp 95–121.

Olney JW. Excitotoxins: an overview. In Fuxe K, Roberts P, Schwarcz R (eds), Excitotoxins. New York: Macmillan, 1983, pp 82–96.

Olney JW, Rhee V, Ho OL. Kainic acid: a powerful neurotoxin analogue of glutamate. Brain Res 77:507–512, 1974.

Olney JW, Sharpe LG, deGubareff T. Excitotoxic amino acids. Soc Neurosci Abstr 1:371, 1975.

Olney JW, Fuller T, deGubareff T. Acute dendrotoxic changes in the hippocampus of kainate treated rats. Brain Res 176:91–100, 1979.

Olney JW, deGubareff T, Labruyere J. Seizure-related brain damage induced by cholinoceptive agents. Nature 301:520–522, 1983a.

Olney JW, deGubareff T, Sloviter RS. "Epileptic" brain damage in rats induced by sustained electrical stimulation of the perforant path. II. Ultrastructural analysis of acute hippocampal pathology. Brain Res Bull 10:699–712, 1983b.

Ommaya A. Mechanisms of cerebral concussion, contusions and other effects of head injury. *In* Youmans J (ed), Youmans Neurological Surgery. Philadelphia: WB Saunders, 1982, Vol 4, pp 1877–1895.

Oppenheimer DR. Microscopic lesions in the brain following head injury. J Neurol Neurosurg Psychiatry 31:299–306, 1968.

Overgaard J, Tweed WA. Cerebral circulation after head injury. I. Cerebral blood flow and its regulation after closed head injury with emphasis on clinical correlations. J Neurosurg 41:531–541, 1974.

Povlishock J. The morphopathologic responses to experimental head injuries of varying severity. *In* Becker D, Povlishock J (eds), Central Nervous System Status Report 1985, sponsored by NINCDS. Richmond VA: Byrd Press, 1985, pp 443–452.

Povlishock J. Traumatically induced axonal damage without concomitant change in focally related neuronal somata and dendrites. Acta Neuropathol 70:53–59, 1986.

Povlishock J, Becker D, Cheng C, Vaughan G. Axonal change in minor head injury. J Neuropathol Exp Neurol 42:225–242, 1983.

Preskorn SH, Hartman BK, Raichle ME, Swanson LW, Clark HB. Central adrenergic regulation of cerebral microvascular permeability and blood flow: pharmacologic evidence. Adv Exp Med Biol 131:127–138, 1980.

Preskorn SH, Irwin GH, Simpson S, Friesen D, Rinne J, Jerkovich G. Medical therapies for mood disorders alter the blood–brain barrier. Science 213:469–471, 1981.

Raichle ME, Eichling JO, Grubb RL Jr, Hartman BK. Central noradrenergic regulation of brain microcirculation. *In* Pappius HM, Feinde W (eds), Dynamics of Brain Edema. New York: Springer, 1976, pp 11–17.

Rimel RW, Giordani B, Barth JT, Boll TJ, Jane JA. Disability caused by minor head injury. Neurosurgery 9:221–228, 1981.

Rimel RW, Giordani B, Barth JT, Jane JA. Moderate head injury: completing the clinical spectrum of brain trauma. Neurosurgery 11(3):344–351, 1982.

Rivlin AS, Tator CH. Objective clinical assessment of motor function after experimental spinal cord injury in the rat. J Neurosurg 47:577–581, 1977.

Robinson SE, Rice MA, Hambrecht KL. Effect of intrastriatal injection of diisopropyl-fluorophosphate on acetylcholine, dopamine, and serotonin metabolism. J Neurochem 46(5):1632–1638, 1986a.

Robinson SE, Saija A, Yamamoto T, Dixon CE, Lyeth BG, Giebel ML, Stonnington HH, Hayes RL. Effects of experimental concussion on cholinergic neurons in specific rat brain regions. Soc Neurosci Abstr 12:966, 1986b.

Rosner MJ, Becker DP. The etiology of plateau waves: a theoretical model with experimental validation. Proc Fifth Int Symp Intracranial Pressure, 1982, p 154.

Rosner MJ, Newsome HH, Becker DP. Mechanical brain injury: the sympathoadrenal response. J Neurosurg 61:76–86, 1984.

Ruge D. The use of cholinergic blocking agents in the treatment of craniocerebral injuries. J Neurosurg 11:77–83, 1954.

Sachs F Jr. Acetylcholine and serotonin in the spinal fluid. J Neurosurg 14:22–27, 1957.

Saija A, Hayes RL, Lyeth BG, Dixon CE, Yamamoto T, Robinson SE. The effect of concussive head injury on central cholinergic neurons. Brain Research 452:303–311, 1988.

Samson F, Pazdernik TL, Cross RS, Churchill L, Gieseler MP, Nelson SR. Brain regional activity and damage associated with organophosphate induced seizures: effects of atropine and benactyzine. Proc West Pharmacol Soc 28:183–185, 1985.

Sargeant AB, Eberhardt LE. Death feigning by ducks in response to predation by red foxes *(Vulpes fulva)*. Am Midland Naturalist 94:108–119, 1975.

Saunders ML, Miller JD, Stablein D. The effects of graded experimental trauma on cerebral blood flow and responsiveness. J Neurosurg 51:18–26, 1979.

Schall-Vess R, Hayes RL, Clifton G, Susskind B. Immunosuppression in the rodent following traumatic brain injury. J Neurosurg, submitted.

Sloviter RS. "Epileptic" brain damage in rats induced by sustained electrical stimulation of the perforant path. I. Acute electrophysiological and light microscopic studies. Brain Res Bull 10:675–697, 1983.

Stalhammar DA, Galinat BJ, Allen AM, Becker DP, Stonnington HH, Hayes RL. A new model of concussive brain injury in the cat produced by extradural fluid volume loading. I. Biomechanical properties. Brain Injury 1:73–91, 1987.

Stockard JJ, Bickford RG, Aung MH. The electroencephalogram in traumatic brain injury. In Vinken PJ, Bruyn GW (eds), Handbook of Clinical Neurology, Vol 23. Amsterdam: North-Holland, 1975, pp 317–368.

Sullivan HG, Martinez J, Becker DP, Miller JD, Griffith R, Wist AO. Fluid-percussion model of mechanical brain injury in the cat. J Neurosurg 45:520–534, 1976.

Takahashi H, Manaka S, Sano K. Changes in extracellular potassium concentration in cortex and brain stem during the acute phase of experimental closed head injury. J Neurosurg 55:708–717, 1981.

Teasdale G. Assessment of head injury. Br J Anaesth 49:761–766, 1976.

Thibault LE, Gennarelli TA. Biomechanics and craniocerebral trauma. In Becker DP, Povlishock JT (eds), Central Nervous System Trauma Status Report, 1985. Sponsored by NINCDS. Richmond, VA: Byrd Press, 1985, pp 379–389.

Thompson RW, Piroch J, Fallen D, Hatton D. A central cholinergic inhibitory system as a basis for tonic immobility (animal hypnosis) in chickens. J Comp Physiol Psychol 87:507–512, 1974.

Tower DB, McEachern D. Acetylcholine and neuronal activity: I. Cholinesterase patterns and acetylcholine in the cerebrospinal fluids of patients with craniocerebral trauma. Can J Res 27:105–119, 1949a.

Tower DB, McEachern D. Acetylcholine and neuronal activity: II. Acetylcholine and cholinesterase activity in the cerebrospinal fluids of patients with epilepsy. Can J Res 27:120–131, 1949b.

Turski WA, Czuczwar SJ, Kleinrok Z, Turski L. Cholinomimetics produce seizures and brain damage in rats. Experientia 39:1408–1411, 1983.

Urca G, Yitzhaky J, Frank H. Different opioid systems may participate in post-electroconvulsive shock (ECS), analgesia and catalepsy. Brain Res 219:385–396, 1981.

Ward A Jr. Atropine in the treatment of closed head injury. J Neurosurg 7:398–402, 1950.

Ward A Jr. The physiology of concussion. In Caveness WS, Walker AE (eds), Head Injury. JB Lippincott, 1966, pp 203–208.

Watkins LR, Mayer DJ. Organization of endogenous opiate and non-opiate pain control systems. Science 216:1185–1192, 1982.

Wei EP, Dietrich WD, Povlishock JT, Navari RM, Kontos HA. Functional, morphological, and metabolic abnormalities of the cerebral microcirculation after concussive brain injury in the cat. Circ Res 46:37–47, 1980.

# III
# Clinical Management, Neurophysiology, and Neuroimaging

# 6

# Complications After Apparently Mild Head Injury and Strategies of Neurosurgical Management

RALPH G. DACEY, JR.

A great deal of information has accumulated on the epidemiology, pathophysiology, and treatment of *severe* head injury. This emphasis on severe head injury reflects the complex treatment it requires and the profound neurological deficits that often occur. However, minor head injury is also a major public health problem (see Kraus and Nourjah, Chapter 2, this volume, for a review of the epidemiology). Patients are often disabled by headache, cognitive problems, and memory disorders seemingly out of proportion to the severity of their injury (Rimel et al., 1981). Another significant problem in minor head injury is that a few patients will develop potentially serious intracranial sequelae such as subdural or epidural hematomas, despite being relatively alert at the time of their initial evaluation. Controversy has therefore arisen regarding the optimal strategy for managing minor head injury, balancing the risks of a few patients' development of neurosurgical complications against the high cost of screening all minor head injury patients for the development of these sequelae. Much of this controversy has focused on the radiological evaluation of minor head injury, specifically on the question of who should have skull films. There is little information on the proper overall management of patients with minor head injury, of which radiological evaluation is only a part.

Two questions can therefore be formulated regarding the neurosurgical management of minor head injury: (1) What is the risk of a potentially serious neurosurgical complication developing after minor head injury? and (2) What is the most effective way to identify those patients most likely to develop such complications?

## ASSESSING THE RISK OF SERIOUS COMPLICATIONS AFTER MINOR HEAD INJURY

The risk of various sequelae of *severe* head injury has been relatively well defined. Approximately 40% of patients will have significant intracranial mass lesions, and about 50% will develop increased intracranial pressure (Becker et al., 1977; Miller et al., 1977, 1981). The incidence of significant neurological deterioration after severe head injury has also been well described. Rose et al. (1977) and Reilly et al. (1975) described patients who "talk and die" after head injury. They found that of 151 patients with fatal head injuries, 58 were capable of speaking at some time after impact. Three-quarters of these patients had intracranial hematomas despite their relative initial alertness. Marshall et al. (1983) described another group of patients studied in the Traumatic Coma Data Bank who "talk and deteriorate," constituting 12% of a group of severely head-injured patients. Thus at least 10% of patients with severe head injury are capable of speech during the interval between impact and treatment, indicating the potential problem with head injuries that appear initially to be relatively minor.

The risk of serious neurosurgical complications in minor head injury has been more difficult to study, however. Mendelow et al. (1982) examined the problem from a somewhat different perspective by describing the incidence of intracranial hematoma in a large consecutive series of 1442 head-injured patients. Intracranial hematomas developed in 3.9% of the patients, and, in a subset of 865 patients who were initially alert and oriented, 1.3% developed intracranial hematomas. In a subsequent population-based study, Mendelow et al. (1983) estimated that 545 (1.5%) of 36,637 patients admitted to primary surgical wards developed intracranial hematomas.

Fischer et al. (1981) retrospectively studied 333 head-injured patients who were alert when evaluated in the emergency room. Eight of these patients (2.4%) subsequently required operative procedures, five for depressed skull fractures and three for subdural hematomas.

At the University of Virginia, 610 minor head injury patients were prospectively identified (Dacey et al., 1986). The goal of this study was to assess the risk of serious neurosurgical complications in a well-defined group of patients. This consecutive series had two inclusion criteria: (1) Patients gave a history of, or were reliably reported to have sustained a cerebral concussion (defined as transient posttraumatic loss of consciousness or other neurological function such as memory, speech, or vision); and (2) a neurosurgeon gave them a Glasgow Coma Scale (GCS) score of 13, 14, or 15 in the emergency room. All patients were managed in a standardized manner, undergoing skull x-rays and a period of in-hospital observation. If patients had a deterioration of neurological condition sufficient to warrant a neurosurgical procedure, they were considered to have developed a significant neurosurgical complication as a study end point. Of the 610 patients entered into the study, 65.4% were males and 34.6% were females. Most patients were between the ages of 11 and 30 (Figure 6–1). About half of the patients had blood alcohol levels greater than

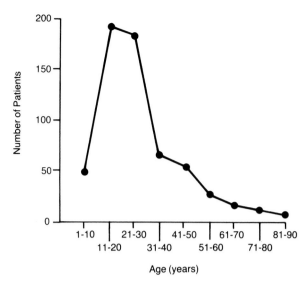

**Figure 6–1**   Age distribution of 610 patients with minor head injury. (Reproduced from Dacey et al., 1986 by permission)

0.10 g/dl. Motor vehicle accidents and bicycle accidents caused 57.9% of injuries, and falls caused 20.0%. Thus the demographic characteristics of the population were similar to those reported for most series of severely head injured patients, in that they tended to be young males in vehicular accidents related to alcohol.

Most of the patients were alert at the time of admission; only 12.6% had detectable muscle weakness on neurological examination. Length of stay in the hospital was related to initial GCS score (Figure 6–2); 72.5% stayed less than 48 hours. Eighteen of the 610 patients (3.0%) required a neurosurgical procedure (Table 6–1). Three patients (0.8%) had intracranial hematomas. One patient rapidly deteriorated under close neurological supervision with an acute subdural hematoma and died despite urgent craniotomy. Intracranial pressure monitoring was performed in seven patients whose level of consciousness decreased, and, despite the presence of high-density lesions on CT scan, all had normal intracranial pressure. This contrasts with the experience in severe head injury where intracranial hypertension is common with high-density CT lesions (Narayan et al., 1982). Compared to the population as a whole, patients who developed serious intracranial complications were more likely to be male, to have had an emergency room GCS of 13 or 14, or to have been injured in a fall.

In summary, a significant number of patients (at least 10%) who become comatose after head injury are capable of speech at some time after impact. The incidence of potentially serious neurosurgical complications after apparently minor head injury ranges between 1% and 3%.

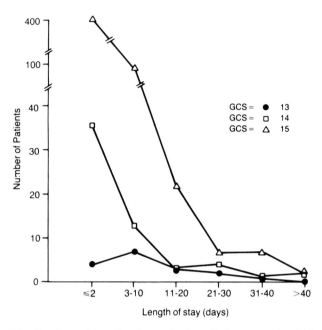

**Figure 6–2** Distribution of length of stay in hospital among the 610 patients with Glasgow Coma Scale (GCS) scores of 13, 14, or 15. (Reproduced from Dacey et al., 1986 by permission)

## RADIOLOGICAL EVALUATION OF PATIENTS WITH MINOR HEAD INJURY

The use of skull radiography as a screening tool for patients with minor head injury is very controversial (Balasubramaniam et al., 1981; Royal College of Radiologists, 1979). Some patients clearly need to have skull x-rays to direct further management. However, it has been difficult to develop appropriate criteria for deciding which patients should have films. Data indicating that skull radiography is overused have come from multiple sources in the United States and in Britain. Bell and Loop (1971) suggested that higher yields of positive findings on skull x-rays could be produced if clinicians would use the presence of one of 21 clinical criteria found to be associated with skull fracture before referring the patients for skull films. They reported 93 fractures in 1,500 patients who had sustained head injuries of varying degrees of severity; 59% of the patients had normal levels of consciousness on admission, whereas 7% were either "semicomatose or comatose." When x-rays were reviewed, 93 fractures were found; 92 of these were in patients who demonstrated one of the 21 criteria. The fracture occurring in the one remaining patient apparently did not change this patient's subsequent management. Bell and Loop suggested that great savings in health care costs could be expected if more selectivity were practiced by clinicians ordering skull x-rays.

Phillips (1979a,b) further extended these studies at the University of Washington and examined the utility of a list of nine "high-yield criteria" for

| Case no. | Age (yr)/sex | Initial GCS | Mechanism of injury[a] | Skull fracture | CT findings[b] | Operative procedure | Injury–operation interval (days) | Outcome GOS[c] |
|---|---|---|---|---|---|---|---|---|
| 1 | 76 M | 13 | fall | yes | EDH and ASDH | craniotomy, removal of clot | <1 | GR |
| 2 | 18 M | 15 | MVA | yes | L. MCA infarct (traumatic cerv. ICA occlusion) | craniotomy, EC–IC anastomosis | <1 | MD |
| 3 | 56 M | 13 | fall | yes | ICH | craniotomy, removal of clot | <1 | GR |
| 4 | 21 M | 15 | MVA | no | m. fossa subarachnoid cyst | craniotomy, removal of membranes | 30 | GR |
| 5 | 28 M | 15 | fall | yes | R. ASDH | craniotomy | <1 | D |
| 6 | 30 M | 15 | MVA | yes | R. EDH | craniotomy | <1 | GR |
| 7 | 39 M | 13 | MVA | no | R. ASDH | craniotomy, removal of clot | <1 | GR |
| 8 | 17 M | 14 | MVA | yes | comp. depressed skull fracture | elevation of fracture | <1 | GR |
| 9 | 18 M | 13 | MVA | yes | R. fr. depressed fracture | craniotomy, elevation depressed fracture | <1 | MD |
| 10 | 28 M | 14 | farm accident | yes | ICH, depressed skull fracture | craniotomy, elevation elevation of fracture, removal of clot | <1 | GR |
| 11 | 67 M | 15 | fall | no | R. CSDH | burr holes | 3 | GR |
| 12 | 55 M | 13 | MVA | no | normal | ICP monitor | <1 | GR |
| 13 | 46 F | 14 | fall | no | R. ICH | ICP monitor | 2 | GR |
| 14 | 44 M | 13 | fall | yes | R. EDH | ICP monitor | <1 | GR |
| 15 | 51 M | 14 | fall | yes | normal | ICP monitor | <1 | GR |
| 16 | 40 F | 15 | MVA | yes | R. fr. contusion | ICP monitor | <1 | GR |
| 17 | 50 M | 15 | assault | yes | normal | ICP monitor | <1 | GR |
| 18 | 35 M | 15 | fall | yes | R. fr. temporal contusion | ICP monitor | <1 | GR |

[a]MVA, motor vehicle accident

[b]ASDH acute subdural hematoma; CSDH, chronic subdural hematoma; EDH, epidural hematoma; ICH, traumatic intracerebral hematoma.

[c]Glasgow Outcome Scale: GR, good recovery; MD, moderate disability; SD, severe disability (D) death.

Source: Modified from Dacey et al. (1986), by permission.

the demonstration of skull fractures after head injury. Phillips noted a progressively increasing rate of posttraumatic skull radiography in his institution prior to his study. He found that when clinicians were required to complete a form indicating the presence or absence of one of the high-yield criteria, the ordering of skull films dropped to 60% of the prestudy rate. He also reported (1979b) that when two hospital emergency rooms were compared, the rate of skull x-ray examinations per 100 patient visits was significantly lower in the ER maintaining the high-yield criteria policy. Although 34% of fractures were missed by the HYC policy, Phillips stated that a subsequent medical record review revealed that in no case did the finding of a skull fracture lead to an "active process" of care for the head injury patients (i.e., it was clinically insignificant).

Other investigators using Phillips's high-yield criteria list have reported somewhat different findings, however. Larsen and Kozial (1979) found that 48% of fractures were missed using the high-yield list. In contrast with the findings of Phillips (1979a,b) and Cummins et al. (1980), 7% of patients in whom fractures were missed needed further care and/or hospitalization. Similarly, DeSmet and his co-workers (1979) found that 35% of fractures were missed when the 21 Bell and Loop high-yield findings were used. All the missed fractures were in children, a finding which suggests that the list should not be applied to children.

Phillips's studies have been criticized. Reynolds (1979) indicated that the retrospective chart reviews used to determine the impact of finding a skull fracture in patients with and without "high yield criteria" were not accurate, and that in fact some patients had been treated less than optimally because of this policy. There was also criticism because the rates of skull x-ray at two very different emergency rooms were used as evidence supporting the conclusion of the studies. Others have been critical of the high-yield criteria (HYC) chosen, finding them restrictive and/or irrelevant (e.g., "craniotomy with shunting tube in place"), especially in their potential for missing compound fractures (Freed, 1980). In a study of physicians' reactions to the HYC policy, Cummins et al. (1980) reported that physicians felt that (1) the list was too narrow, (2) it did not complement their problem-solving strategies, (3) it did not allow them to respond to familial and patient expectations, and (4) it interfered with their routine approach to such problems. The rate of compliance with the HYC list ranged from 20% to 50% (Cummins et al., 1980; Phillips 1979b).

Despite criticism of Phillips's studies, similar data came from Eyes and Evans (1978) in a review of 504 patients who presented to the casualty department in Liverpool. Skull fractures were found in 2%, and no correlation was found between x-ray findings and need for hospital admission. Only 25% of these patients were admitted to hospital, and only 13% had a period of unconsciousness. This indicates that, overall, these were a mildly injured group of patients. These authors felt that scalp lacerations and/or hematomas are not sufficient indication for skull radiography when they exist alone.

A larger study, conducted in nine centers in Britain, was reported by the Royal College of Radiology (1981). In 4,829 patients with "uncomplicated" head injury, 67 fractures were found: 64 vault, 2 basal, and 1 frontal. Four intracranial hematomas occurred in this group, and three of these would have been detected even if no skull x-rays had been taken. The authors estimated that only one patient with an intracranial hematoma would have been sent home without definitive care if skull x-rays had not been ordered. They reported that the cost of detecting this one patient was extremely high, and suggested that clinicians be more selective in ordering skull x-rays, basing the decision primarily on symptoms or signs found at the time of presentation. Subsequently, these data were reexamined by the Royal College of Radiology (1981) to determine the effect of six alternative patient selection guidelines. The most conservative approach resulted in skull x-rays being performed on 94% of patients with skull fractures and all patients with significant complications. The least conservative approach (in which the patient would be admitted if no x-ray capability were available) resulted in only 58% of the fractures being detected, and one patient with a serious outcome (intracranial hematoma) being sent home. The costs of radiology were reduced 21.3% and 72.9%, respectively, by these schemes.

Clinical indications for posttraumatic skull x-rays may be different in *children* with minor head injury (Bruce and Shut, 1980; DeSmet et al., 1979). Leonidas and his associates (1982) studied 354 infants and children who had undergone skull radiography; 42% had fractures and none had a serious intracranial complication. One patient underwent elevation of a depressed vault fracture as a result of the skull x-rays. In no other case was the treatment plan altered by the finding of a skull fracture. A disproportionate incidence of skull fracture occurred in infants: 14% of children less than one year old had fractures, compared to 3% of older children. These investigators suggested that the high-yield criteria of Phillips were not as applicable to children since only 9 of 15 fractures would have been detected using this scheme—a sensitivity of 60%. They recommended adding to the list cephalohematoma, drowsiness, and age under one year, in order to increase its senstivity in children.

Thornbury and his co-workers (1984) changed the emphasis somewhat in determining which patients should be x-rayed, by reviewing 1,845 patients originally reported by Masters (1980) and developing a list of "low yield criteria." They reported that patients who were asymptomatic or had headaches, dizziness, scalp hematomas, or scalp lacerations were not at increased risk for intracranial complications if they were found to have a fracture. They contended that if this approach were to be used, a substantial reduction in post-traumatic skull radiography could be effected without failing to detect serious intracranial sequelae.

Cooper and Ho (1983) approached the problem from another new perspective. They studied 202 patients with known traumatic intracranial masses to determine the impact of the discovery of a skull fracture specifically in alert patients without neurological deficits. Skull fractures were found in 37% of these patients, and 92% had an altered level of consciousness at the time of presentation. Sixteen patients were alert, and 6 of these had skull fractures. The 10 alert patients without skull fracture were all admitted because of neurological deficits or nausea and vomiting. One patient who had a skull fracture was completely intact neurologically and was discharged from the emergency room. He later returned with neurological deterioration secondary to an epidural hematoma, and recovered after the hematoma was removed. Cooper and Ho hence concluded that the identification of linear fractures is not a cost-effective determinant of the need for hospital admission after minor head injury.

A significant amount of information thus suggests that skull x-rays are overused in head injury evaluation, and that the numbers of patients x-rayed could be safely decreased. On the other side of the skull x-ray controversy, however, a significant amount of data suggests that the finding of a skull fracture is an important part of the clinical picture in evaluating head injuries. This finding is said to be important for two reasons: (1) A simple linear skull fracture significantly increases the risk that an alert patient will subsequently deteriorate as a result of an intracranial complication; and (2) compound depressed skull fractures can be missed on clinical examination, resulting in complications caused by infection (Jennett, 1980; Jennett and Bond, 1985).

Much of the information regarding the importance of fracture detection has come from Scotland. Miller and Jennett (1968), discussing complications in 400 patients with depressed skull fracture, observed that about half these patients had been only briefly unconscious; 26% suffered complications of their fracture; 11% had infections, and 7% had intracranial hematomas. In 38 of the cases complicated by infection, the presence of a depressed fracture was unsuspected on clinical grounds. Miller and Jennett noted that failure to recognize a depressed fracture was sometimes due to failure to obtain skull x-rays and was not infrequently a cause of avoidable posttraumatic complications.

Jennett and others (Guidelines . . . , 1984; Jennett, 1980; Jennett and Bond, 1985) have been advocates of obtaining skull x-rays on all patients who present with a history of unconsciousness or amnesia at any time, neurological symptoms or signs, CSF leaks, suspected penetrating injury, and scalp bruising or swelling. These recommendations are much less selective than those proposed by most radiologists, and are based on the premise that finding a skull fracture is important (Jennett, 1980), principally to detect compound injuries and to decide whether a mildly injured patient should be admitted to the hospital. Jennett (1980) reported that two-thirds of severely injured patients had fractured skulls. Basal fractures were found in only 45% of patients who had clinical signs of such a fracture, and clinical signs were present in 87% of patients with a radiological fracture. Fractures were also usually found in patients who had such serious intracranial complications as epidural hematomas (90% had fractures) or subdural hematomas (75% had fractures) (Gibson, 1983; Jennett, 1980). Among patients admitted after head injury to Scottish primary surgical wards (usually for observation), the incidence of fracture ranged from 6% to 9%. Among all those seen in accident and emergency departments in Britain, the incidence was much lower (about 1–3% of that portion of the population who were x-rayed).

According to Jennett (1980), a fracture in a less seriously injured patient significantly increases the likelihood of secondary intracranial complications, especially hematoma and infection. The latter can usually be prevented by appropriate management, whereas recovery from the former depends on early recognition and rapid surgical intervention. The clinician who knows that his or her patient has a fracture is better able to anticipate these complications, which can occur in patients whose initial injury is mild. It may not be obvious that admission for observation is necessary. Indeed some patients who have fractures and develop these complications prove "not even to have sought medical advice immediately after injury" (Miller and Jennett, 1968). Jennett (1980) calculates that the risk that a hematoma will develop in a mildly injured patient is increased about 400 times by the finding of a skull fracture. Eighty-five percent of skull fractures occur in patients who have had only a brief period of unconsciousness or have never lost consciousness after injury. Because about 15% of patients with intracranial hematomas that require operation have no initial loss of consciousness, there is a risk that the severity of injury can be underestimated.

Jennett (1980) argues that important clinical decisions depend on the skull x-ray findings, such as whether to admit the mildly injured patient or transfer him or her to a neurosurgical facility, and whether to perform formal debridement on a patient who has a possible compound depressed fracture under a scalp laceration. Jennett's contention that fracture detection after recent head injury is important has been supported by other studies. Jones and Jeffreys (1981) found that the presence of a fracture in a patient admitted for neurological observation increased by a factor of 24 the risk of subsequent neurological deterioration. Similarly, Fischer et al. (1981) found no incidence of later neurological complications in a series of 333 alert head-injured patients admitted for observation when there was no fracture. Dacey et al. (1986) reported 610 prospectively identified minor head injury patients whose risk of subsequently needing a neurosurgical operation was increased by a factor of 20 by the finding of a skull fracture. Young and Schmidek (1982) examined the importance of recognizing occipital skull fractures; they noted that 37% of patients either died or had neurological deficits when occipital skull fracture was present.

Mendelow et al. (1983) described a large number of Scottish head injury patients in terms of two easily obtained pieces of clinical data: whether or not the patient was alert, and whether or not the patient had a skull fracture. These authors compiled data from several series to estimate the risk of an intracranial hematoma developing in patients who presented to accident and emergency departments and in patients admitted to primary surgical wards. In Britain, patients with minor head injuries needing a period of neurological observation are usually admitted to primary surgical wards. Of the 545 patients with intracranial hematomas presenting during the study period, 15.4% were alert initially and 75.6% were found to have fractures. Thirty-five percent of the patients with intracranial hematomas who initially were oriented had no skull fracture. It was estimated that of the 189,432 patients with a complaint of head injury attending accident and emergency departments during the study period, 92.5% were oriented and 1.7% had a skull fracture, whereas the corresponding features in the group of 36,637 patients admitted to primary surgical wards were 76.1% and 8.4%, respectively. It was estimated that the risk of intracranial hematoma ranged between 1 in 5,983 and 1 in 4 for patients attending accident

**Table 6-2**   Absolute Risk of Intracranial Hematoma After Head Injury

|  | Number (%) of patients with hematomas | Absolute risk (emergency dept.) | Absolute risk (primary surgical ward) |
|---|---|---|---|
| No skull fracture: |  |  |  |
| Oriented | 29 ( 5.3%) | 1:5983 | 1:906 |
| Not oriented | 104 (19.1%) | 1:121 | 1:70 |
| Skull fracture: |  |  |  |
| Oriented | 55 (10.1%) | 1:32 | 1:29 |
| Not oriented | 357 (65.5%) | 1:4 | 1:4 |

*Source:* Modified from Mendelow et al. (1983), by permission.

and emergency wards, and 1 in 906 and 1 in 4 in primary surgical wards, depending on whether or not the patient was alert and whether or not the patient had a skull fracture (see Table 6-2). Mendelow and his colleagues concluded that both an assessment of the patient's level of consciousness and a determination of the presence of skull fracture are crucial pieces of information in evaluating head-injured patients. These investigators advocated using the presence or absence of skull fracture to decide whether a minor head injury patient with a normal level of consciousness should be admitted for further observation or discharged.

The most recent compilation of data bearing on the utilization of posttraumatic skull radiography examined data from three studies (Masters, 1980; Masters et al., 1987; Royal College of Radiologists, 1981). The authors concluded that "most patients with a fracture do not have an associated intracranial lesion and many patients with an acute traumatic intracranial lesion do not have a fracture" (Masters et al., 1987). The authors further analyzed information on these patients and concluded that if patients were to be managed according to the strategy in Table 6-3, the likelihood of missing an intracranial injury because of failure to diagnose an occult skull fracture would be about 1 in 2,500 (Masters et al., 1987).

The controversy surrounding posttraumatic skull radiography is therefore not totally resolved, although it appears that the recommendations of those who are most active in investigating this problem are coming closer together. In fact, the only major difference between the indications for skull x-ray as determined by a group of British neurosurgeons (Guidelines . . . , 1984) and those in the moderate- and high-risk groups of the Food and Drug Administration (FDA) panel (Masters et al., 1987) is that the group in Britain would x-ray the patient with a scalp bruise or swelling, whereas the FDA panel would not. A more significant difference in approach is that the British neurosurgeons would use skull x-rays to determine whether some alert patients without neurological symptoms could be safely sent home despite having had loss or alteration in consciousness at the time of injury. The clinical information suggesting a change in consciousness at the time of injury would place the patient in the FDA panel's moderate-risk group, for which they recommend extended

**Table 6–3**  Management Strategy for Radiographic Imaging in Head Trauma

| Low-risk group[a] | Moderate-risk group[a] | High-risk group |
|---|---|---|
| 1. Asymptomatic | 1. History of change of consciousness at time of injury or subsequently | 1. Depressed level of consciousness not clearly due to alcohol, drugs, or other cause (e.g., metabolic and seizure disorders) |
| 2. Headache | 2. History of progressive headache | 2. Focal neurological signs |
| 3. Dizziness | 3. Alcohol or drug intoxication | 3. Decreasing level of consciousness |
| 4. Scalp hematoma | 4. Unreliable or inadequate history of injury | 4. Penetrating skull injury or palpable depressed fracture |
| 5. Scalp laceration | 5. Age less than 2 years (unless injury very trivial) | |
| 6. Scalp contusion/abrasion | 6. Posttraumatic seizure | |
| 7. Absence of moderate or high-risk criteria | 7. Vomiting | |
| | 8. Posttraumatic amnesia | |
| | 9. Multiple trauma | |
| | 10. Serious facial injury | |
| | 11. Signs of basilar fracture | |
| | 12. Possible skull penetration or depressed fracture | |
| | 13. Suspected physical child abuse | |
| Observation alone; discharge with head sheet to reliable environment; watch for signs of high- or moderate-risk groups | Extended close observation; watch for signs of high-risk group. Consider for CT examination or plain skull radiography; may require neurosurgical consult | Candidate for neurosurgical consult and/or emergency CT examination |

[a]Physician assessment of the severity of injury may warrant reassignment to a higher-risk group. Any single criterion from a higher-risk group warrants assignment of the patient to the highest-risk group applicable.

*Source:* Modified from Masters et al. (1987), by permission.

close observation. The implications of this management approach are discussed below.

## CT SCANNING IN MINOR HEAD INJURY

Since CT became available in the 1970s, it has had a great impact on the management of head injury. Most of the emphasis in studies of CT utilization in head trauma has been focused on patients with severe injuries. CT scanning is clearly the most direct means of obtaining information about intracranial sequelae of severe head injury. Some neurosurgeons have suggested that CT scanning of minor head injury patients could be used in certain situations to exclude significant intracranial injury, thereby allowing the discharge of patients who might otherwise be admitted for observation (Becker et al., 1982).

French and Dublin (1977) found that 13% of their alert and neurologically normal patients had abnormal CT scans. They noted that abnormal scans in this group were likely to follow a blow from a small object, or to be found in an elderly patient with atrophy. Despite the abnormal scans, no patient in this group required craniotomy.

Bruce and Schut (1980) have outlined their indications for CT scanning in children after head injury. In children under one year of age, CT scans should be obtained on those with prolonged unconsciousness, full fontanelle, bradycardia, and skull radiographs showing splitting of the sutures. The indications for scanning in children older than one year who are conscious when first seen are progressive disturbance of consciousness, focal neurological deficit, and depressed skull fracture. These authors note that children who have sustained a localized blow to the head as a result of being hit by a baseball bat or a stone, for example, should have skull x-rays to exclude a depressed skull fracture. Another difficulty in treating head injury in this age group is that children often respond to mild head injury with more prominent lethargy, nausea, and vomiting than is seen in adults, and a great deal of clinical judgment must be exercised in determining which of them should undergo scanning. This occurred in 42 of 967 consecutive pediatric patients (4.3%) reviewed by Snoek et al. (1984). Three of these patients died of severe increased intracranial pressure, and one had a hematoma. Thus, although the syndrome of delayed deterioration can be extremely serious, most children recover uneventfully.

In the series of 610 minor head injury patients reported by Dacey et al. (1986), 11.1% had CT scans. Thirty-four percent of those scanned had either intracranial air or high- or low-density intracranial lesions. The relationship between skull x-ray findings and CT findings is shown in Figure 6–3. Patients with skull fractures were more likely to have intracranial abnormalities on CT scan. However, in almost 80% of patients with skull fractures, CTs were either normal or were not performed. This CT scan/skull fracture relationship is remarkably similar to that reported by Zimmerman et al. (1978), despite the fact that only 43% of their patients had minimal to moderate disturbance of consciousness. These investigators found that the incidence of skull fracture in

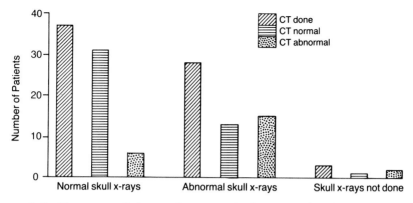

**Figure 6–3** Frequency of abnormal computerized tomography (CT) scans among the 610 patients with minor head injury in whom skull x-ray films were either normal, abnormal, or not obtained. (Reproduced from Dacey et al., 1986, by permission)

adults with positive versus negative CT scans was 67% and 23%, respectively. The incidence of positive CT findings in minor head injury is therefore about 3–5% in patients who require hospital admission. Whether CT should be integrated into future management schemes is discussed in the following section on observation and treatment. Recent data from Liesegang et al. (1984) suggest, however, that early CT findings may significantly underestimate the degree of brain injury.

## MANAGEMENT OF MINOR HEAD INJURY: OBSERVATION AND TREATMENT

The objective in treatment of minor head injury is the same as that for severe head injury: to achieve an optimal outcome by preventing further secondary brain injury due to intracranial mass lesions and increased intracranial pressure. Scalp lacerations, maxillofacial fractures, and other associated injuries must be detected and appropriately treated. In patients who have neurological deficits or an obvious open injury, detection of intracranial complications is not usually a problem since CT scans are almost always obtained on these patients. A more difficult situation arises when the patient has sustained a relatively mild concussive injury. Because serious neurosurgical complications are unusual in these patients (Dacey et al., 1986; Jones and Jeffreys, 1981), most physicians rely on a period of close observation. It is expected that latent serious injuries will become apparent during this observation, which is usually carried out in the hospital or in an area of the emergency facility where intracranial mass lesions and increased intracranial pressure can be treated rapidly once they become apparent. From a procedural point of view, therefore, a crucial decision to be made initially is whether to admit a patient who has sustained a minor head injury. Criteria for admission after mild head injury vary

**Table 6-4**    Recommendations of a Group of British Neurosurgeons Regarding Management of Minor Head Injury

Indications for skull x-ray examination after recent head injury
1. Loss of consciousness or amnesia at any time
2. Neurological symptoms or signs
3. Cerebrospinal fluid or blood from the nose or ear
4. Suspected penetrating injury
5. Scalp bruising or swelling

Indications for admission to a general hospital[a]
1. Confusion or any other depression of the level of consciousness at the time of examination
2. Skull fracture
3. Neurological symptoms or signs
4. Difficulty in assessing the patient—for example, alcohol, epilepsy, or other medical condition
5. Lack of a responsible adult to supervise the patient; other social problems

[a]Brief amnesia after trauma with full recovery is not sufficient indication for admission. Relatives and friends of patients sent home should receive written advice about changes that would require the patient to be returned urgently to hospital.
*Source:* Modified from Guidelines . . . (1984), by permission.

throughout the United States and Europe, but it is clear that patients who have altered levels of consciousness, neurological deficits, or obvious open or penetrating injuries should be admitted for further treatment, evaluation, or observation.

## CLINICAL MANAGEMENT OF MINOR HEAD INJURY

The goals of management of patients with minor head injury are generally the same as those for more severe head injuries: (1) early detection and treatment of intracranial mass lesions and increased intracranial pressure; (2) early detection and appropriate treatment of compound depressed fractures, cerebrospinal fluid (CSF) leaks, and penetrating injuries; and (3) detection of injury patterns suggesting child abuse. To accomplish these objectives, it is usually necessary to use a period of careful neurological observation and/or selective use of skull x-rays or CT scanning. The most difficult aspect of caring for patients with apparently minor head injuries is to develop protocols that facilitate the detection of all potential complications and are not extremely inconvenient for the patient or prohibitively expensive.

A group of British neurosurgeons recommended the list of indications for skull radiography and hospital admission after minor head injury shown in Table 6-4 (Guidelines . . . , 1984). This strategy is based on the belief that almost all of the small number of patients who deteriorate after minor head injury will have a skull fracture and hence will have been admitted to the hospital where their complication can be rapidly dealt with. The work of Mendelow et al. (1982, 1983) supports this approach by estimating that the risk that an intracranial hematoma will occur in an alert patient without a skull fracture is about 1 in 6,080. Jennett argues that a more selective admissions policy where alert patients are admitted only if they have a skull fracture allows optimal utilization of scarce bed and nursing resources in minor head injury (Jennett, 1980).

A somewhat different approach has recently been suggested by a multidisciplinary group of family physicians, pediatricians, emergency physicians, and neurosurgeons, empaneled by the FDA to make recommendations on the use of diagnostic radiology after head injury (Masters et al., 1987). In making their recommendations, they also covered the guidelines regarding which patients should be admitted for observation or referred for a neurosurgical consultation. Their recommendations were based on the relationship between skull fracture and intracranial injury shown in Tables 6–5 and 6–6. Although they note that skull fracture is associated with a higher risk of intracranial injury, the data they reviewed show that most patients with fractures have no intracranial complications, and that intracranial complications can occur in the absence of a fracture. They recommend that physicians use "careful clinical evaluation" to identify patients at risk for intracranial complications. Their recommended management strategy, based on clinical criteria, is presented in Table 6–3. Patients in the low-risk group should have observation alone (presumably in a reliable outpatient setting, although this is not explicitly stated). Patients in the moderate-risk group should have extended close observation and may benefit from skull x-rays or CT scans if these will contribute to therapeutic management. Patients in the high-risk group need emergency CT scans and usually require neurosurgical attention.

These recommendations appear to represent a consensus among those most often called upon to see a minor head injury patient. They provide guidelines that are applicable to most of these patients. However, they do not deal with several controversial areas. First, some neurosurgeons (particularly in

**Table 6–5** Incidence of Fractures Versus Intracranial Injury (CI) in Patients Who Had Skull X-Ray Examiantions

| | Study | | | | |
|---|---|---|---|---|---|
| Findings | Masters | FDA[a] | Royal College of Radiologists | Jones | Total |
| No. of patients undergoing skull x-ray examinations | 1,845 | 4,068 | 5,850 | 10,295 | 22,058 |
| Fracture with ICI | 7 (9)[b] | 20 (22) | 8 (7) | 32 (7) | 67 (9) |
| Fracture without ICI | 72 (91) | 70 (78) | 114 (93) | 435 (93) | 691 (91) |
| Total fractures | 79 (4) | 90 (2) | 122 (2) | 467 (5) | 758 (3) |
| ICI with fracture | 7 (21) | 20 (56) | 8 (89) | 32 (53) | 67 (49) |
| ICI without fracture | 26 (79) | 16 (44) | 1 (11) | 28 (47) | 71 (51) |
| Total ICI | 33 (2) | 36 (0.9) | 9 (0.2) | 60 (0.6) | 138 (0.6) |

*Note:* All patients in the low-, moderate-, and high-risk groups who underwent radiography are included.

[a]FDA Head Injury Study described in the text.

[b]Number of patients (%).

*Source:* Masters et al. (1987), by permission.

**Table 6–6**  Incidence of Fractures and Intracranial Injury in Patients with Head Injuries Who Met Only Low-Risk Criteria

| | | | Study | | |
|---|---|---|---|---|---|
| | Masters | FDA[a] | Royal College of Radiologists | Balasubramaniam et al. | Total |
| No. of patients undergoing skull x-ray examinations | 1,845 | 4,068 | 5,850 | 1,186 | 12,949 |
| No. of patients in the low risk group | 499 | 2,795 (5,254)[b] | 3,327[c] | 685 | 7,306 (9,765)[b] |
| No. of simple fractures in the low-risk group (%) | 8 (1.6) | 12 (0.4) | 22 (0.7)[c] | 11 (1.6) | 53 (0.7) |
| No. of intracranial injuries in the low-risk group | 0 | 0 | 0[c] | 0 | 0 |

[a]FDA Head Injury Study described in the text.

[b]Although 2,795 of the patients who had skull x-ray films were at low risk, a total of 5,254 low-risk patients were identified.

[c]An additional patient who was assaulted with a hammer was originally classified as "uncomplicated, clinically negative" in the Royal College of Radiologists study. According to our management strategy (Table 6–3), this patient was classified as being at moderate risk and is therefore not included in this table of low risk patients.

*Source:* Masters et al. (1987), by permission.

Britain) would object to the implied recommendation that all patients who have completely recovered from a change in consciousness at the time of injury should be admitted, whether or not they have undergone skull x-rays (Totten and Buxton, 1979). In the subset of patients with a history of concussion without skull fracture, this may result in much unnecessary hospitalization (Jennett, 1980; Jennett and Teasdale, 1981; Jones and Jeffreys; 1981). Second, the FDA panel's recommendations would permit the discharge of the extremely rare patient who fits into the low-risk group, has a skull fracture, and is discharged, only to deteriorate subsequently with an intracranial complication. Jones and Jeffreys (1981) estimate that in Scotland, England, and Wales there would be 163 such patients each year. The FDA panel (Masters et al., 1987) estimates this risk at about 1 in 2,500. Third, the possibility exists for missing an occasional compound depressed fracture not associated with the findings that usually indicate the presence of such a fracture. For example, 62% of the depressed fractures reported by Miller and Jennett (1968) were caused by vehicular, industrial, or sporting accidents—factors not usually considered to put patients at high risk for depressed fracture. Despite these possible shortcomings, the management strategy outlined by this panel appears to be a reasonable compromise between the pressures for reducing posttraumatic skull radiology and those advocating a more selective admissions approach for minor head injury.

Dacey et al. (1986) examined the potential cost implications of alternative admissions and diagnostic imaging strategies in minor head injury. They pro-

**Table 6-7**  Alternative Management Schemes for Minor Head Injury

| | |
|---|---|
| *Scheme A:* | Hospitalize all concussion patients for observation. |
| | Obtain no skull x-rays in patients with GCS = 15, except to detect open injuries. |
| *Scheme B:* | Hospitalize all concussed patients with altered level of consciousness (GCS = 13 or 14). |
| | Obtain skull x-rays on all patients (including those with GCS = 15). |
| | Discharge only those patients with GCS = 15d and normal skull x-ray. |
| *Scheme C:* | Hospitalize all concussed patients with altered level of consciousness (GCS = 13 or 14). |
| | Obtain CT scans on patients with GCS = 15. |
| | Discharge only those patients with GCS = 15 and normal skull x-ray. |

*Source:* Modified from Dacey et al. (1986), by permission.

spectively identified 610 patients admitted for observation or treatment after apparently minor head injury. Using the costs generated by each of the patients, they estimated the total cost of care under each of three management plans (see Table 6-7): (1) Hospitalize for observation all postconcussion patients; (2) perform skull x-rays on all postconcussion patients, hospitalizing only those who have a fracture or altered level of consciousness; (3) perform CT scans on all alert patients (GCS score 15), hospitalizing only those who have altered level of consciousness, neurological deficit, or abnormal CT scans. The latter two plans, if applied, would have resulted in a 50% reduction in total management costs (Dacey et al., 1986). It should be noted that in both the latter two alternative plans, a very small number of patients could still be sent home with a potentially life-threatening complication. These approaches remain to be tested in large prospective trials of alternative management policies for head injury.

In summary, an optimal strategy for managing mild head injury in the acute stage has not yet been developed. However, selective referral of patients for either CT scan or skull x-ray based on clinical findings should be incorporated into overall management (Masters et al., 1987). A period of neurological observation should be used to identify the 1–3% of mild head injury patients who will develop serious immediate intracranial complications (Dacey et al., 1986).

# REFERENCES

Balasubramaniam S, Kapadia T, Campbell J, Jackson TL. Efficacy of skull radiography. Am J Surg 142:366–369, 1981.

Becker DP, Miller JD, Ward JD, Greenberg RP, Young HF, Sakalas R. The outcome from severe head injury with early diagnosis and intensive management. J Neurosurg 47:491–502, 1977.

Becker DP, Miller JD, Young HF, Selhorst JB, Kishore PRS, Greenberg RP, Rosner

MJ, Ward JD. Diagnosis and treatment of head injury in adults. *In* Youmans JR (ed), Neurological Surgery, 2nd ed, Vol 4. Philadelphia: WB Saunders, 1982, p 1938.

Bells RS, Loop JW. The utility and futility of radiographic skull examination for trauma. N Engl J Med 284:236–239, 1971.

Bruce DA, Shut L. The value of CAT scanning following pediatric head injury. Clin Pediatr (Phila) 19:719–725, 1980.

Cooper PR, Ho V. Role of emergency skull x-ray films in the evaluation of the head-injured patient: a retrospective study. Neurosurgery 13:136–140, 1983.

Cummins RO, LoGerfo JP, Inui TS, Weiss NS. High-yield criteria for posttraumatic skull roentgenography. JAMA 244:673–676, 1980.

Dacey RG, Alves W, Rimel R, Jane JA. The risk of serious neurosurgical complications after apparently minor head injury. J Neurosurg 65:203–210, 1986.

DeSmet AA, Fryback DG, Thornbury JR. A second look at the utility of radiographic skull examination for trauma. AJR 132:95–99, 1979.

Eyes B, Evans AF. Post-traumatic skull radiographs: time for a reappraisal. Lancet 2:85–86, 1978.

Fischer RP, Carlson J, Perry JF. Postconcussive hospital observation of alert patients in a primary trauma center. J Trauma 21:920–924, 1981.

Freed HA. Skull x-ray criteria endorsed by the Food and Drug Administration: Some flaws and proposed modifications. Neurosurgery 7:636–638, 1980.

French BN, Dublin AB. The value of computerized tomography in the management of 1000 consecutive head injuries. Surg Neurol 7:171–183, 1977.

Gibson TC. Skull x-rays in minor head injury: a review of their use and interpretation by casualty officers. Scott Med J 28:132–137, 1983.

Guidelines for initial management after head injury in adults: suggestions from a group of neurosurgeons. Br Med J 288:983–985, 1984.

Jennett B. Skull x-rays after recent head injury. Clin Radiol 31:463–469, 1980.

Jennett B, Bond M. Assessment of outcome after severe brain damage. Lancet 1:480, 1985.

Jennett B, Teasdale G. Management of Head Injuries. Philadelphia: FA Davis, 1981.

Jones JJ, Jeffreys RV. Relative risk of alternative admission policies for patients with head injuries. Lancet 2:850–852, 1981.

Larsen KT, Kozial DF. High yield criteria and emergency department skull radiography: two community hospitals' experience. JACEP 8:393–395, 1979.

Leonidas JC, Ting W, Binkiewicz A, Vaz R, Scott RM, Pauker SG. Mild head trauma in children: when is a roentgenogram necessary? Pediatrics 69:139–143, 1982.

Liesegang J, Siggelkow C, Weichert HC. Computertomographische und neurologische verlaufsbeobachtungen in der akutphase gedeckter schadelhirnverletzungen. Neurochirurgia (Stuttg) 27:62–65, 1984.

Marshall LF, Toole BM, Bowers SA. National Traumatic Coma Data Bank: Part 2. Patients who talk and deteriorate: implications for treatment. J Neurosurg 59:285–288, 1983.

Masters SJ. Evaluation of head trauma. Efficacy of skull films. AJR 135:539–547, 1980.

Masters SJ, McClean PM, Arcarese JS, Brown RF, Campbell JA, Freed HA, Hess GH, Hoff JT, Kobrine A, Koziol DF, Marasco JA, Merten DF, Metcalf H, Morrison JL, Rachlin JA, Shaver JW, Thornbury JR. Skull x-ray examinations after head trauma. Recommendations by a multidiciplinary panel and validation study. N Eng J Med 316:84–91, 1987.

Mendelow AD, Campbell DA, Jeffrey RR, Miller JD, Hessett C, Bryden J, Jennett B. Admission after mild head injury: benefits and costs. Br Med J 285:1530–1532, 1982.

Mendelow AD, Teasdale G, Jennett B, Bryden J, Hessett C, Murray G. Risks of intracranial haematoma in head injured adults. Br Med J 287:1173–1176, 1983.

Miller JD, Jennett WB. Complications of depressed skull fracture. Lancet 2:991–995, 1968.

Miller JD, Becker DP, Ward JD, Sullivan HG, Adams WE, Rosner MJ. Significance of intracranial hypertension in severe head injury. J Neurosurg 47:503–516, 1977.

Miller JD, Butterworth JF, Gudeman SK, Faulkner JE, Choi SC, Selhorst JB, Harbison JW, Lutz HA, Young HF, Becker DP. Further experience in the management of severe head injury. J Neurosurg 54:289–299, 1981.

Narayan RK, Kishore PRS, Becker DP, Ward JD, Enas GG, Greenberg RP, DaSilva AD, Lipper MH, Choi SC, Mayhall CG, Lutz HA III, Young HF. Intracranial pressure: to monitor or not to monitor? A review of our experience with severe head injury. J Neurosurg 56:650–659, 1982.

Phillips LA. Emergency services utilization of skull radiography. Neurosurgery 4:580–582, 1979a.

Phillips LA. Comparative evaluation of the effect of a high yield criteria list upon skull radiography. JACEP 8:106–109, 1979b.

Reilly PL, Graham DI, Adams JH, Jennett B. Patients with head injury who talk and die. Lancet 2:375, 1975.

Reynolds AF. Letter to the editor. J Neurosurg 4:200, 1979.

Rimel RW, Giordani B, Barth JT, Boll TJ, Jane JA. Disability caused by minor head injury. Neurosurgery 9:221–228, 1981.

Rose J, Valtonen S, Jennett B. Avoidable factors contributing to death after head injury. Br Med J 2:615–618, 1977.

Royal College of Radiologists. Costs and benefits of skull radiography for head injury. A National Study by the RCR. Lancet 2:791–795, 1981.

Royal College of Radiologists. Patient selection for radiographic skull examination for trauma: a national study by the RCR. AJR 132:95–99, 1979.

Snoek JW, Minderhoud JM, Wilmink JT. Delayed deterioration following mild head injury in children. Brain 107:15–36, 1984.

Thornbury JR, Campbell JA, Masters SJ, Fryback DG. Skull fracture and the low risk of intracranial sequelae in minor head trauma. AJR 143:661–664, 1984.

Totten J, Buxton R. Were you knocked out? Lancet 1:369–370, 1979.

Young HA, Schmidek HH. Complications accompanying occipital skull fracture. J Trauma 22:914–920, 1982.

Zimmerman RA, Bilaniuk LT, Genaralli T, Bruce D, Dolinskas C, Uzzell B. Cranial computed tomography in diagnosis and management of acute head trauma. AJR 131:27–34, 1978.

# 7

# Mild Head Injury in Children

J. W. SNOEK

Head trauma is a major cause of morbidity and mortality in children. Each year about 100,000 children younger than 15 years of age are admitted to U.S. hospitals, over 90% of these for mild head injuries (Kraus et al., 1987). Most children who have sustained minor head injury do not represent significant diagnostic and management problems, apart perhaps from assessment of the severity of injury in the acute stage, and make a good recovery without specific treatment. Every emergency doctor, however, is familiar with the atypical child who suddenly develops alarming signs following an injury that at first had appeared minor or even trivial.

## ASSESSMENT OF SEVERITY OF INJURY

Triage decisions are often difficult to make in the acute stage following injury, especially in young children. It is obvious that children with a depressed level of consciousness and/or focal neurological signs have sustained significant brain injury and should be admitted promptly for specialized investigation and monitoring. The same holds for patients with depressed fractures and penetrating injuries, with or without signs of cerebrospinal fluid (CSF) leaks, and for vomiting and irritable children who are too sick to be sent home. Diagnostic problems are posed by children who are "not 100%" on initial evaluation, especially when uncertainty exists about the severity of the primary injury. It is often difficult to assess the actual content of consciousness (the verbal score of the Glasgow Coma Scale; Teasdale and Jennett, 1974) in children who are fearful and restless in the unfamiliar setting of the emergency department; in preverbal children it is impossible. Nonmassive hemispheric contusions do not alter consciousness, but may cause focal neurological signs, which are often difficult to demonstrate in uncooperative children. The loss of consciousness in cerebral concussion is by definition transient, but historical evidence of more than momentary loss implies significant brain dysfunction by the impact. Linear or depressed fractures and focal brain injuries may be associated with concussion, and these may lead to secondary brain damage due to intracranial complications. In the conscious patient, assessment of the severity of the sustained injury rests on an adequate history, which is often difficult to obtain in children. Many children sustain head injury in the presence of parents or playmates, but the usefulness of their firsthand accounts is often hampered by an inability to recall the exact events. Many children themselves are unable to give a history of loss of consciousness. It is obvious that assessment of posttraumatic amnesia, which is a good measure of the severity of primary brain damage, is even more difficult in most cases.

In the absence of (1) a reliable history, (2) any direct signs of brain damage (such as altered level of consciousness and/or focal neurological signs), or (3) indirect signs (such as scalp lacerations or a depressed fracture), the only clue to there having been violence to the head of significant impact may be the presence of a fracture of the skull. There is, at present, considerable controversy regarding the efficacy of obtaining routine skull radiographs in patients with head injury. Recently, the recommendations of a multidisciplinary panel of medical experts have been published (Masters et al., 1987), which identified two groups of patients for which skull series are not recommended. The *low-risk group* consists of patients with head trauma whose injuries are trivial and who have virtually no likelihood of intracranial injury. Fractures in this group of patients are rarely, if ever, associated with intracranial injury and therefore do not need to be identified. Patients in the *high-risk group* have clearly suffered major brain damage and should be referred for prompt neurosurgical consultation, emergency CT scanning, or both. Skull series are considered unnecessary in these patients, as positive results will not influence management, and negative results never rule out intracranial hemorrhage. The panel also identified an intermediate, *moderate-risk group,* for which they regard skull series as possibly helpful. Selection criteria for this group include (1) a history of change of consciousness at the time of injury or subsequently; (2) an unreliable or inadequate history of injury; (3) posttraumatic seizures; (4) age less than 2 years; and (5) suspected physical child abuse. By incorporating the latter selection criteria into its moderate-risk group, the panel acknowledged the existing differences between pediatric and adult head injuries in regard to the method of injury, the nature of injury, and the response to injury.

## INITIAL MANAGEMENT

Following the first evaluation in the emergency room, the head-injured child may suffer from either too much or too little care. If the risk of complications after a mild head injury is overestimated, an unnecessary (and often psychologically traumatic) admission may be the result. If, on the contrary, real risks are overlooked, irreversible brain damage may result.

Children should be allowed to go home if, from all available evidence, no significant injury to the nervous system can be deduced. In practice, this means (1) no history of loss of consciousness exceeding five minutes; (2) no abnormalities on neurological examination; (3) no vegetative disturbances; and (4) no skull fracture (if appropriate). Reliable parents should be informed about the nature of signs of deterioration and instructed to contact the emergency department should any of these signs occur. If there is doubt about the severity of the insult or if the parents cannot guarantee regular observation at home, admission is necessary.

The overwhelming majority of children with mild head injury will rapidly return to normal function: In most children, minor head injury is indeed minor (Casey et al., 1986). A small proportion, however, will deteriorate and may then represent significant diagnostic and treatment problems. The following sections deal with the different clinical pictures presented by children with such delayed deterioration following mild head injury. This overview is based on a series from the University Hospital of Groningen, the Netherlands, originally described by Snoek et al. (1984) in *Brain*. This series consisted of 42 children who developed neurological signs after a lucid or symptom-free period following a seemingly minor injury. In the majority of cases (31; 74%), a fall had been the cause of injury; 5 children had been struck by some object (12%), whereas only 6 patients (14%) had either been involved in a car accident or had been hit by a car. In 40 patients, the injury was "trivial" according to the criteria of Jennett (1962, 1975) (no amnesia, hematoma, or skull fracture, or linear fracture only); in 2 cases there was a history of a brief loss of consciousness (not exceeding five minutes). This group constituted 4.3% of 967 consecutive patients aged 2 months to 17 years who were seen at the emergency department during the years 1978–81. Only primary referrals have been taken into account. The characteristics of the 967 patients are presented in Figure 7–1. Figure 7–2 shows the age distribution of the 42 patients with delayed deterioration.

## INTRACRANIAL HEMATOMA

Only one patient in our series had a hematoma:

> *Case 1.* A 10-year-old boy struck his head against a wall while being tossed by his friends. He was briefly unconscious, probably less than one minute, but recovered quickly. On admission, he opened his eyes on request, obeyed commands, and was fully orientated. There was a small occipital fracture. He deteriorated slowly over the following day. Laboratory screening revealed a clotting disorder, which was found to be a variant of von Willebrand–Jürgens disease. A CT scan showed a hyperdense area in the posterior fossa, which on exploration proved to be a venous extradural hematoma. He made a slow but excellent recovery.

The risk of developing a life-threatening intracranial hematoma following mild head injury is probably small for children in comparison with adults. In

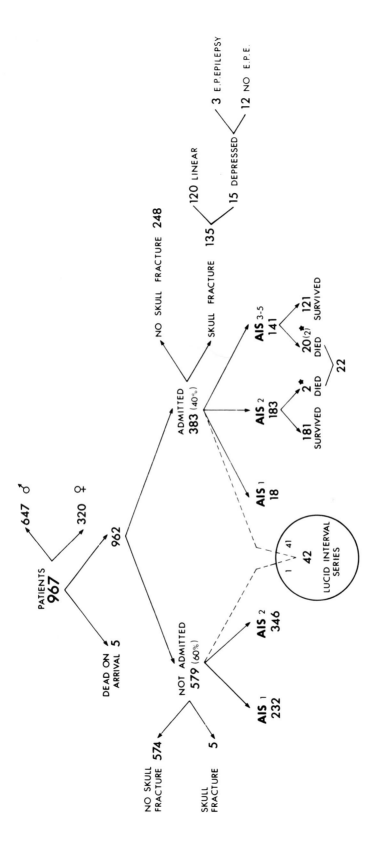

**Figure 7-1**  Characteristics of the group of 967 consecutive patients, aged 2 months to 17 years. AIS, Abbreviated Injury Scale (Ommaya, 1979): AIS code 1, minor degree of injury; 2, moderate; 3, severe (not life-threatening); 4, severe (life-threatening); 5, critical (survival uncertain); E.P.E., early posttraumatic epilepsy. *Death attributable primarily to extracranial injuries. For details, see source reference. (Reproduced from Snoek et al., 1984, by permission)

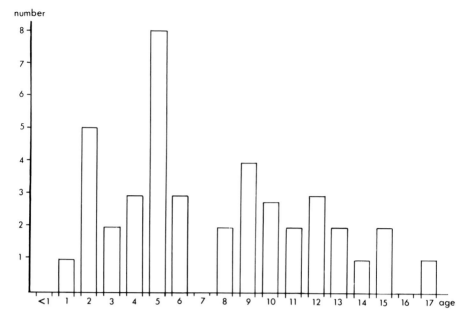

**Figure 7–2**    Age distribution of 42 children with a lucid interval following mild head injury.

a recent prospective series of 610 patients with apparently minor head injury, none of 18 patients (3%) requiring a neurosurgical procedure were under 17 years of age (Dacey et al., 1986). However, in the period covered by our study, an intracranial hematoma with a history of a lucid interval was diagnosed and operated upon in 7 children. Six of these were secondary referrals (i.e., they had previously been admitted to another hospital) and have therefore not been included in the series.

Of all intracranial hematomas occurring in patients under the age of 20, 40% are extradural, compared with less than 10% of hematomas in patients over 40 years, who more often have intradural hematomas (Jamieson and Yelland, 1968, 1972a,b). In recent series, extradural hematomas were found in 2.6–3.4% of admitted head-injured children under 15 years of age (Choux et al., 1975; Dhellemmes et al., 1985; Mazza et al., 1982). Children with extradural hematomas have often suffered relatively minor head injury, as stressed by Choux et al. (1975), who noted that the majority of their patients with this type of hematoma had had no disturbance of consciousness at the time of injury. Extradural hematomas may occur in the absence of a skull fracture in children, whereas most adult patients with such hematoma have a fracture (Galbraith, 1973). Choux et al. (1975) reported a rather high percentage (81%) of skull fractures in their series, as compared with 40% in the series described by Hendrick et al. (1963), for example.

Extradural hematoma of the posterior fossa is more common in children than in adults. In a recent series of 7 patients, 6 were younger than 17 years (Garza-Mercado, 1983). Four of these patients had not been unconscious following the impact; 3 patients had been unconscious for less than 10 minutes. An occipital fracture was found in every patient. The hematoma was believed to be venous in all patients. Similar findings have been reported by others (e.g., Ammirati and Tomita, 1984; Kushner and Luken, 1983).

Acute subdural hematomas unaccompanied by contusion of the brain are rarely encountered in children, except after birth injury (Shapiro, 1987). Recently, however, a Japanese series of 26 infants has been reported, who demonstrated an acute subdural hematoma, in all cases apparently due to minor head injury and not associated with cerebral contusion (Aoki and Masuzawa, 1984). The most common cause of injury was a fall backward. The majority of patients were between 7 and 10 months old and most of the patients had been taken to hospital because of generalized convulsions. All patients were found to have retinal and preretinal hemorrhages. Unfortunately, CT scanning was performed in only 7 patients, the remaining patients having been diagnosed by cerebral angiography and subdural tapping. The basic nature of this type of injury has been challenged by Rekate (1985), who expressed the view that most, if not all, of these infants were victims of child abuse as a more likely explanation. Finding retinal hemorrhages in a child under 1 year old is regarded as almost pathognomonic of the "shaking injury" of child abuse (Bruce, 1984).

Traumatic chronic subdural hematomas are rare in children (Shapiro, 1987).

CT scanning (Figure 7-3) is the most reliable way to diagnose or exclude an intracranial hematoma, and it is considered part of good medical practice to make every effort to secure a CT scan in any patient whose clinical state even raises the possibility of this treatable complication (Jennett and Teasdale, 1981).


## CONVULSIVE CASES

Thirteen children (31%) in our series had early posttraumatic seizures. Their mean age was 7.3 years (range, 1–17). Seven of these patients (mean age, 3.5 years; range, 1–8) presented with a focal or generalized status epilepticus, which necessitated intubation and controlled ventilation in six.

> *Case 2.* A 5-year-old boy fell off his bicycle. He did not lose consciousness and resumed cycling immediately. One hour after injury he developed focal seizures involving the right hand and arm. On admission one hour later, the boy was in a generalized status epilepticus, which reacted promptly to intravenous diazepam. A CT scan, performed within three hours after injury, showed no abnormalities. An EEG, performed within 24 hours, showed asymmetry with localized slow activity in the left temporal region. There were multifocal isolated spikes and sharp slow-wave complexes, maximal in both temporal and parietal areas. Several hours after admission, the patient was fully alert, recalling all details of the injury. He was discharged after two days. Two EEGs, performed one and five months after injury, respectively, were normal. The past medical history of this patient revealed that he was premature and dysmature at birth. During his first 14 days

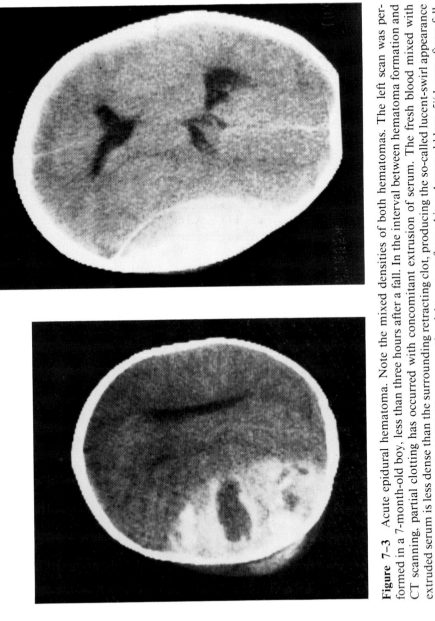

**Figure 7–3**  Acute epidural hematoma. Note the mixed densities of both hematomas. The left scan was performed in a 7-month-old boy, less than three hours after a fall. In the interval between hematoma formation and CT scanning, partial clotting has occurred with concomitant extrusion of serum. The fresh blood mixed with extruded serum is less dense than the surrounding retracting clot, producing the so-called lucent-swirl appearance (Zimmerman and Bilaniuk, 1982). The scan on the right was performed in a 4-year-old boy, 5½ hours after a fall. At this stage, the hematoma has a more homogeneous appearance.

of life, cyanosis had been observed on several occasions. Serial EEGs had not shown any abnormality at that time. He had been treated with anticonvulsants up to the age of 5. Psychomotor development was normal.

*Case 3.* A 17-year-old girl struck her head during gym. Immediately she noted "flashes," lasting several seconds only. She resumed the lesson, but moments later she fell off the flying-rings and had a generalized convulsion. She was taken home, where she had two more convulsions. On admission, she was alert. No skull fracture was found. An EEG, performed on the following day, demonstrated intermittent slow activity in the right frontotemporal region. No epileptic discharges were observed.

More than half of the patients developed their seizures within one hour after injury, 12 out of 13 within two hours, and only 1 after a longer period (28 hours). The family history for epilepsy was negative in all patients. Five patients, however, had a past medical history that may have predisposed them to developing seizures (febrile convulsions, rhesus incompatibility, mental retardation, or prematurity; 1 patient had had an identical episode of convulsions after a previous trivial injury). One patient possibly had a rubella infection and was readmitted with a second episode of status epilepticus a week later, at which time an increased rubella titer was found.

Early posttraumatic seizures occurred in 16 head-injured children of the total series of 967 (1.7%). The 3 patients not having had a lucid interval all had a depressed fracture (Figure 7–1). In the lucid interval series, 5 out of 13 patients with early epilepsy had a skull fracture (38%). One or more EEGs were performed in 11 cases, usually within 24 hours after injury. The EEG findings were variable, and there was no relation between EEG abnormalities and the type of seizure. Recently, similar findings have been reported by others (Enomoto et al., 1986). Early seizures are generally reported more frequently in children than in adults. Hauser (1983) reviewed the literature and reports frequencies ranging from 1% to 30%—the highest percentages occurring in severely head-injured children. Most series report an incidence of 5%, but in some series the incidence is twice as high in children under 5 years of age (Hendrick and Harris, 1968; Jennett, 1962, 1975). According to Jennett, seizures rarely follow a trivial injury except in children under 5 years. In our series, the occurrence of early posttraumatic seizures was not limited to the under-5 age group, as 6 of the 13 patients were between 6 and 17 years of age. A similar age distribution has been described by Grand (1974), who described five cases of early posttraumatic status epilepticus in childhood and stressed the minor nature of injury in these children. He contrasts this with the clinical significance of early posttraumatic status in adults, which is thought to be an ominous sign. Similar observations have been made by Livingston and Mahloudji (1969). Jennett (1973) also explicitly stated that early seizures may draw attention to certain complications such as intracranial hematoma, but that they are never the only signs of such a development. Posttraumatic status epilepticus itself, however, may result in death (Reilly et al., 1975; Rose et al., 1977; Small and Woolf, 1957). According to Jennett, the major significance of early posttraumatic seizures is the risk of late epilepsy, which he found to be 25%. Only the occurrence of focal early seizures in children did not significantly increase the risk of late epilepsy (Jennett, 1962, 1973, 1975). Except for the child that was readmitted in a second episode of status epilepticus one week after the accident, no recurrence of seizures was noted during the follow-up period in our series (regular follow-up: six months to two years; review of the hospital records in 1987 revealed that none of these patients had developed late posttraumatic epilepsy).

## NONCONVULSIVE CASES: PATIENTS WITH A TRANSIENT SYNDROME OF (SUB)ACUTE ONSET

In 22 children there was a history of acute or subacute deterioration (i.e., from a level of no signs, the full clinical picture was reached within 15 minutes), whereas the signs in most cases ended also quickly, if not abruptly, mostly after a short period (never exceeding 12 hours). These signs consisted of loss of consciousness with (9 patients) or without (7 patients) focal neurological signs; focal neurological signs only (1 patient); or a period of severe restlessness or confusion following a period of normal behavior (5 patients). The mean age of these patients was 6 years (range, 2–13). A skull fracture was found in 5 patients. The onset of neurological signs was between 5 and 30 minutes after injury in 12 patients, between 30 and 60 minutes in 4, and between 1 and 2 hours in 5; only in 1 patient did signs occur with a considerable interval following injury (36 hours). Duration of signs ranged from 15 to 30 minutes in 5 patients, from 30 minutes to 2 hours in 2, and between 2 and 12 hours in 15. Vomiting occurred at the onset of signs in 21 patients (95%). The past medical history was unremarkable in all but 3 cases. One girl (aged 12 years) was known to have behavioral problems and EEG abnormalities (bilateral synchronous spike and wave complexes) without history of seizures. There was a family history of epilepsy but no history of seizures in another boy (aged 6 years) whose EEG subsequently showed spike and wave complexes. One patient was admitted with fever, the CSF showing no abnormalities.

## DISTURBANCE OF SENSORY LEVEL ONLY

In seven patients a disturbance of conscious level occurred following a lucid interval. In our series, sleepiness in itself was not regarded as a sign of secondary deterioration. Of course many, if not most, children will fall asleep some time after the shock of an injury and the subsequent examination and treatment in an unfamiliar hospital setting. In these children, the deterioration of conscious level occurred rather abruptly, in all cases accompanied by vomiting and sometimes by evident pallor.

> *Case 4.* A 2½-year-old boy tripped and fell down four steps. He struck his occiput on the ground. He cried immediately and had no loss of consciousness. With a latent interval of 30 minutes, during which the child was alert and behaved normally, the conscious level deteriorated quickly and he vomited once. Within minutes the boy was totally unresponsive. He was rushed to hospital. When exam-

ined, 30 minutes after the onset of signs, he had regained consciousness. No bruises were noted and no neurological abnormalities were found. There was no skull fracture.

This *pediatric concussion syndrome* or *posttraumatic stupor* (Schnitker, 1949) is seen rather frequently in infants and young children (Plum and Posner, 1980). Mealy (1968) gives the following description:

> In younger children, who were not unconscious immediately after the blow or only dazed momentarily, the triad of excessive somnolence or lethargy, irritability and vomiting is characteristic. The onset of these symptoms may be delayed for an hour or more after an initial period of well-being. Often these children will not talk, tend to withdraw from the examiner, and merely cry when disturbed. When not aroused they promptly drift off into a sleep-like state. They either remain listless in any position they are placed or lie up curled upon their sides. This pattern of response to head trauma is sufficiently stereotyped and seen often enough to be considered a definite syndrome representative of concussion in infants and young children.

In Schnitker's series, 6 out of 11 children were those of physicians who became unduly alarmed, realizing the possible complications of a head injury (Schnitker, 1949). Todorow and Feller (1982) described 49 children with mild posttraumatic stupor. This "sleepy state," which lasted for three to five hours, occurred in 9% of all children admitted after a minor head injury. The lucid interval ranged from 15 minutes to three hours. In almost one-third of the patients minor neurological signs were noted (i.e., pupillary abnormalities, pyramidal tract signs or ataxia), whereas EEG abnormalities were found in half. These EEG abnormalities consisted mostly of slight to moderate slowing of background frequency and, in many cases, persisted for a considerable time (from five days to six weeks) after the clinical signs had subsided. Vitzthum et al. (1986) described 12 children with similar signs. This *delayed encephalopathy* occurred in 2% of all admitted head-injured children. It seems likely that the actual incidence of this type of deterioration following mild head injury is much higher: In only a minority of affected children, signs of such severity occur that these children will come under medical care. The same holds for the following entity, which appears to be closely related.

## DISTURBANCES OF SENSORY LEVEL WITH FOCAL NEUROLOGICAL SIGNS, OR FOCAL NEUROLOGICAL SIGNS ONLY

The most frequently observed focal neurological signs in our series were pupillary abnormalities (in 4 out of 10 patients), followed by conjugate deviation and hemiparesis. Transient blindness occurred in two patients, in one case without deterioration of conscious level. There were remarkable differences in the severity of the presenting clinical picture, as is illustrated by the following two case histories:

> *Case 5.* A 2-year-old boy fell down some stairs. He cried immediately. One hour later, he became unresponsive within a few minutes. On admission he was obtunded with a left hemiparesis. A CT scan, performed within three hours of

injury, was normal. Within four hours after injury the hemiparesis disappeared and the level of consciousness became normal. Two days later, the boy was discharged. An EEG, performed on the same day, showed slow waves over the whole of the right hemisphere.

*Case 6.* A 5-year-old boy was struck by a car. He was unconscious for less than five minutes. In the ambulance, the right pupil dilated while he was talking. He subsequently became comatose with bilaterally dilated unreactive pupils. On admission, one hour after the accident, he was awake with normally reacting pupils. The EEG (day 5) showed only slight diffuse abnormalities. He was discharged after six days.

Early descriptions of the alarming signs in children or adolescents following apparently mild head injury have been presented by Walton (1898), Prick (1936), Schnitker (1949), Pickles (1949), and Biemond (1970, covering the period 1929–41). As early as 1897, Walton and Brooks stated:

It is not uncommon in children to find localized paralysis following blows upon the head, closely simulating the results of hemorrhage, but completely disappearing in the course of a week or two, a fact which has to be borne in mind in making the diagnosis of middle meningeal or other hemorrhage in early life.

Biemond (1970) wrote:

These symptoms disappear just as rapidly as they come on. One or two days after the occurrence of the alarming cerebral episode (for which these children are usually admitted to hospital as surgical emergencies), the little patients are quite normal again, play in their beds, and bestow a friendly smile upon the worried physician, and all this without any therapeutic intervention at all.

## CORTICAL BLINDNESS

Two patients demonstrated transient blindness:

*Case 7.* A 4-year-old boy fell from the shoulders of an older friend and struck his head on the pavement. He cried immediately. One hour later he suddenly yelled that he could not see anymore and vomited. He complained about an occipital headache. The period of total blindness lasted about half an hour and vision returned abruptly afterwards. On admission the boy was drowsy and uncooperative. Vision, pupils, and fundi were normal. Skull radiographs showed a small right occipital fracture. The boy remained drowsy and vomited on postural change for one day, but subsequently made a quick recovery.

*Case 8.* A 5-year-old boy fell on ice and struck his forehead. He did not lose consciousness. Minutes later he said that he could not see anymore and behaved accordingly. During this period of blindness he was examined by a general practitioner who noted normal pupillary reactions. Full vision reappeared rather abruptly after one hour and was not followed by headache or vegetative signs. Upon admission no neurological abnormalities were found. The boy could recall all events. Skull series were normal. He was kept overnight and discharged on the following day.

Similar cases have been reported by others (Bodian, 1964; Gjerris and Mellemgaard, 1969; Greenblatt, 1973; Griffith and Dodge, 1968; Haas et al., 1975; Hochstetler and Beals, 1987; Sacher and Klöti, 1987). Bodian (1964) considered that this transient traumatic blindness is caused by dysfunction of the optic nerves, chiasma, or tracts, possibly due to vasospasm. In contrast, Gjerris and Mellemgaard (1969) and most later authors considered dysfunction of the occipital cortex, probably edema, or a combination of contusion and edema to be the cause. Greenblatt (1973) and later Haas et al. (1975) proposed a relationship between these attacks and migraine. This alleged relationship will be discussed in a later section. Permanent total blindness with subsequent optic atrophy following minor head injury in a 10-year-old girl was reported by Venable et al. (1978). The blindness occurred immediately following a fall on the forehead. In contrast to the patients with cortical blindness, both pupils were dilated and unreactive to light. Partial third nerve paresis was noted on the right side. The cause of the blindness was considered to be vasospasm or occlusion of small vessels supplying the optic nerves or chiasma. The child had a past history of recurrent migraine and a family history suggestive of migraine, and, according to the authors, this may have increased the risk for the effects of minor trauma to the visual system.

## CONFUSION

Five children demonstrated a period of acute confusion following a period of normal behavior. In all but one patient, the onset of confusion was accompanied by vomiting.

> *Case 9.* A 6-year-old boy was struck by a falling gate. He was not unconscious. He went to school where he told his teacher what happened. One hour later, with unobtrusive behavior in the meantime, the boy acutely started to cry, became confused, was disorientated and did not recognize the teacher anymore. On examination, two hours after the accident, the boy was extremely agitated and combative. He was disoriented and perseverated. Memory for new information was defective. In between periods of restless behavior he repeatedly fell asleep, only to wake up screaming. He did not vomit. No focal neurological signs were noted on examination. The disorientation persisted for four hours, after which he fell asleep for several hours. Ten hours after admission he behaved quite normally. There was amnesia for the preceding hours, but not for the accident. An EEG, performed 24 hours after the accident, showed slow activity in the posterior regions, more on the left than on the right side. This was considered normal for age.

Haas et al. (1975) described different juvenile head trauma syndromes. Their type 2 attacks consisted of somnolence and irritability, usually in combination with vomiting. They noted the similarities with juvenile migraine attacks presenting as an acute confusional state (Gascon and Barlow, 1970; Ehyai and Fenichel, 1978). Irritability or restless confusion occurred in 11 out of 37 children, with transient neurological disorders occurring in the acute stage of trivial head injury in another series (Oka et al., 1977).

## NONCONVULSIVE CASES: PATIENTS WITH SLOW DETERIORATION AND GRADUAL SPONTANEOUS IMPROVEMENT

In three patients (aged 10, 12, and 15 years, respectively), the signs developed slowly over a period of time after a lucid interval and then gradually resolved. In two patients, these symptoms consisted of slowly progressive confusion with focal abnormalities in both the EEG and CT scan, located in the frontal region in one patient and in the left temporal region in the other. In the third case, the deterioration consisted of more severe confusion, with signs of uncal herniation:

> *Case 10.* A 12-year-old boy was hit by a car. He did not lose consciousness. On admission he was lucid but nauseated. There was no skull fracture. Twelve hours after the accident, he started to deteriorate with confusion and an enlarged pupil on the right side. Angiography (because of unavailability of the CT scanner) showed a shift of the midline vessels with signs of a swollen right temporal lobe. No avascular mass was discovered. Several hours later, his level of consciousness started to improve and the pupils became normal. The boy remained drowsy for two more days, after which he recovered quickly. An EEG, performed four days after injury, showed diffuse slowing together with a local area of slow activity in the right temporal region.

## FATAL CASES

There were three deaths in our series. One patient died following a rapid deterioration:

> *Case 11.* An 8-year-old boy jumped from a slow moving cart and fell on his head. He got up immediately, walked towards his father and said "I feel so funny in my head." He then became flaccid. His mother, a nurse, subsequently stated that she had noticed dilated pupils at the time. On admission one hour later, the boy was in shock and respiration was shallow. He was unresponsive and both pupils were dilated and fixed. No bruises were found on the head, and there was no skull fracture. Echoencephalography showed no midline shift. The boy was intubated and ventilated. Soon after admission, massive pulmonary edema developed. It was felt that the situation was hopeless, and no attempts were made at further investigation. He died within hours of admission. Permission for donor nephrectomy was granted by his parents; unfortunately, no attempts were made to obtain permission for autopsy.

Two patients died following a slow deterioration:

> *Case 12.* A 13-year-old girl fell off her bicycle. She did not lose consciousness at the time. On examination, three hours after the accident, she was lucid but nauseated. No neurological abnormalities were found. There was no skull fracture. She was sent home. Several hours later, she developed a left hemiparesis and became drowsy. A CT scan showed compression of the ventricles and a marked midline shift to the left. No abnormalities in the brain parenchyma were detected. An angiogram, performed in order to exclude an isodense hematoma, showed slowed intracerebral circulation but no avascular mass. The girl was intubated

and ventilated; high doses of corticosteroids were given, together with mannitol. She deteriorated over the next few hours and died on the following day. Permission for autopsy was refused. The past medical history of this girl revealed that she had been allergic, having reacted to all kinds of stimuli with severe angioneurotic edema.

*Case 13.* A 9-year-old boy fell off his skateboard. He resumed playing immediately, not having lost consciousness. Later that day he watched television for several hours and then went to bed. The next morning he complained of a headache and told his mother that he had difficulty in walking. Some time later, he became stuporous and vomited. On admission, 16 hours after the accident, he did not open his eyes to painful stimuli, but he located these adequately while moaning. A bruise was noted in the right parietal area. There was no skull fracture. The left pupil was dilated, the right somewhat smaller; neither reacted to light. While the patient was being examined, both pupils started to react to light spontaneously. As the CT scanner was not available, an angiogram had been scheduled. It was felt, however, that the spontaneous improvement made an expanding intracranial mass less likely. Without having further deteriorated in the meantime, the boy suddenly developed fixed dilated pupils and apnea. He was immediately taken to the operating room where multiple bilateral burr holes revealed a tight, swollen brain but no extradural or intradural hematoma. Brain needling excluded the presence of hydrocephalus. The boy died 15 hours after admission. Permission for autopsy was refused.

Lindenberg et al. (1955) described the postmortem findings of children dying from blunt head injuries. Diffuse cerebral swelling was the most consistent finding. They concluded that this posttraumatic brain swelling is markedly more common in children than in adults and that it may develop after seemingly minor head trauma without subsequent loss of consciousness. As an example of this, they mention the case of a 1½-year-old boy who slipped in the bathroom and fell on his forehead. He was all right for the first few minutes, but after 15 minutes he turned pale, became drowsy, then stuporous, and he died about 30 minutes after the accident. At autopsy, the only external traumatic lesion was a subcutaneous hemorrhage over the forehead. The brain showed severe generalized swelling. Microscopically, only ischemic lesions in both thalami were seen, which were attributed to compression of brainstem branches of the posterior cerebral arteries as a result of this generalized brain swelling. Biemond (1970) described three children who died following a mild head injury. In all children an exploratory craniotomy was performed, yielding negative results. Postmortem examination showed diffuse cerebral swelling with microscopic findings of hyperemia in the smaller arteries and precapillaries. He considered the brain swelling to be the primary event, probably attributable to diencephalic lesions. In a study of CT and histopathology, Snoek et al. (1979) described the postmortem findings of six children with the CT appearance of diffuse cerebral swelling. All these children, however, had suffered severe head injury. The ventricles were small in all of the cases in whom the CT scan had shown compressed ventricles. Three of these children had neuropathological evidence of diffuse damage to white matter; in two there were signs of moderate or severe hypoxic brain damage, but the sixth case could only be classified as an example of "idiopathic brain swelling," with absence of distinct abnormalities on histological examination.

Unfortunately, autopsy was not performed in the three cases of the mild head injury series. However, the clinical course and radiological and (in one case) surgical findings, strongly suggest that death was due to "malignant brain swelling" in all these cases.

## POSSIBLE MECHANISMS RESPONSIBLE FOR DETERIORATION FOLLOWING MILD HEAD INJURY IN CHILDREN

In the literature, several explanations have been offered for such delayed deterioration. Secondary deterioration not due to intracranial hematoma has been attributed to:

1. Cerebral edema (Biemond, 1970; Gjerris and Mellemgaard, 1969; Pickles, 1949; Schnitker, 1949; Walton and Brooks, 1897)
2. Local contusion with subsequent brain swelling and serous exudation into the subarachnoid space (Walton, 1898)
3. Diffuse cerebral swelling possibly due to cerebral hyperemia (Bruce et al., 1979, 1981a,b; Gennarelli 1987; Langfitt and Bruce, 1975)
4. Convulsions (Grand, 1974; Livingston and Mahloudji, 1961; Reilly et al., 1975; Rose et al., 1977; Small and Wolf, 1957)
5. Cerebral arterial vasospasm (Bodian, 1964; Haas and Sovner, 1969; Venable et al., 1978)
6. Stretch of perforator arteries resulting in basal ganglia infarction (Maki et al., 1980)
7. A migrainous mechanism (Haas et al., 1975; Guthkelch, 1977)
8. Spreading depression of Leão (Oka et al., 1977)
9. A functional disturbance of the rostral brainstem (Todorow and Feller, 1982)
10. A mechanically or chemically induced disturbance of the periaqueductal gray matter at the region of the fourth ventricle (Bruce, 1984)

Several authors considered both convulsive and nonconvulsive signs as part of one syndrome and have attempted to give an explanation for its occurrence, whereas others have confined themselves to giving an explanation for the occurrence of convulsions or of nonconvulsive signs only. Two speculative pathophysiological entities will be described in more detail in the following section.

## FOCAL OR GENERALIZED BRAIN SWELLING, DUE EITHER TO RAPID EDEMA FORMATION OR TO CEREBRAL HYPEREMIA

For almost a century, there have been reports of clinical findings in head-injured children and adolescents suggesting the presence of an intracranial hematoma, but with these findings apparently being due to some other condition. The first case studies were reported by Walton and Brooks (1897) and Walton (1898). Walton and Brooks described a young woman who fell off a horse, striking her head forcefully against a fence. From their description of signs, she did in fact suffer a very severe head injury that rendered her unconscious from the moment of impact. She deteriorated on the following day, after a mild, transient improvement. On trepanation, a tense and nonpulsating dura was found and clear fluid under pressure was relieved when this was incised. The reported postmortem findings suggest that this woman had suffered severe diffuse axonal injury (DAI) (Adams et al., 1977), with small hemorrhagic areas throughout the white matter. The authors, however, for the first time drew attention to the differences between the steady deterioration of conscious level in cases of intracranial hematoma, as compared with the fluctuating course when such hematoma is not the cause of deterioration. Walton (1898) described two patients with a lucid interval following injury. Spontaneous improvement in the first case led to postponement of surgery, whereas in the second case "overcrowding in the Boston City Hospital" caused a delay of 12 hours, when improvement was noted rendering the intended surgery superfluous. Walton attached great value to the combination of brain swelling and the (apparent) hygroma that had been found in the horsewoman. In order to assess whether evident progress has been made in the past 90 years regarding the theories about the pathophysiological processes underlying such transient deterioration, it is appropriate to recite his conclusions:

*First.* A severe blow on the head may result, either directly or by contrecoup, in a local bruising, congestion and swelling of the brain tissue, with serous exudation into the subarachnoid space, either with or without oedema of the brain substance.

*Second.* If this accumulation of fluid occurs over the motor centres it may be imprisoned so as to cause focal pressure symptoms, simulating meningeal hemorrhage.

*Third.* This accumulation of fluid is not compensatory, but represents an ineffectual effort toward relief of tension, as shown by the swollen condition of the underlying brain substance when exposed by operation. The mechanism is probably analogous to if not identical with that of the so-called serous meningitis of Quincke.

*Fourth.* The lesion is self-limiting, the resulting paralysis disappearing in the course of a few days.

*Fifth.* This condition may be mistaken for middle meningeal or middle cerebral hemorrhage. The diagnosis is difficult and sometimes impossible. Factors in the diagnosis are (a) an atypical course, (b) absence of steadily increasing coma, and (c) the appearance of sensitiveness to pain on manipulation of the head, even after the consciousness is so great that questions are not answered. The general symptoms (restlessness, stupor, headache, and moderate febrile movement) may be the same in both conditions.

*Sixth.* The mere presence of paralysis following a blow upon the head is not necessarily an indication for immediate operation, and in the absence of steadily deepening unconsciousness and of steady progression of other cerebral symptoms, it will be often wise to postpone surgical interference, though generally speaking an exploratory operation is always justified in case of focal paralysis following head injury.

*Seventh.* This lesion is to be particularly borne in mind in the case of children and young adults, and perhaps in alcoholic patients. In elderly patients the same set of symptoms points more decidedly toward hemorrhage.

Pickles (1949) concluded that transient acute cortical edema, with associated capillary anemia, best explained the rapid and complete recovery without operation.

In recent years, posttraumatic cerebral swelling is a matter of great controversy, both regarding its nature as well as its clinical significance. At least part of the problem appears to be that terms such as *brain edema* and *brain swelling* are ambiguous in the clinical context (Jennett, 1981) and are often used interchangeably. Cerebral swelling is an abnormal increase in the volume of cerebral tissue, whereas cerebral edema is a particular form of brain swelling in which there is an increase in tissue fluid within brain substance (Clasen and Penn, 1987; Clasen et al., 1986). Until recently, posttraumatic brain swelling has always been attributed to brain edema, but the crucial evidence for this cause is inconclusive. Galbraith et al. (1984), employing the microgravimetric method, measured directly the water content of the white matter of brain tissue taken from severely head injured patients during operation. It was found to be elevated in both diffuse and mass lesions, but there was no relationship between the brain water content and intracranial pressure in patients with a diffuse lesion. Bullock et al. (1985), using a similiar technique, comfirmed the presence of reduced perifocal specific gravity in patients with focal injuries, suggesting that brain edema is present around such lesions. In contrast to the results reported by Galbraith et al., these authors found normal white matter specific gravity values in patients with diffuse injury, suggesting that brain edema was not present in these patients. The concept of brain edema causing diffuse cerebral swelling has now been replaced by the alternative explanation of increased cerebral blood volume (CBV). Bruce et al. (1979, 1981a,b) and Zimmerman et al. (1978) described the CT appearance of diffuse cerebral swelling, which they considered to be the commonest CT finding in head-injured children. This picture consists of obliteration or narrowing of the lateral and third ventricles and perimesencephalic cisterns (Figure 7–4). According to these authors, the most likely explanation for this cerebral swelling is an increase in intracerebral blood rather than an increase in brain water content. This increase in cerebral blood is due either to a true increase in cerebral blood volume or to a redistribution of intracranial blood from the pial to the intraparenchymal vessels. The arguments in favor of a vascular cause of brain swelling are threefold:

1. Cerebral attentuation values (measured in the deep frontal white matter) are higher on CT scans demonstrating cerebral swelling than on follow-up scans (mean increase about 3 Hounsfield units). In addition, these values are also higher than the normal range defined from values measured on normal pediatric CT scans and certainly than would be expected if brain edema were the cause of this cerebral swelling, as an increase in water content of the brain is linearly related to an increase in attenuation numbers (Zimmerman et al., 1978; Bruce et al., 1979, 1981a,b).
2. An increased cerebral blood flow (CBF) has been demonstrated in children who showed this CT pattern of diffuse cerebral swelling. It is suggested that these two

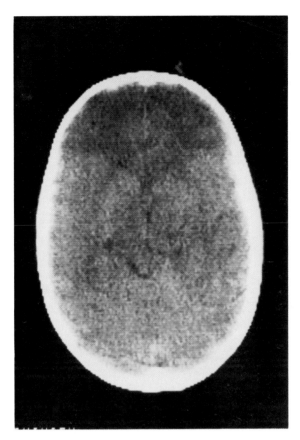

**Figure 7–4**    Diffuse cerebral swelling. Example of CT section at the level of the anterior horns and the mesencephalon. Note the narrow aspect of the ventricular horns. The quadrigeminal cistern is partly obliterated.

findings are related, and the cerebral swelling is therefore ascribed to cerebral hyperemia (Zimmerman et al., 1978; Bruce et al., 1979, 1981a,b). Langfitt et al. (1966) introduced the concept of *vasomotor paralysis*. They postulated an acute reduction in vasomotor tone, resulting in cerebral vasodilatation and increased cerebral blood volume. If this condition of increased CBV continues for a long enough period, vascular permeability may be increased, resulting in true edema formation and elevated intracranial pressure (ICP). Obrist et al. (1979, 1984) performed cerebral metabolism studies in patients who exhibited cerebral hyperemia and found evidence for the existence of true *luxury perfusion*. Bruce (1984), however, reports an increase in cerebral metabolic rate for oxygen ($CMR_{O_2}$) in children with diffuse swelling (despite low Glasgow Coma scores), suggesting increased metabolic activity in these children. Unilateral cerebral swelling, which has been described as occurring within 20–30 minutes after trauma, has also, on the basis of attenuation measurements, been ascribed to cerebral vasodilatation (Kobrine et al., 1977; Waga et al., 1979).

3. An often used argument in favor of a vascular mechanism in the pathogenesis of brain swelling is the rapidity with which it can develop, as the only compartment that can increase at such a rate must be the intravascular space.

The cause of the cerebral vasodilatation, which allegedly leads to cerebral swelling, is as yet unknown. Meyer et al. (1971) found in their animal model that the areas causing increases in CBF when stimulated were located in the pontine and midbrain reticular formation, the thalamus, and the hypothalamus. Raichle et al. (1978) assumed that locus coeruleus stimulation may change both CBF and cerebral capillary permeability, probably through central vascular aminergic pathways. Bruce (1984) argued that excitation of the floor of the fourth ventricle and periaqueductal gray matter results in increased cerebral metabolic activity and increased cerebral blood flow and volume. He suggests that this excitation is caused either by delayed effects of mechanical trauma or by the effect of some chemical mediator that percolates through the brain and ventricular system until it reaches the region of the fourth ventricle.

The evidence for this vascular cause of cerebral swelling is as yet rather weak, however. *First,* the significance of rather marginal variations in mean CT attenuation numbers has been challenged on the basis of the normal range of CT numbers in children (Snoek et al., 1984). *Second,* although the reported increase of 3 Hounsfield units (HU) in CT attenuation numbers is relatively small in the context of other variable factors influencing the measurements, it represents a large shift if it is to be explained solely on the basis of an increase in blood content (Snoek et al., 1984). Clasen et al. (1986) calculated that doubling the cerebral blood volume would increase the CT number only by 0.7 HU. *Third,* the same authors calculated that cerebral blood volume must be tripled to account for ventricular collapse, whereas the maximal allowable increase in cerebral blood volume (CBV) due to congestion, under pathological conditions is about 100%, and therefore, vascular congestion cannot account for the ventricular collapse seen in diffuse cerebral swelling. In fact, determination of CBV by emission tomography in four head-injured children belonging to the series of Bruce et al. (1981a) showed a decrease in CBV in three of them (Kuhl et al., 1980). Recently, Arvigo et al. (1985) demonstrated global depression of cerebral perfusion of both hemispheres in mild contusion patients, the majority of whom were under 20 years of age.

Thus, if it is not cerebral hyperemia, what is it? Recently, Clasen et al. argued that there is compelling evidence that diffuse traumatic edema rather than cerebral congestion is the cause of cerebral swelling (Clasen and Penn, 1987; Clasen et al., 1986). As yet, the matter appears not to have been settled, and further studies employing new techniques are urgently needed to solve this problem. Nuclear magnetic resonance imaging (MRI) and positron emission tomography (PET) are likely to revolutionize concepts of brain swelling and brain edema resulting from head injury. Recently, the first promising results of MRI studies have been published, dealing with experimental (Barnes et al., 1986) and tumor-related (Bell et al., 1987) cerebral edema.

Likewise, the problem of the clinical significance of the finding of a CT appearance suggesting diffuse cerebral swelling is as yet unresolved. The crucial question is whether such a swelling is the cause of the deterioration in head-injured children, or whether in most patients it is an epiphenomenon caused by the same processes that lead to the clinical deterioration. Cold and Jensen (1980) found that hyperemia following head injury is a common phenomenon in children, that this hyperemic phase lasts for some days to several weeks, and that it is of no prognostic importance. The CT pattern of diffuse cerebral swelling suggests a grave prognosis when it is observed in the acute stage of severe head injury (Teasdale et al., 1984; Toutant et al., 1984), but its prognostic significance is less clear when it is observed in later stages, especially after mild head injury. According to Gennarelli (1987), brain swelling can accompany any type of head injury, and the magnitude of the swelling does not correlate well with the severity of injury.

The CT appearance of diffuse cerebral swelling was reported to be present in 29% of head-injured children and adolescents (Bruce et al., 1981a). All these children had suffered an acceleration/deceleration type of head injury (in contrast to the patients of our series, in whom a simple fall was the most common cause of injury). There was a higher incidence in patients with a low score on the Glasgow Coma Scale (41% with a score of 8 or less) than in patients with a score greater than 8 (15%). These authors did not specifically mention the rate of occurrence of this CT pattern in children with a lucid interval. Conversely, in the clinical description of their group of 63 juvenile patients with the CT pattern of diffuse cerebral swelling, 37% had experienced some form of lucid interval. Within the latter group two subgroups were described. In a typical case of the first subgroup (eight cases), there was a lucid interval with a period of talking and complete consciousness from minutes to hours after injury, followed by the onset of vomiting, headache, and frequently pallor and sweating, associated with decreased alertness. These patients exhibited evidence of decreased spontaneous motor activity and loss of spontaneous speech and of eye opening. No mention is made of focal neurological signs. None of these patients progressed to coma according to the criteria of Teasdale and Jennett (1974), and all made a good recovery. The other subgroup consisted of 15 patients who had been unconscious following trauma and then had an interval associated with recovery of eye opening, occasional words, and more spontaneous motor function. Within minutes to hours after injury, rapid deterioration occurred, manifesting itself by a deteriorating level of consciousness, loss of eye opening, and worsening motor responses, frequently with intermittent pupillary dilatation. Four of these patients had early seizures. In one of the patients extracerebral collections of CSF density were found, which resolved without therapy. One of the patients died as a result of delayed brain swelling. The others all made a good recovery, with a reported mean hospital stay in this group of patients of 14 days.

According to Gennarelli (1987), mild degrees of delayed diffuse cerebral swelling may be the cause of posttraumatic lethargy following a lucid interval in pediatric head injury, but the severe form of such delayed swelling causes coma leading to death or to a very prolonged illness. In the typical case he describes, there is a more or less completely lucid interval immediately after injury. The child then becomes lethargic and lapses into coma, often in association with an early posttraumatic seizure. The CT scan by then has the appearance of diffuse cerebral swelling. The intracranial pressure (ICP) is elevated, and, if adequate control of ICP is accomplished, the swelling begins to diminish a week or more after the injury, to such a degree that extracerebral collections occur, which disappear spontaneously by one month after injury. At that time, some degree of neurological recovery from deep coma has occurred and the CT appearance by then is that of cerebral atrophy. The brain resumes its normal configuration over the next six to nine months. However, according to Bruce et al. (1981a), this sequence of clinical and radiological events is almost without exception observed in children with the immediate onset of unconsciousness following severe rather than mild head injury.

Most of the patients of our series showed a benign, often shortlasting syndrome. As a result, few CT scans have been performed. In only one out of four scans, performed in children with a rapid deterioration consisting of either convulsive or nonconvulsive signs, was the typical CT appearance consistent with diffuse cerebral swelling observed; the time course in this patient (a 12-year-old girl with a shortlasting alarming picture, consisting of deep coma with bilaterally unreactive pupils) was different from that in all others, as these signs occurred very late (36 hours) after injury. Apparently, in the majority of cases deterioration is not associated with such cerebral swelling. At present, therefore, when the CT pattern of diffuse cerebral swelling is observed in a case of deterioration following mild head injury in a child, it is not clear whether this swelling causes the deterioration or not. There is no doubt, however, that in some patients severe and often uncontrollable unilateral or diffuse brain swelling may occur, even following injuries in which acceleration/deceleration plays no role or only a minor one. This form of brain swelling may well be an aspecific reaction of the pediatric brain to a variety of stimuli (Eiben, 1967; Lyon et al., 1961), among which head injury is just one.

## A MIGRAINOUS MECHANISM

In known migraineurs, especially in children and adolescents, attacks may be triggered by mild head injury (Barlow, 1984a; Behrman, 1977; Blau, 1985; Fitzsimons and Wolfenden, 1985; Guthkelch, 1977; Morris, 1972; Whitty, 1986). There are also many reports of cases in which migraine apparently commenced after a mild head injury (Ashworth, 1985; Barlow, 1984a; Behrman, 1977; Espir et al., 1972; Guthkelch, 1977; Haas and Ross, 1986; Haas and Sovner, 1969; Haas et al., 1975; Matthews, 1972; Wilkinson, 1986).

> *Case 14* (not included in the *Brain* series). The first attack of this boy, born in 1973, occurred in 1975 when he fell down several stairs. He cried immediately, but minutes later he became drowsy and very irritable. His mother noted a weakness of the right arm and leg, but on examination four hours after the fall, no hemiparesis was found. Within hours after admission he became alert and cooperative.
>
> In 1979, he was admitted elsewhere because of the acute onset of hemiparesis and aphasia within minutes after bumping his head. A third, similar, attack occurred in 1981.
>
> In 1983, he was admitted because of the spontaneous onset of severe frontal headache, hemiparesis, aphasia, and vomiting. A CT scan showed a small hypodense area in the left temporal region. The CSF was normal, but one day later

mild pleocytosis was noted. Serial EEGs, performed over the next fortnight, successively revealed slow activity in the left frontotemporal area, periodic discharges in the same area, diffuse abnormalities, and a combination of focal slow activity in the right posterior regions in combination with diffuse abnormalities. On the second day, a right hemianopsia was noted, and on the third day a partial seizure occurred, with deviation of the head to the right and twitching of the right side of the face. In view of the CSF, CT, and EEG abnormalities, a provisional diagnosis of herpes simplex (HSE) encephalitis was made and treatment with vidarabine was started. Laboratory investigations later on proved to be negative for HSE, however. Within a week after admission all signs had disappeared. A second CT scan was normal. An angiogram, performed 1½ week later, was suggestive of mild vasospasm in the territory of the left middle cerebral artery. This angiogram provoked a severe confusional state, aphasia, and (probably) visual disturbances, which lasted for two days.

A fifth attack occurred in 1984, when he struck his head during gym, which was followed by aphasia and vomiting, lasting several hours.

Since 1986, he has had several spontaneously occurring attacks consisting of blurring of vision, clumsiness of the right hand, and sensory symptoms spreading from his right hand to his mouth in several minutes, followed by severe throbbing headache.

The family history revealed that his mother's sister suffers from common migraine.

Some authors regard the *pediatric concussion syndrome* as nothing but a particular manifestation of a migraine attack triggered by head trauma (Guthkelch, 1977; Haas and Lourie, 1984). Haas and Sovner (1969) described six children with repeated trauma-triggered attacks of transient neurological phenomena which preceded or accompanied typical migraine headaches. In all but one case, there was a family history of similar attacks and of migraine headaches. In accordance with the prevailing view about the pathophysiology of migraine (Wolff, 1963), traumatic cerebral arterial spasm was postulated as the initial event in the attacks. In a later paper (Haas et al., 1975), 50 attacks were described, occurring in 25 patients; 40 of these attacks occurred in children under 14 years of age. All attacks developed after a latent interval, generally of 1–10 minutes. Attacks were grouped into four clinical types: (1) hemiparesis; (2) somnolence, irritability, and vomiting; (3) blindness; and (4) brainstem signs. Two patients had a seizure. Eleven of the patients had more than one attack (not necessarily the same each time), and five of the children later had spontaneous attacks which resembled their triggered attacks closely enough to be considered the same experience. In this series, the family history of migraine was not as conspicuous as in their earlier series, but there was a remarkably high parenteral incidence of migraine with neurological signs (12%), and there appeared to be a tendency for trauma-triggered attacks to occur in siblings. In the series of children with nonconvulsive deterioration described by Guthkelch (1977), a strong family history of migraine was also present, but others either have reported a low prevalence of migraine in relatives of such patients (Ashworth, 1985; Behrman, 1977), or have explicitly excluded cases with a positive family history of migraine (Oka et al., 1977).

In our retrospective series, it was difficult to retrieve the family history of migraine. Many hospital records, however, contained a detailed past history and family history. If there would have been a strong tendency for complicated migraine to occur in the children or their relatives, this would undoubtedly have been noted in at least several instances, but this was not the case. Only one patient (a convulsive case) had had an identical episode of convulsions after a previous trivial injury. Review of the records in 1987 (follow-up of six to nine years) revealed that none of the patients had been subsequently investigated for migraine attacks in our or in other hospitals. Although this finding of course does not exclude the possibility that indeed many of these patients had developed repeated migraine attacks, this appears to be most unlikely. A formal follow-up with recording of a detailed family history of migraine will be executed in 1989, when most of the patients will have reached or passed puberty.

The so-called periodic syndrome (i.e., attacks of headache, abdominal pain, and associated autonomic disturbances occurring in children), which bears a relationship with both migraine and epilepsy, is often triggered by mild head injury (Kellaway et al., 1960). According to these authors, the EEGs of children with this syndrome consistently show the 14 and 6 per second positive spike pattern. It is interesting to note that most recently, Gibbs and Gibbs (1987) reported a very high prevalence of this particular EEG finding in head-injured children, and they regard this pattern as a characteristic delayed reaction to mild head injury in childhood. The significance of this spike pattern, however, is an extremely controversial question (Jay, 1981; Niedermeyer, 1982). No clear examples of this EEG finding were observed in our patients—a fact that is hardly surprising as most EEGs have been performed in the waking state, when it is usually absent.

The question is whether isolated transient, benign posttraumatic syndromes are in fact migraine or migraine-related attacks, even if they occur in children or adolescents with an absent personal or family history of migraine. This may well be the case. If there is sufficient provocation, both migraine and seizures may be expressed in anyone, and heredity is just one factor influencing the excitability threshold (Barlow, 1984b; Welch, 1987).

Oka et al. (1977) described a series of 37 children in whom transient neurological disorders occurred in the acute stage of trivial head injury. The ages of their patients ranged from 10 months to 21 years, but the majority were under 14 years of age. Cases in which the family or past history revealed seizures or migraine were excluded. Of these 37 children, 28 developed convulsive attacks, and 9 children demonstrated nonconvulsive signs consisting of headache, nausea and vomiting, pallor, somnolence, irritability and restlessness, stupor, hemiparesis, and aphasia. These authors considered the nonconvulsive signs to be the primary and basic disturbance, and they regarded the convulsive attacks as secondary phenomena. Most of the convulsive patients were under 8 years of age. The fact that the nonconvulsive disturbance was followed by convulsions in the younger children was ascribed to a maturational factor. Identical observations have been made by Guthkelch (1977), who independently drew the same conclusions.

According to Oka et al., both nonconvulsive and convulsive phenomena can be explained as manifestations of the experimental phenomenon designated as *cortical spreading depression of Leão*. Leão (1944) found that a variety of stimuli, including mechanical stimulation of the exposed cerebral cortex, elicit a characteristic response, consisting of a marked enduring reduction of the spontaneous electrical activity of the cortex, spreading at a rate of 3 mm/min across the cortical surface. At the front of the moving wave, vigorous spike discharge takes place. Under certain experimental conditions, spreading depression leads to paroxysmal activity or "spreading convulsion," which may explain the existence of certain migraine–epilepsy syndromes (Andermann, 1987).

Although there are serious difficulties in extrapolating from experimental spreading depression in animals to migraine and related disorders in humans (Gloor, 1986; Pearce, 1985), Leão's spreading depression is now widely believed to be the pathophysiological substrate underlying migraine (Lauritzen, 1987a–c; Olesen, 1986, 1987; Olesen et al., 1982; Shinohara et al., 1979). This is based not only on similarities between neurological abnormalities (i.e., somatosensory and motor deficits and signs of involvement of the hypothalamus) that accompany spreading depression in rats and migraine in humans (Lauritzen, 1987a), but also on the similarities of cerebral blood flow changes during classic migraine and experimentally induced spreading depression (for reviews, see Lauritzen, 1987c; Olesen, 1986).

It is tempting to try to develop a unifying concept that takes into account the relevant facts and theories described in the preceding paragraphs of this section. Blau and Solomon (1985) drew attention to the possibility that the brain swells during migraine attacks. They described a 26-year-old patient with two congenital skull defects who noted protuberances from these defects during a severe attack of migraine, which disappeared when the attack was over. A similar observation had been made 50 years earlier in a patient who, during a prolonged migraine attack, had had a craniectomy for suspected brain tumor, yielding negative results (Goltman, 1935/6). At craniotomy the dura was found to be very tense and not pulsating. When the dura was opened, CSF escaped under increased pressure. After the operation this patient had recurrent attacks of common migraine during which the normally depressed area over the craniotomy filled up, apparently as a result of brain swelling. CT evidence of massive hemisphere swelling occurring during migraine attacks has been reported by others as well (Fitzsimons and Wolfenden, 1985; Harrison, 1981). All these patients were adolescents or young adults. As the pediatric brain is even more liable to react to various stimuli with swelling, it is likely that such a phenomenon may play an even greater role in childhood.

As yet, disagreement exists about the changes in cerebral blood flow during migraine attacks. According to the group of Olesen and Lauritzen (Copenhagen), a consistent decrease is observed during classic migraine attacks (i.e., *spreading hypoperfusion*), which is not followed by an increase during the headache phase. In contrast, many others have consistently noted such hyperemia in migraine patients during their headaches (Mathew et al., 1976; Meyer et al., 1984, 1986; Norris et al., 1975; Sakai and Meyer, 1979; Skinhøj, 1973). Most recently, Olesen and co-workers have also noted hyperperfusion, occurring after an interval of six or more hours after the period of hypoperfusion *(reactive hyperemia)* and bearing no relation with headache (Andersen et al., 1988). Thus, both brain swelling and hyperemia appear to play a role in migraine. If one combines these findings, the similarities between delayed brain swelling (apparently due to cerebral hyperemia) occurring following mild head injury in children and during migraine attacks become apparent. At present, however, this possible pathophysiological relation between certain posttraumatic syndromes in children and migraine attacks is only speculative.

## MANAGEMENT OF THE DETERIORATING HEAD-INJURED CHILD

Obviously, whether or not to secure an immediate CT scan in a child that has deteriorated after a mild head injury depends on the clinical findings encountered on the first assessment following this deterioration. If, at that time, the child is alert after a single seizure or a transient nonconvulsive deterioration, CT scanning is unnecessary in the majority of cases. If, on the other hand, the neurological deterioration is still continuing or if the child is in a status epilepticus not reacting promptly to intravenous diazepam, resuscitation should be started and general intensive care measures should be taken (i.e., anticonvulsant administration, endotracheal intubation, hyperventilation to a $P_aCO_2$ of 25–30 torr, appropriate treatment of pulmonary problems in the case of aspiration, etc., followed by urgent CT scanning. If the presence of a hematoma is demonstrated, prompt evacuation of the clot is lifesaving. If the CT scan shows unilateral or diffuse cerebral swelling, the child should be maintained on moderate hyperventilation for 24–48 hours, which should be sufficient in most cases. In a few patients, monitoring of intracranial pressure with treatment of any rise when present may be necessary. According to some authors, mannitol is contraindicated in patients with diffuse cerebral swelling, as it may further increase the cerebral blood volume, and they recommend that its use be avoided for the first 24 hours after head injury in these patients (Bruce et al., 1981b). It is our policy not to prescribe antiepileptics in case of a single seizure in mildly head-injured patients. In the case of repeated seizures, however, antiepileptic treatment should be started.

## CONCLUSIONS

Mild or even trivial injuries in children are not infrequently followed by a deterioration that is preceded by a lucid or symptom-free period and is usually transient. On clinical grounds it is possible to differentiate between several distinct pictures, characterized by either focal or generalized cerebral dysfunction, both with and without seizures. At this moment, it can only be speculated whether or not these different clinical pictures reflect different pathophysiological entities. There appear to be intriguing, but at this time rather speculative, clinical and pathophysiological similarities with migraine.

In any deteriorating head-injured child who was symptom-free previously, the possibility of an expanding intracranial mass will have to be excluded, preferably by CT scanning, although few hematomas will be found. The remaining patients show a benign and shortlasting syndrome followed by a spontaneous and full recovery in most, but not in all cases.

## REFERENCES

Adams JH, Mitchell DE, Graham DI, Doyle D. Diffuse brain damage of immediate impact type. Brain 100:489–502, 1977.

Ammirati M, Tomita T. Posterior fossa epidural hematoma during childhood. Neurosurgery 14:541–544, 1984.

Andermann F. Migraine and epilepsy: an overview. *In* Andermann F, Lugaresi E (eds), Migraine and Epilepsy. Stoneham, MA: Butterworths, 1987, pp 405–422.

Andersen AR, Friberg L, Skyhøj E, Olsen T, Olesen J. Delayed hyperemia following hypoperfusion in classic migraine. Single photon computed tomographic demonstration. Arch Neurol 45:154–159, 1988.

Aoki N, Masuzawa, H. Infantile acute subdural hematoma: clinical analysis of 26 cases. J Neurosurg 61:273–280, 1984.

Arvigo F, Cossu M, Fazio B, Gris A, et al. Cerebral blood flow in minor cerebral contusion. Surg Neurol 24:211–217, 1985.

Ashworth B. Migraine, head trauma and sport. Scott Med J 30:240–242, 1985.

Barlow CF. Traumatic headache syndromes. *In* Barlow CF (ed) Headaches and Migraine in Childhood. Oxford: Blackwell, 1984a, pp 181–197.

Barlow CF. Migraine with seizures, stroke and syncope. *In* Headaches and Migraine in Childhood. Oxford: Blackwell, 1984b, pp 126–154.

Barnes D, McDonald WI, Tofts PS, Johnson G, Landon DN. Magnetic resonance imaging of experimental cerebral oedema. J Neurol Neurosurg Psychiatry 49:1341–1347, 1986.

Behrman S. Migraine as a sequela of blunt head injury. Injury 9:74–76, 1977.

Bell BA, Kean DM, MacDonald HL, Barnett GH, et al. Brain water measured by magnetic resonance imaging: correlation with direct estimation and changes after mannitol and dexamethasone. Lancet 1:66–69, 1987.

Biemond A. Closed craniocerebral traumata. *In* Brain Diseases. Amsterdam: Elsevier, 1970, Chapter 73, pp 771–785.

Blau JN. Pathogenesis of migraine headache: initiation. J R Coll Physicians Lond 19:166–168, 1985.

Blau JN, Solomon F. Migraine and intracranial swelling: an experiment of nature [Letter]. Lancet 2:718, 1985.

Bodian M. Transient loss of vision following head trauma. NY State J Med 64:916–920, 1964.

Bruce, DA. Delayed deterioration of consciousness after trivial head injury in childhood. Br Med J 289:715–716, 1984.

Bruce DA, Raphaely RC, Goldberg AI, Zimmerman RA, et al. Pathophysiology, treatment and outcome following severe head injury in children. Child's Brain 5:174–191, 1979.

Bruce DA, Alavi A, Bilaniuk LT, Dolinskas C, et al. Diffuse cerebral swelling following head injuries in children: the syndrome of "malignant brain edema." J Neurosurg 54:170–178, 1981a.

Bruce DA, Sutton LN, Schut L. Acute brain swelling and cerebral edema in children. *In* de Vlieger M, de Lange SA, Beks JWF (eds), Brain Edema. New York: John Wiley, 1981b, pp 125–145.

Bullock R, Smith R, Favier J, du Trevou M, Blake G. Brain specific gravity and CT scan density measurements after human head injury. J Neurosurg 63:64–68, 1985.

Casey R, Ludwig S, McCormick MC. Morbidity following minor head trauma in children. Pediatrics 78:497–502, 1986.

Choux M, Grisoli F, Peragut J-C. Extradural hematomas in children: 104 cases. Child's Brain 1:337–347, 1975.

Clasen RA, Guariglia P, Stein RJ, Pandolfi S, Lobick JJ. Histopathology and computerized tomography of human traumatic cerebral swelling. *In* Baethmann A, Go KG, Unterberg A (eds), Mechanisms of Secondary Brain Damage. New York: Plenum, 1986, pp 29–45.

Clasen RA, Penn RD. Traumatic swelling and edema. *In* Cooper PR (ed), Head Injury, 2nd ed. Baltimore: William & Wilkins, 1987, pp 285–312.

Cold GE, Jensen FT. Cerebral blood flow in the acute phase after head injury. I. Correlation to age of the patients, clinical outcome and localisation of the injured region. Acta Anaesthesiol Scand 24:245–251, 1980.

Dacey RG, Alves WM, Rimel RW, Winn R, Jane JAJ. Neurosurgical complications after apparently minor head injury: assessment of risk in a series of 610 patients. J Neurosurg 65:203–210, 1986.

Dhellemmes P, Lejeune J-P, Christiaens J-L, Combelles G. Traumatic extradural hematomas in infancy and childhood: experience with 144 cases. J Neurosurg 62:861–864, 1985.

Ehyai A, Fenichel GM. The natural history of acute confusional migraine. Arch Neurol 35:368–369, 1978.

Eiben RM. Acute brain swelling (toxic encephalopathy). Pediatr Clin North Am 14:797–808, 1967.

Enomoto T, Ono Y, Nose T, Maki Y, Tsukada K. Electroencephalography in minor head injury in children. Child's Nerv Syst 2:72–79, 1986.

Espir MLE, Hodge ILD, Matthews PHN. Footballer's migraine [Letter]. Br Med J 3:352, 1972.

Fitzsimons RB, Wolfenden WH. Migraine coma. Meningitic migraine with cerebral oedema associated with a new form of autosomal dominant cerebellar ataxia. Brain 108:555–577, 1985.

Galbraith SL. Age-distribution of extradural haemorrhage without skull fracture. Lancet 1:1217–1218, 1973.

Galbraith SL, Cardoso E, Patterson J, Marmarou A. *In* Go KG and Baethmann A (eds), Recent Progress in the Study and Therapy of Brain Edema. New York: Plenum, 1984, pp 323–330.

Garza-Mercado R. Extradural hematoma of the posterior cranial fossa. Report of seven cases with survival. J Neurosurg 59:664–672, 1983.

Gascon G, Barlow C. Juvenile migraine presenting as an acute confusional state. Pediatrics 45:628–635, 1970.

Gennarelli TA. Cerebral concussion and diffuse brain injuries. *In* Cooper PR (ed), Head Injury, 2nd ed. Baltimore: William & Wilkins, 1987, pp 108–124.

Gibbs FA, Gibbs EL. Electroencephalographic study of head injury in childhood. Clin Electroencephalogr 18:10–11, 1987.

Gjerris F, Mellemgaard L. Transitory cortical blindness in head injury. Acta Neurol Scand 45:623–631, 1969.

Gloor P. Migraine and regional cerebral upflow [Letter]. Trends Neurosci 9:21, 1986.

Goltman AM. The mechanism of migraine. J Allergy 7:351–355, 1935/6.

Grand W. The significance of post-traumatic status epilepticus in childhood. J Neurol Neurosurg Psychiatry 37:178–180, 1974.

Greenblatt SH. Posttraumatic transient cerebral blindness. JAMA 225:1073–1076, 1973.

Griffith JF, Dodge PR. Transient blindness following head injury in children. N Eng J Med 278:648–651, 1968.

Guthkelch AN. Benign post-traumatic encephalopathy in young people and its relation to migraine. Neurosurgery 1:101–106, 1977.

Haas DC, Lourie H. Delayed deterioration of consciousness after trivial head injury in childhood [Letter]. Br Med J 289:1625, 1984.

Haas DC, Ross GS. Transient global amnesia triggered by mild head trauma. Brain 109:251–257, 1986.

Haas DC, Sovner RD. Migraine attacks triggered by mild head trauma, and their relation to certain post-traumatic disorders of childhood. J Neurol Neurosurg Psychiatry 32:548–554, 1969.

Haas DC, Pineda GS, Lourie H. Juvenile head trauma syndromes and their relationship to migraine. Arch Neurol 32:727–730, 1975.

Harrison MJG. Hemiplegic migraine [Letter]. J Neurol Neurosurg Psychiatry 44:652–653, 1981.

Hauser WA. Post-traumatic epilepsy in children. In Shapiro K (ed), Pediatric Head Trauma. New York: Futura, 1983, pp 271–287.

Hendrick EB, Harris L. Post-traumatic epilepsy in children. J Trauma 8:547–556, 1968.

Hendrick EB, Harwood-Hash DCF, Hudson AR. Head injuries in children: a survey of 4465 consecutive cases at the Hospital for Sick Children, Toronto, Canada. Clin Neurosurg 11:46–65, 1963.

Hochstetler K, Beals, RD. Transient cortical blindness in a child. Ann Emerg Med 16:218–219, 1987.

Jamieson KG, Yelland JDN. Extradural haematoma. Report of 167 cases. J Neurosurg 29:13–23, 1968.

Jamieson KG, Yelland JDN. Surgically treated traumatic subdural haematomas. J Neurosurg 37:137–149, 1972a.

Jamieson KG, Yelland JDN. Traumatic intracerebral haematoma. Report of 63 surgically treated cases. J Neurosurg 37:528–532, 1972b.

Jay GW. Epilepsy, migraine and EEG abnormalities in children: a review and hypothesis. Headache 22:110–114, 1981.

Jennett WB. Epilepsy after non-missile head injuries. London: Heinemann, 1962 (1st ed), 1975 (2nd ed).

Jennett B. Trauma as a cause of epilepsy in childhood. Dev Med Child Neurol 15:56–62, 1973.

Jennett B. Clinical brain swelling: edema or engorgement. In de Vlieger M, de Lange SA, Beks JWF (eds), Brain Edema. New York: John Wiley, 1981, pp 61–65.

Jennett B, Teasdale G. Intracranial hematoma. In Management of Head Injuries. Philadelphia: FA Davis, 1981, pp 153–191.

Kellaway P, Crawley JW, Kagawa N. Paroxysmal pain and autonomic disturbances of cerebral origin: a specific electro-clinical syndrome. Epilepsia 1:466–483, 1960.

Kobrine AI, Timmins E, Rajjoub RK, Rizzoli HV, Davis DO. Demonstration of massive traumatic brain swelling within 20 minutes after injury. Case report. J Neurosurg 46:256–258, 1977.

Kraus JF, Fife D, Conroy, C. Pediatric brain injuries: the nature, clinical course, and early outcomes in a defined United States' population. Pediatrics 79:501–507, 1987.

Kuhl DE, Alavi A, Hoffman EJ, Phelps ME, et al. Local cerebral blood volume in head-injured patients. Determination by emission computed tomography of 99mTc-labeled red cells. J Neurosurg 52:309–320, 1980.

Kushner MJ, Luken, MG. Posterior fossa epidural hematoma. A report of three cases diagnosed with computed tomography. Neuroradiology 24:169–171, 1983.

Langfitt TW, Bruce DA. Microcirculation and brain edema in head injury. In Vinken PJ, Bruyn GW (eds), Handbook of Clinical Neurology, Vol 23: Injuries of the Brain and Skull. Amsterdam: North Holland, 1975, pp 133–161.

Lauritzen M. Cortical depression as a putative migraine mechanism. Trends Neurosci 10:8–12, 1987a.

Lauritzen M. Cerebral blood flow in migraine and spreading depression. In Andermann F, Lugaresi E (eds), Migraine and Epilepsy. Stoneham, MA: Butterworths, 1987b, pp 325–337.

Lauritzen M. Cerebral blood flow in migraine and cortical spreading depression. Acta Neurol Scand 76 (Suppl 113), 1987c.

Leão AAP. Spreading depression of activity in cerebral cortex. J Neurophysiol 7:359–390, 1944.

Lindenberg R, Fisher RS, Durlacher SH, Lovitt WV, Freytag E. The pathology of the brain in blunt head injuries of infants and children. In Proceedings of the Second International Congress of Neuropathology, Part 2. Amsterdam: Excerpta Medica, 1955, pp 477–479.

Livingston KE, Mahloudji M. Delayed focal convulsive seizures after head injury in infants and children. A syndrome that may mimic extradural hematoma. Neurology (Minn) 11:1017–1020, 1969.

Lyon G, Dodge PR, Adams RD. The acute encephalopathies of obscure origin in infants and children. Brain 84:680–708, 1961.

Maki Y, Akimoto H, Enomoto T. Injuries of basal ganglia following head trauma in children. Child's Brain 7:113–123, 1980.

Masters SJ, McClean PM, Arcarese JS, Brown RF, et al. Skull x-ray examinations after head trauma. Recommendations by a multidisciplinary panel and validation study. N Eng J Med 316:84–91, 1987.

Mathew NT, Hrastnik F, Meyer JS. Regional cerebral blood flow in the diagnosis of vascular headache. Headache 15:252–260, 1976.

Matthews WB. Footballer's migraine. Br Med J 2:326–327, 1972.

Mazza C, Pasqualin A, Feriotti G, Da Pian R. Traumatic extradural haematomas in children: experience with 62 cases. Acta Neurochir (Wien) 65:67–80, 1982.

Mealy J. Closed head injury. In Pediatric Head Injuries. Springfield, IL: Thomas, 1968, pp 53–87.

Meyer JS, Teraura T, Sakomoto K, Kondo A. Central neurogenic control of cerebral blood flow. Neurology (Minn) 21:247–262, 1971.

Meyer JS, Hata T, Imai A, Zetusky WJ. Migraine and intracranial swelling [Letter]. Lancet 2:1308–1309, 1984.

Meyer JS, Zetusky W, Jonsdottir M, Mortel K. Cephalic hyperemia during migraine headaches. A prospective study. Headache 26:388–397, 1986.

Morris AM. Footballer's migraine [Letter]. Br Med J 2:770, 1972.

Niedermeyer E. Abnormal EEG patterns (epileptic and paroxysmal). In Niedermeyer E, Lopes da Silva F, Electroencephalography: Basic Principles, Clinical Applications and Related Fields. Baltimore: Urban and Schwarzenberg, 1982, pp 155–177.

Norris JW, Hachinski VC, Cooper PW. Changes in cerebral blood flow during a migraine attack. Br Med J 3:676–677, 1975.

Obrist WD, Gennarelli TA, Segawa H, Dolinskas CA, Langfitt TW. Relation of cerebral blood flow to neurological status and outcome in head-injured patients. J Neurosurg 51:292–300, 1979.

Obrist WD, Langfitt TW, Jaggi JL, Cruz J, Gennarelli TA. Cerebral blood flow and metabolism in comatose patients with acute head injury. J Neurosurg 61:241–253, 1984.

Oka H, Kako M, Matsushima M, Ando K. Traumatic spreading depression syndrome. Review of a particular type of head injury in 37 patients. Brain 100:287–298, 1977.

Olesen, J. The pathophysiology of migraine. In Clifford Rose F (ed), Handbook of Clinical Neurology, Vol. 48: Headache. Amsterdam: Elsevier Science, 1986, pp 59–83.

Olesen J. The ischemic hypotheses of migraine. Arch Neurol 44:321–322, 1987.

Olesen J, Lauritzen M, Tfelt-Hansen P, Henriksen L, Larsen B. Spreading cerebral oligemia in classical- and normal cerebral blood flow in common migraine. Headache 22:242–248, 1982.

Ommaya K. Indices of neural trauma: an overview of the present status. In Popp AJ, Bourke RS, Nelson LR, Kimelberg HK (eds), Neural Trauma. New York: Raven Press, 1979, pp 205–216.

Pearce JMS. Is migraine explained by Leão's spreading depression? Lancet 2:763–766, 1985.

Pickles W. Acute focal edema of the brain in children with head injuries. N Engl J Med 240:92–95, 1949.

Plum F, Posner JB. Supratentorial lesions causing coma. In The Diagnosis of Stupor and Coma, 3rd ed. Philadelphia: FA Davis, 1980, pp 87–151.

Prick JJ. Ervaringen over trauma cerebri bij kinderen. Mndschr Kindergen 5:324–334, 1936.

Raichle ME, Grubb RL Jr, Phelps ME, Gado MH, Caronna JJ. Cerebral hemodynamics and metabolism in pseudotumor cerebri. Ann Neurol 4:104–111, 1978.

Reilly PL, Graham DI, Adams JH, Jennett, B. Patients with head injury who talk and die. Lancet 2:375–377, 1975.

Rekate HL. Subdural hematomas in infants [Letter]. J Neurosurg 62:316, 1985.

Rose J, Valtonen S, Jennett B. Avoidable factors contributing to death after head injury. Br Med J 2:615–618, 1977.

Sacher P, Klöti J. Die transitorische posttraumatische zerebrale Blindheit. Schweiz Med Wochenschr 117:656–659, 1987.

Sakai F, Meyer JS. Abnormal cerebrovascular reactivity in patients with migraine and cluster headache. Headache 19:257–266, 1979.

Schnitker MT. A syndrome of cerebral concussion in children. J Pediatr 35:557–560, 1949.

Shapiro K. Special considerations for the pediatric age group. In Cooper PR (ed), Head Injury, 2nd ed. Baltimore: William & Wilkins, 1987, pp 367–389.

Shinohara M, Dollinger B, Brown G, Rapoport S, Sokoloff L. Cerebral glucose utilization: local changes during and after recovery from spreading cortical depression. Science 203:188–190, 1979.

Skinhøj E. Hemodynamic studies within the brain during migraine. Arch Neurol 29:95–98, 1973.

Small JM, Woolf AL. Fatal damage to the brain by epileptic convulsions after a trivial injury to the head. J Neurol Neurosurg Psychiatry 20:293–301, 1957.

Snoek JW, Jennett B, Adams JH, Graham DI, Doyle D. Computerised tomography after recent severe head injury in patients without acute intracranial haematoma. J Neurol Neurosurg Psychiatry 42:215–225, 1979.

Snoek JW, Minderhoud JM, Wilmink JT. Delayed deterioration following mild head injury in children. Brain 107:15–36, 1984.

Teasdale G, Jennett B. Assessment of coma and impaired consciousness. A practical scale. Lancet 2:81–84, 1974.

Teasdale E, Cardoso E, Galbraith S, Teasdale G. CT scan in severe diffuse head injury: physiological and clinical correlations. J Neurol Neurosurg Psychiatry 47:600–603, 1984.

Todorow S, Feller A-M. Benign secondary disturbance of consciousness (posttraumatic stupor) in children after cerebral trauma. Z Kinderchir 36:83–87, 1982.

Toutant SM, Klauber MR, Marshall LF, Toole BM, et al. Absent or compressed basal cisterns on first CT scan: ominous predictors of outcome in severe head injury. J Neurosurg 61:691–694, 1984.

Venable HP, Wilson S, Allan WC, Prensky AL. Total blindness after trivial frontal head trauma: bilateral indirect optic nerve injury. Neurology (Minn) 28:1066–1068, 1978.

Vitzthum H-E, Willenberg E, Lampe J, Minda R. Delayed encephalopathy. Zentralbl Neurochir 47:131–133, 1986.

Waga S, Tochio H, Sakakura M. Traumatic cerebral swelling developing within 30 minutes after injury. Surg Neurol 11:191–193, 1979.

Walton GL. Subarachnoid serous exudation productive of pressure symptoms after head injuries. Am J Med Sci 116:267–275, 1898.

Walton GL, Brooks JR. Observations on brain surgery suggested by a case of multiple cerebral hemorrhage. Boston Med Surg J 136:301–305, 1897.

Welch KMA. Migraine: a biobehavioral disorder. Arch Neurol 44:323–327, 1987.

Whitty CWM. Familial hemiplegic migraine. In Clifford Rose F (ed), Handbook of Clinical Neurology, Vol. 48: Headache. Amsterdam: Elsevier Science, 1986, pp 141–153.

Wilkinson M. Clinical features of migraine. In Clifford Rose F (ed), Handbook of Clinical Neurology, Vol. 48: Headache. Amsterdam: Elsevier Science, 1986, pp 117–133.

Wolff, HG. Headache and Other Head Pain, 2nd ed. New York: Oxford University Press, 1963.

Zimmerman RA, Bilaniuk LT. Computed tomographic staging of traumatic epidural bleeding. Radiology 114:809–812, 1982.

Zimmerman RA, Bilaniuk LT, Bruce DA, Dolinskas C, et al. Computed tomography of pediatric head trauma: acute general cerebral swelling. Radiology 126:403–408, 1978.

# 8

# Computed Tomography and Magnetic Resonance Imaging in Mild to Moderate Head Injury

HOWARD M. EISENBERG
AND HARVEY S. LEVIN

In this chapter we discuss two methods of defining brain pathology in patients with mild to moderate head injuries: computed tomography (CT) and magnetic resonance imaging (MRI). It is clear that in mild/moderate injuries, abnormalities are much more frequently found by MRI than by CT. Two important questions, then, are what is the significance of these MRI abnormalities, and what do they suggest with regard to our concepts of the pathology of these kinds of injuries?

Mild injuries are only rarely associated with abnormal CT scans, whereas, according to Rimel and co-workers (1982), about one-fourth of patients admitted for moderate injuries have a positive CT scan. This lack of demonstrable pathology, in dramatic contrast to the situation in more severe head injuries, has supported the belief that in most cases of mild/moderate injury, gross focal lesions are uncommon. For example, in an ongoing study, the National Institutes of Health Traumatic Coma Data Bank, which by the spring of 1987 had accumulated data on approximately 600 patients with severe closed injury, only 5% of cases had scans that were considered normal in all respects. Signs of mass effect (shift of midline structures or compressed midbrain cerebrospinal fluid cisterns) were common in these patients and, more important to this discussion, nearly one-third of these patients had focal lesions greater than 15 cc in volume and approximately 50% had smaller lesions (Eisenberg et al., 1988).

The first MRI studies in patients with head trauma included patients with mild/moderate injuries (Gandy et al., 1984; Han et al., 1984; Snow et al., 1986). These studies were descriptive and left open the possibility that the few MRI abnormalities found in the less severely injured patients could be inci-

**Table 8-1**  Neurobehavioral Procedures Used in the MRI Study of Mild/Moderate Head Injury

---

*Executive functions (frontal lobes)*
Oral Word Association—Verbal Fluency (Benton and Hamsher, 1978)
Figural Fluency (Jones-Gotman and Milner, 1977)
Modified Card Sorting (Nelson, 1976)

*Memory (temporal lobes)*
Verbal Selective Reminding (Buschke and Fuld, 1974)
Visuospatial Selective Reminding (Levin and Larrabee, 1983)

---

dental lesions. At that stage in our understanding of MRI, unexpected findings were often attributed to the coincidence of other conditions, particularly subclinical multiple sclerosis or other unknown, possible technical factors producing "artifacts." The 1986 paper by Jenkins and his co-workers, presented at the Institute for Neurologic Sciences in Glasgow, was the first published report that used a more rigorous approach to examine MRI scans of head-injured patients. They related the severity of impact, as indexed by the degree of altered consciousness, to the number and location of MRI abnormalities. Particularly interesting was their finding that the depth (i.e., distance from the inner table of the skull) of an abnormality was associated with the degree of altered consciousness. In addition, Jenkins et al. found that patients with deep lesions generally had more superficial lesions as well. This distribution of lesions and its correlation with behavior is consistent with the widely accepted concept of traumatic brain injury; that is, the brain is injured concentrically from superficial to deep, the depth being dependent on the severity of impact (Ommaya and Gennarelli, 1974). The distribution of MRI abnormalities found by Jenkins et al. then indicated that these abnormalities are actually related to the injury. Our group has replicated the findings obtained in Glasgow and has extended the previous work by showing that the depth of parenchymal lesion visualized by MRI is related also to the duration of impaired consciousness and quality of outcome (Levin et al., 1988).

We were also interested in the distribution of MRI abnormalities in our patients with mild/moderate injuries whom we imaged in a prospective study comparing CT and MRI findings (Levin et al., 1987). Most importantly, we sought to correlate MRI findings with neuropsychological function both in the acute period and during recovery. When we were designing this study, we noticed that the distribution of MRI abnormalities in mild to moderate patients was similar to the distribution of CT focal lesions in severely injured patients; that is, frontal and temporal locations predominated. It was clear, then, that the classic neurological examination would not be sufficient for determination of behavioral correlates of injury in these sites. One of the first steps then was to develop a neurobehavioral battery that would be efficient for identifying the functional correlates of these injuries and, to the extent possible, for discriminating frontal and temporal impairments separately. The battery we chose then emphasized executive functions and memory tests, as outlined in Table 8–1.

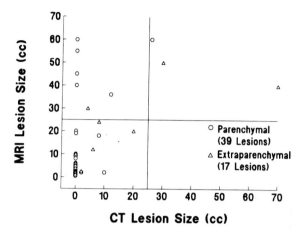

**Figure 8–1** Size of intracranial lesion visualized by computerized tomography (CT) as compared with magnetic resonance imaging (MRI). Vertical and horizontal lines demarcate potentially surgical lesions that were at least 25 cc in volume. The findings were obtained in the total series of 20 patients with minor or moderate head injury. (Reproduced from Levin et al., 1987, by permission)

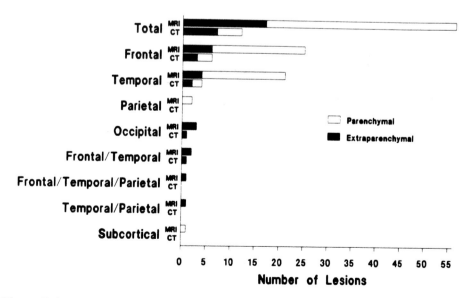

**Figure 8–2** Intrahemispheric locus of lesion revealed by computerized tomography (CT) versus magnetic resonance imaging (MRI) in 20 patients with minor or moderate head injury. (Reproduced from Levin et al., 1987, by permission)

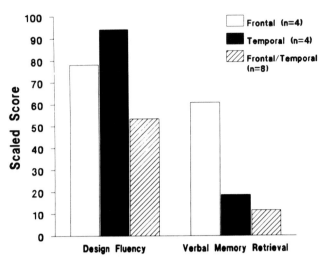

**Figure 8–3**  Neuropsychological test performance in head-injured patients with focal lesions visualized by MRI in the frontal and/or temporal regions. To permit direct comparison of design fluency (a measure of frontal lobe functioning) with verbal memory retrieval (a measure primarily of temporal lobe functioning), the performance of the subgroups of patients is plotted as a scaled score in which the mean and standard deviation of the control group are equivalent to 100 and 10, respectively. Accordingly, a scaled score of 100 is equivalent to the mean of the control group, whereas a scaled score of 80 signifies a level of performance that falls 2 standard deviations below the control group mean. Reproduced from Levin et al., 1987, by permission)

Twenty consecutively admitted patients with mild/moderate injuries (Glasgow Coma Scale [GCS] score - 9–15) and meeting the other entry criteria of the study were investigated (Levin et al., 1987). To compare the size of focal abnormalities on CT or MRI, we measured the area of each lesion and, using slice thickness, determined lesion volume by summing the area × slice thickness for all consecutive scan slices showing the lesion. Because we did not use smoothing formulas (i.e., mathematical manipulations that smooth out the boundaries of a lesion), the calculated volumes may be slightly overestimated.

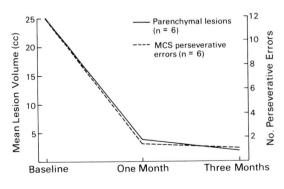

**Figure 8–4**  Mean volume of all lesions present on MRI and mean number of perseverative errors on the Modified Card Sorting (MCS) Test for six patients studied at baseline, one month, and three months.

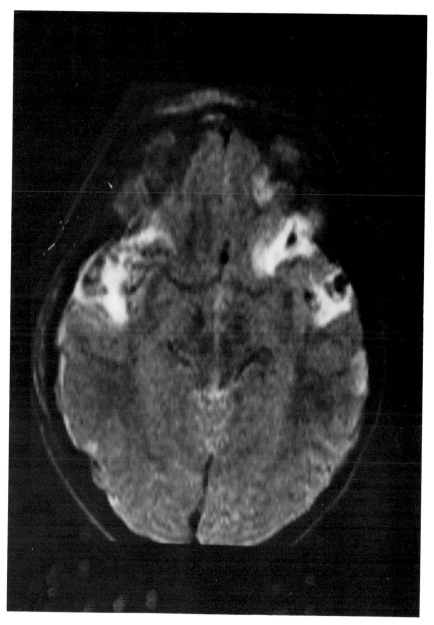

**Figure 8–5** MRI scan of a 16-year-old student (patient N.B.) who sustained a mild head injury (GCS score = 14) four days earlier. In contrast to normal CT findings, MRI revealed bitemporal and left frontal areas of high intensity which were interpreted as multiple small contusions accompanied by some degree of subarachnoid hemorrhage.

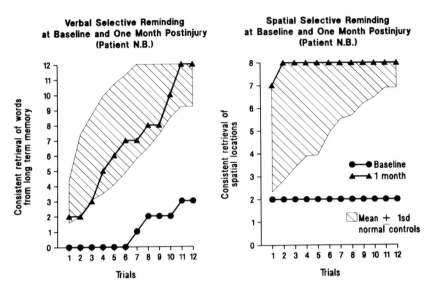

**Figure 8–6** Verbal and visuospatial memory scores of patient N.B., plotted against trials at four days (baseline) and one month after she sustained a mild head injury. Note the initial impairment on both verbal and visuospatial memory, which improved to within the range of normal controls (hatched region).

However, the same methods were used for determining volumes from both CT and MRI scans.

Figure 8–1 compares CT and MRI lesions by volume for the 20 patients. As shown, several patients had focal abnormalities, some greater than 25 cc, detected by MRI but not by CT. Further, in virtually every case where MRI and CT showed an abnormality in the same location, the volume of the MRI abnormality was larger than that shown by CT. Figure 8–2 shows the distribution of MRI and CT abnormalities by anatomical location. As we had expected, there was a predominance of frontal and temporal lobe sites. The most important finding of this study was that neurobehavioral impairments could be related to the size and location of MRI abnormalities and that the resolution of these MRI abnormalities was paralleled by improvement in function.

Figure 8–3 shows the relationship between neurobehavioral test scores and location of lesions for tests of design fluency (frontal lobe test) and verbal memory (temporal lobe test). The group of patients with both frontal and temporal lobe lesions combined had the lowest scores, but patients with lesions confined to the frontal lobe(s) performed most poorly on design fluency (i.e., frequent perseverative errors) and those with focal temporal lobe abnormalities had more difficulty on memory (i.e., temporal lobe) tests. Further, when patients were tested again at one month and three months post injury, their test scores improved at least to the normal range. This improvement in test scores coincided with the resolution of MRI abnormalities (Figure 8–4).

Although the results of the study have been published (Levin et al., 1987), the relatively few patients in each group (i.e., frontal or temporal lobe injury alone) makes some of our conclusions preliminary, and at this point we feel that information from individual patients is interesting. For example, in one case (patient N.B.) with only temporal MRI findings (Figure 8-5) and no CT abnormalities, impairment was present initially on tests of memory (verbal and visuospatial Selective Reminding) (Figure 8-6). Improvement in N.B.'s memory over three months paralleled resolution of her MRI abnormalities. In contrast, N.B.'s tests of frontal lobe function were normal both at baseline and at follow-up.

In contrast to patient N.B., a second case (patient T.C.) with an MRI

**Figure 8-7** MRI scan of patient T.C. four days after she sustained a mild head injury (GCS score = 15, on admission) when she struck her head on a diving board. In comparison with CT which revealed a questionable lesion in the left frontal region, MRI showed a large left frontal lesion with heterogeneous signal intensity. This parenchymal lesion resolved over one month and was paralleled by improvement in her verbal fluency. In contrast to patient N.B., neurobehavioral findings revealed no evidence of a memory disturbance in T.C.

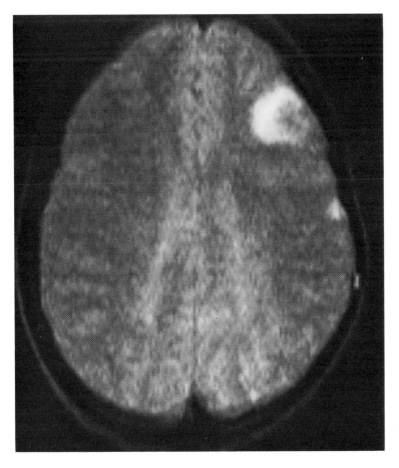

abnormality confined to the left frontal lobe (Figure 8–7) had consistently normal memory test scores. However, this patient had reduced verbal fluency (primarily a frontal lobe function) at baseline. The patient's verbal output increased to the normal range and the MRI abnormality resolved during the three months of study.

On the basis of these data from the 20 patients, we suggest that the location of MRI abnormalities is related to specific neurological dysfunction and that these abnormalities then indicate the site of focal pathology. We believe that these MRI abnormalities represent secondary injuries—possibly increased tissue water—although acknowledging that the primary pathology in these cases is unknown. However, if our assumptions are correct, the pathology of mild to moderate injury involves not only diffuse insult but also multifocal lesions located predominantly in frontal and temporal lobes.

### ACKNOWLEDGMENTS

Research summarized in this chapter was supported by NIH grant NS 21889 and Moody Foundation Grant 84-152. The authors are indebted to Eugenio G. Amparo, M.D., Faustino C. Guinto, Jr., Ph.D., Walter M. High, Jr., Ph.D., and David H. Williams for their contributions to the studies summarized herein, and to Liz Zindler for manuscript preparation.

### REFERENCES

Benton AL, Hamsher K. Manual for the Multilingual Aphasia Examination. Iowa City, IA: University of Iowa, 1978.

Buschke H, Fuld PA. Evaluating storage, retention, and retrieval in disordered memory and learning. Neurology (Minn) 24:1019–1025, 1974.

Eisenberg HM, Gary HE Jr, Jane JA, Marmarou A, Marshall LF, Young H. CT scan findings in a series of 595 patients with severe closed head injury: a report from the NIH Traumatic Coma Data Bank. Paper presented at the American Association of Neurologic Surgeons Meeting, April, 1988, Canada.

Gandy SE, Snow RB, Zimmerman RD, Deck MDF. Cranial nuclear magnetic resonance imaging in head trauma. Ann Neurol 16:251–257, 1984.

Han JS, Kaufman B, Alfidi RJ, et al. Head trauma evaluated by magnetic resonance and computed tomography: a comparison. Radiology 150:71–77, 1984.

Jenkins A, Teasdale G, Hadley MDM, MacPherson P, Rowan JO. Brain lesions detected by magnetic resonance imaging in mild and severe head injuries. Lancet 2:445–446, 1986.

Jones-Gotman M, Milner B. Design fluency: the invention of nonsense drawings after focal cortical lesions. Neuropsychologia 15:653–674, 1977.

Levin HS, Larrabee GJ. Disproportionate decline in visuospatial memory in human aging. Soc Neurosci Abstr 9:918, 1983.

Levin HS, Amparo EG, Eisenberg HM, Williams DH, High WM Jr, McArdle CB, Weiner RL. Magnetic resonance imaging and computerized tomography in relation to the neurobehavioral sequelae of mild and moderate head injuries. J Neurosurg 66:706–713, 1987.

Levin HS, Eisenberg HM, Amparo EG, Williams DH, High WM Jr, Crofford MJ. Depth of parenchymal lesions visualized by magnetic resonance imaging in relation to level of consciousness after closed head injury. Paper presented at the American Association of Neurological Surgeons Meeting, April, 1988, Canada.

Nelson HE. A modified card sorting test sensitive to frontal lobe defects. Cortex 12:313–324, 1976.

Ommaya AK, Gennarelli TA. Cerebral concussion and traumatic unconsciousness: correlation of experimental and clinical observations on blunt head injuries. Brain 97:633–654, 1974.

Rimel RW, Giordani B, Barth JT, et al. Moderate head injury: completing the clinical spectrum of brain trauma. Neurosurgery 11:344–351, 1982.

Snow RB, Zimmerman RD, Gandy SE, et al. Comparison of magnetic resonance imaging and computed tomography in the evaluation of head injury. Neurosurgery 18:45–52, 1986.

# 9

# Neurophysiological Assessment of Mild Head Injury

RUDOLF SCHOENHUBER
AND MASSIMO GENTILINI

Head injury embraces all degrees of severity, from an apparently symptomless blow on the head to irreversible traumatic brain damage. Clinical methods are used to measure the severity of trauma. The best known of them, the Glasgow Coma Scale (GCS, Teasdale and Jennett, 1974), enables us to differentiate severe, moderate, and mild head injury according to eye opening, and verbal and motor responses. In patients with severe or moderate head injuries, the GCS is sensitive and has a high prognostic value for the final outcome. The newer neuroimaging techniques such as computed tomography (CT) and magnetic resonance imaging (MRI) are also useful for detecting structural brain lesions, which are found almost exclusively in severe or moderate head injuries.

Fortunately, the great majority of head-injured patients suffer from mild head injuries. They usually are slightly drowsy at hospital admission, but no focal abnormalities can be detected at clinical examination. Most patients recover rapidly and soon return to work. However, many of them complain for months or even years of symptoms such as headache, dizziness, loss of memory and concentration, causing them social and economic distress.

In these patients suffering from mild head injury, an exact quantification of impairment would be particularly important, also in view of medicolegal problems. Clinical methods are not sensitive enough. As an alternative, neuropsychological methods have been proposed. Although sensitive, they are not routinely used in the clinical setting. Of the neuroimaging techniques, only MRI has shown some usefulness; however, its cost-efficiency still has to be proven.

## EEG IN MILD HEAD INJURY

The value of electroencephalography (EEG) for monitoring severe head injuries has already been established. Its sensitivity for hemispheric lesions and its capacity to reflect immediately (on line) the functional modifications of brain activity as they occur, makes EEG a valuable complement to clinical and neuroimaging methods in severe or moderate head injuries. These advantages and the widespread availability of EEG at relatively low cost suggested since its earliest use that EEG could be applied in mild head injuries (MHI) as well, in both experimental and clinical settings (Dow et al., 1944; Walker et al., 1944).

In mild head injury, only subtle EEG alterations can be expected, and their detection is limited by the large intersubject variability of normal EEG and the relatively imprecise nature of conventional visual analysis. In most patients, the EEG recorded hours or days after a mild head injury is normal. In some patients, however, slight diffuse abnormalities such as unstable background activity and increased low-frequency activity are recorded. Focal abnormalities are typically not present after cerebral concussion. These minor abnormalities usually decrease after several days and disappear within two weeks.

In about 10% of patients examined more than three months after cerebral concussion, however, slight diffuse abnormalities persist. Two EEG patterns—low-voltage EEG and posterior theta rhythm—were formerly considered to be posttraumatic sequelae (Courjon, 1972). However, low-voltage EEG has the same incidence in patients examined after cerebral concussion as in the normal population, as already shown in 1953 by Jung and Meyer-Mickeleit, working independently. Low-voltage activity—often associated with fast-frequency components—is considered a psychophysiological correlate of anxiety and has been named "psychogenic alpha suppression" by Scherzer (1966). Low-voltage EEG is also a normal inherited variant of normal electrical activity (Vogel, 1963; Vogel et al., 1961).

Posterior theta rhythm or 4-Hz rhythm, the second EEG pattern considered typical for the chronic posttraumatic stage, is also considered a normal inherited EEG variant, and has the same incidence as in the normal population (Vogel, 1963).

The main goal for the extensive use—or better, abuse—of EEG in MHI has always been to relate even the most aspecific EEG changes to subjective posttraumatic symptoms reported at a later time after a slight head or neck trauma. Most EEGs that are recorded in our outpatient laboratory are requested to evaluate patients suffering from headache and dizziness, usually of posttraumatic origin. As we would expect, almost all tracings are normal EEG variants.

Even in patients recovering from moderate or severe head injuries, there is no correlation between persistent EEG abnormalities and subjective complaints. These results were reported by Duensing as early as 1948. In 1962, Courjon stressed the lack of specific EEG changes in this subjective syndrome and the great number of normal tracings found in these patients. Radermecker (1961) warned explicitly against any attempt to objectify postconcussional syndrome (PCS) by means of EEG. Even pronounced EEG abnormalities do not necessarily prove the existence of an organic basis for a patient's complaints, nor do normal tracings allow the conclusion that trauma-induced symptoms must be absent (Ladurner and Lorenzoni, 1970; Lorenzoni, 1963).

If, as usual, EEG recordings are available only from the late posttraumatic stage, it is difficult to determine whether or not a given EEG abnormality is the sequela of cerebral trauma. In the only study on patients who for neurological or psychiatric problems had had an EEG before a head injury, Lorenzoni (1970) discovered that of 72 patients 37 (51%) had abnormal EEG even *before* injury!

This is not to deny the value of EEG in dealing with MHI patients. A first EEG recorded after a mild head injury can be useful in at least three possible situations (Goetze and Wolter, 1957):

1. It can disclose a focus due to cerebral contusion, even in an apparently concussive trauma.
2. It can locate a nontraumatic brain lesion such as a tumor.
3. It can predict the possibility of late posttraumatic complications such as epilepsy, abscess, or hematoma.

It is therefore not surprising that the report of auditory brainstem responses (ABRs) abnormalities in postconcussion dizziness seemed promising for those interested in objective assessment of MHI.

## AUDITORY BRAINSTEM RESPONSES IN MILD HEAD INJURY

ABRs are a quantitative technique, developed in 1967 by Sohmer and Feinmesser, the clinical relevance of which became clear in the late 1970s. At the same time, cost-efficient equipment became available. The technique basically involves recording "far field potentials" obtained by averaging 2,000 or more responses to clicks of 100-$\mu$sec duration delivered to one ear through an earphone. The response (ABR) is easily recorded and consists of a sequence of seven vertex-positive peaks, of which peaks I, III, and V are the most stable and easily recognized. In stable, normal subjects, ABRs are stable over time, and interindividual differences are relatively small (Stockard et al., 1977).

The neural generators of these peaks are still under discussion, but studies on abnormal ABR recordings, when correlated with CT scans or with postmortem studies, are consistent with a peripheral, cochlear origin of peak I, pontine origin of peak III, and mesencephalic origin of peak V. The absolute latency depends on stimulation intensity; therefore, in the neurological setting, interpeak latencies are preferred to absolute peak values. Thus an increased interpeak latency I–III reflects a more peripheral (i.e., VIII nerve or lower pons) involvement, whereas an increased III–V latency reflects a higher pons or mesencephalic involvement (Starr, 1985, 1987).

The main advantage of ABR in comparison to EEG is that it is a quantitative method with clear criteria of abnormality.

In the past few years, there have been at least four papers published on the usefulness of ABR in patients suffering from PCS (Table 9-1). The prevalence

**Table 9–1** Published Data on ABR Abnormalities in Postconcussion Syndrome

| Reference | No. of patients | Days from trauma | Pathological ABR (%) |
|-----------|-----------------|------------------|----------------------|
| Rowe and Carlsson, 1980 | 27 | 1–240 | 9% |
| Noseworthy et al., 1981 | 11 | 35–1825 | 0% |
| Benna et al., 1982 | 55 | ≤90 | 27% |
| Rizzo et al., 1983 | 57 | 14–180 | 5% |

of ABR alterations reported in the literature ranges from zero to 27%, reflecting the scarce homogeneity of the relatively small groups thus far described. The duration of unconsciousness, as a measure of the severity of head injury, varies from zero to several hours. Moreover, in some patients ABR recordings were made months or even years after head injury, whereas in others they were recorded during the first few days.

The value of ABR in PCS has therefore been questioned (Jones, 1982; Shubert, 1982; Williams, 1982). The incidence of ABR abnormalities after head injury, their specificity and time course, their relation to other indices of trauma severity, and—most importantly—their prognostic value for late complications, including subjective complaints, are only some of the problems related to the use of ABR in mild head injuries.

In a prospective study dealing with the incidence of ABR abnormalities after mild head injury, we studied 165 patients referred to the University Hospital of Modena, from November 1982 to September 1983 (Schoenhuber et al., 1985). Criteria for admission to our study were:

1. Loss of consciousness for less than 20 minutes
2. An initial score on the Glasgow Coma Scale of 13–15
3. Hospitalization of less than four days
4. Negative neurological examination upon admission and discharge, and no medical complications

Patients younger than 12 or older than 75 years were excluded from the study.

For each patient, ABR was recorded within 48 hours after trauma. Rarefaction clicks of 0.1-msec duration were delivered monoaurally at 70 dB sound level (SL). The evoked responses were recorded with a bandpass of 3.2 to 3,200 Hz on a MEDELEC M6 system. Interpeak latencies I–III, III–V, and I–V were calculated and considered abnormal if they exceeded by 3 standard deviations the corresponding mean of 37 normal subjects with similar age distribution. Upper normal limits for interpeak I–III, III–V, and I–V were 2.56, 2.47, and 4.69 msec, respectively (Schoenhuber et al., 1985).

At least one prolonged interpeak latency (of six possible for every patient) was found in 16 of 165 patients (about 10%). In a similar study on head-injured patients, the same incidence was found in the subgroup of 100 MHI cases (Geets and Louette, 1983). No specific pattern of ABR abnormalities could be detected. Interpeak latency I–III was most often affected, however.

**Table 9–2**   Incidence of ABR Abnormalities Versus Other Indices of Severity (Skull Fracture and PTA Duration)

|  | Normal ABR | Abnormal ABR | Total | $\chi^2$ | $p$ |
|---|---|---|---|---|---|
| Skull fracture | 35 | 5 | 40 | .572 | ns[a] |
| No fracture | 114 | 11 | 125 |  |  |
| PTA | 112 | 10 | 122 | 2.841 | ns |
| No PTA | 39 | 4 | 43 |  |  |

[a]ns, not significant.

No relation was found between abnormal ABR and other data related to the severity of trauma, such as the presence of skull fracture, or the duration of posttraumatic amnesia in our series of 165 MHI patients (Table 9–2; see also Schoenhuber and Gentilini, 1986).

In 119 patients, it was possible to make two ABR recordings—the first within 48 hours from trauma and the second after one month—with the aim of studying the time course of ABR abnormalities after MHI. When the mean values of all 119 patients were compared, no significant differences for each interpeak latency could be found between the first and second recording (Table 9–3). When each patient was considered separately, the incidence of abnormal ABR was 10.9% in the first and 8.4% in the second recording. The difference was not significant ($\chi^2 = .4331648$; 1 $d.f.$)

Most MHI patients showed stable ABR recordings; that is, normal recordings remained normal ($n = 100$), and ABR alterations persisted for at least one month after injury ($n = 4$). There were exceptions, however: Of the 13 with initially pathological ABR, 9 improved and became normal; of the 106 with a normal first ABR, 6 showed pathological recordings at follow-up.

This increase of ABR latencies is indeed surprising. Interestingly, it is also reported in another published longitudinal ABR study, in which the conduction time I–V increased in 8 out of 26 patients between the first recording and at the control six weeks later (McClelland, 1985; Montgomery et al., 1984). A possible explanation might be a delayed response to nerve trauma, or to damage of the nerve vasculature resulting in delayed arterial spasm or arterial or

**Table 9–3**   Mean Values and Standard Deviations of Interpeak Latencies (Pooled for Both Sides of Stimulation) Found Within 48 Hours from Trauma and One Month Later

|  | First recording | Second recording | $t^a$ | $p$ |
|---|---|---|---|---|
| I–III | 2.14 ± 0.23 | 2.18 ± 0.25 | 1.74 | ns |
| III–V | 1.90 ± 0.27 | 1.85 ± 0.29 | 1.87 | ns |
| I–V | 4.04 ± 0.25 | 4.02 ± 0.31 | 0.70 | ns |

[a]t, Student's t-test

**Table 9-4** Incidence of Abnormal ABR in Patients Claiming at Least
One or at Least Two Posttraumatic Symptoms

| | No symptoms | One or more symptoms | Total |
|---|---|---|---|
| Normal ABR | 19 | 77 | 96 |
| Pathol. ABR | 1 | 6 | 7 |
| Total | 20 | 83 | 103 |

| | One or no symptoms | Two symptoms or More | Total |
|---|---|---|---|
| Normal ABR | 32 | 64 | 96 |
| Pathol. ABR | 1 | 6 | 7 |
| Total | 33 | 70 | 103 |

venous thrombosis. There may also be external compression by expanding hematoma fluid or by edema. In these cases, nervous fiber continuity may be intact, but compression for long periods may result in partial degeneration, leading to persistent ABR abnormalities.

In a subgroup of 30 patients, no relation could be found between altered ABR and the presence of neuropsychological impairment one month after trauma. On a battery of six tests evaluating intelligence, attention, and memory, no differences were obtained between the 6 patients with abnormal ABR and the other 24 with normal ABR (Schoenhuber and Gentilini, 1986).

The most relevant question, concerning the prognostic value of ABR for late subjective complaints, has been approached by sending the same initial 165 MHI patients a letter six months to one year after the trauma, in which they were asked whether they had suffered from headache, dizziness, depression, anxiety, subjective loss of memory and concentration, or irritability for at least six months after the trauma. Of 103 patients responding to the questionnaire, 7 initially had had pathological ABR recordings. Seventy-seven patients reported at least one long-lasting symptom, and 64 reported at least two. Irritability, subjective memory deficits, and depression were the most frequently claimed. The incidence of pathological ABRs in MHI patients claiming at least one or at least two symptoms was the same as in the remaining patients (respective $\chi^2$ values = 0.0194 and 0.3883, 1 $d.f.$, corrected according to Yates—see Table 9-4). No symptom seemed significantly associated with any of the reported symptoms (Figure 9-1).

Our data seem to lead to the same disappointing and frustrating conclusions as those referred to in relation to the use of EEG in MHI patients: These data show that even after mild head injury, slight impairment of cerebral function is detectable in a small proportion of patients; however, it is impossible to relate these minor abnormalities to neuropsychological dysfunction, or to subsequent social maladjustment or even to psychiatric symptoms.

Thus the optimistic initial reports on the usefulness of ABR in mild head

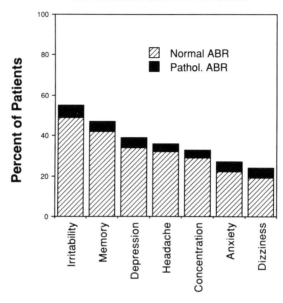

**Figure 9-1**   Late complaints in 103 mild head injury (MHI) patients in relation to ABR results.

injury have not been confirmed by our studies. Many factors may be considered as possible causes of this failure, for example:

1. There is no clear direct proof of brainstem dysfunction in cerebral concussion. The loss of consciousness and the posttraumatic amnesia are probably related to momentary dysfunction affecting the cerebral cortex more diffusely than the brainstem.
2. It should be noted that ABR reflects impulse transmission in a system of parallel channels within the brainstem. Slight dysfunctions may therefore be well compensated.
3. Even if there is slight brainstem dysfunction, it is very difficult to suggest a possible mechanism for PCS or altered higher nervous activity. Patients with abnormal ABR due to localized vascular, demyelinating, or tumoral lesions do not show the same symptoms as those with PCS or neuropsychological impairment.

## CONCLUSIONS

Even if both conventional EEG and ABR have given no acceptable results, there still is a necessity for neurophysiological methods in neurotraumatology. It should be noted that other current methods are equally insufficient. The

Glasgow Coma Scale (GCS) is not sensitive enough for scoring MHI patients and has no prognostic value for early or late complications. Likewise, skull fractures have no value. The significance of PTA is still unclear, and its quantification is also very difficult. Neuroimaging techniques are too expensive for routine use.

The application of clinical neurophysiology to MHI will, in the future, depend heavily on more precise knowledge of the pathophysiology. Experimental mild head injury and clinical assessment of acute CNS dysfunction may be approached with the same methods. Cortical impairment may well be documented by quantitative EEG, and possible changes in excitability may be studied with electrically evoked and recorded reflexes.

On the other hand, functions more relevant to patients' complaints may be measured with neurophysiological methods at a later stage after trauma. Quantitative EEG will probably renew the interest in EEG, since it is a valuable index for vigilance. Event-related responses and their topographical mapping may combine the yield of reaction-time studies with that of clinical neurophysiology, particularly in the field of attention. In a totally different approach, abnormalities of vegetative functions, which are often part of PCS, may be easily quantified through heart rate and blood pressor responses. Dizziness may also be assessed quantitatively be means of neuro-otological and posturographical recordings.

## REFERENCES

Benna P, Bergamasco B, Bianco C, Gilli M, Ferrero P, Pinessi L. Brainstem auditory evoked potentials in postconcussion syndrome. Ital J Neurol Sci 4:281–287, 1982.

Courjon J. La place de l'électroencéphalographie en traumatologie cranienne. Cah Méd Lyon 38:315–317, 1962.

Courjon J. Traumatic disorders. In Rémond A (ed) Handbk Electroencephalogr Clin Neurophysiol, Vol 14, Part 8. Amsterdam: Elsevier Scientific, 1972, pp 66–67.

Dow RS, Ulett G, Raak J. Electrencephalographic studies immediately following head injury. Am J Psychiatry 101:174–183, 1944.

Duensing F. Erfahrungen mit der Elektroenkephalographie bei Schaedelschussverletzungen. Dtsch Z Nervenheilk 159:514–536, 1948.

Geets W, Louette N. EEG et potentiels évoqués du tronc cerebral dans 125 commotions récentes. Rev Electroencephalogr Neurophysiol Clin 13:253–258, 1983.

Goetze W, Wolter M. Grenzen der Hirnstromuntersuchung bei der Begutachtung von Hirntraumafolgen. Med Sachverst 53:104–109, 1957.

Jones RK. Postconcussion syndrome. Arch Neurol 39:257, 1982.

Jung R. Neurophysiologische Untersuchungsmethoden. In von Bergmann G et al (eds), Handbuch der inneren Medizin, Berlin: Springer, 1953, pp 1206–1420.

Ladurner G, Lorenzoni E. Electroencephalographic findings in post-traumatic psychiatric syndrome. Electroencephalogr Clin Neurophysiol 28:326, 1970.

Lorenzoni E. Der Wert des EEG beim Schaedelhirntrauma. Wien Med Wochenschr 42/43:787–789, 1963.

Lorenzoni E. Electroencephalographic studies before and after head injuries. Electroencephalogr Clin Neurophysiol 28:216, 1970.

McClelland RJ. A neuropsychological investigation of minor head injury. *In* Papakostopulos D, Butler S (eds), Clinical and Experimental Neuropsychophysiology. London: Croon Helm, 1985, pp 615–634.

Meyer-Mickeleit RW. Das Elektroenzephalogramm nach gedeckten Kopfverletzungen. Dtsch Med Wochenschr 1:480–484, 1953.

Montgomery A, Fenton GW, McClelland RJ. Delayed brainstem conduction time in post-concussion syndrome. Lancet 1:1011, 1984.

Noseworthy JH, Miller J, Murray TJ, Regan D. Auditory brainstem responses in postconcussion syndrome. Arch Neurol 38:275–278, 1981.

Radermecker J. La valeur médico-légale de l'électroencéphalographie dans les séquelles subjectives des traumas cranio-cérébraux fermés: synthèse et conclusions. Acta Neurol Belg 61:468–476, 1961.

Rizzo PA, Pierelli F, Pozzessere G, Floris R, Morocutti C. Subjective posttraumatic syndrome. Neuropsychobiology 9:78–82, 1983.

Rowe MJ, Carlson C. Brainstem auditory evoked potentials and postconcussion dizziness. Arch Neurol 37:679–683, 1980.

Scherzer E. Das flache EEG als bioelektrischer Ausdruck der Erwartungsspannung (psychogene Alphareduktion). Psychiatr Neurol 152:207–212, 1966.

Schoenhuber R, Bortolotti P, Malavasi P, Di Donato G, Gentilini M, Nichelli P, Merli GA, Tonelli L. Brainstem acoustic evoked potentials in 165 patients examined within 48 hours of a minor head injury. *In* Morocutti C, Rizzo PA (eds), Evoked potentials: Neurophysiological and Clinical Aspects. Amsterdam: Elsevier Science, 1985, pp 237–241.

Schoenhuber R, Gentilini M. Auditory brain stem responses in the prognosis of late postconcussional symptoms and neuropsychological dysfunction after minor head injury. Neurosurgery 19:532–534, 1986.

Shubert DL. Postconcussion syndrome. Arch Neurol 39:257, 1982.

Sohmer H, Feinmesser M. Cochlear action potentials recorded from the external ear in man. Ann Otorhinolaryngol 76:427–438, 1967.

Starr A. Auditory pathway origins of scalp-derived auditory brainstem responses. *In* Morocutti C, Rizzo PA (eds), Evoked Potentials: Neurophysiological and Clinical Aspects. Amsterdam, Elsevier Science, 1985, pp 133–143.

Starr A. Auditory brainstem potentials: their theory and practice in evaluating neural function. *In* Halliday AM, Butler SR, Paul R (eds), *A Textbook of Clinical Neurophysiology.* New York: John Wiley, 1987, pp 383–414.

Stockard JE, Stockard JJ, Westmoreland BF, Kobayashi RM. Brainstem auditory evoked responses. Normal variation as a function of stimulus and subject characteristics. Arch Neurol 136:823–831, 1977.

Teasdale G, Jennet B. Assessment of coma and impairment of consciousness: a practical scale. Lancet 2:81–84, 1974.

Vogel F. Genetische Aspekte des Elektroenzephalogramms. Dtsch Med Wochenschr 88:1748–1759, 1963.

Vogel F, Goetze W, Kubicki S. Wert von Familienuntersuchungen für die Beurteilung des Niederspannungs-EEG nach geschlossenen Schaedelhirntraumen. Dtsch Z Nervenheilk 182:337–354, 1961.

Walker AE, Kollros JS, Case TJ. Physiological basis of concussion. J Neurosurg 1:103–116, 1944.

Williams JM. Postconcussion syndrome. Arch Neurol 39:257, 1982.

# IV
# Neuropsychological Sequelae

# 10

## Cumulative and Persisting Effects of Concussion on Attention and Cognition

DOROTHY GRONWALL

The model of concussion that prevailed until the end of the 1960s and beyond was that of a transitory alteration of consciousness which was completely reversible. Until the past decade or so, there was no evidence to contradict this view. Nor was there any evidence to contradict the view (e.g., Miller, 1961) that those who persisted in complaining of the symptoms that make up the "postconcussion syndrome" were other than neurotics and malingerers.

Until the development of magnetic resonance imaging (MRI), none of the available techniques for measuring CNS damage unequivocally showed that concussion had any effect on brain structures. It is now possible, however, to document the brain changes that accompany the behavioral changes after mild head injury (see Eisenberg and Levin, Chapter 8, this volume).

These behavioral changes are rarely apparent on standard neuropsychological test batteries, but these tests were developed to detect localized brain damage, whereas head injury produces a reduction in information processing capacity (Gronwall and Sampson, 1974; Gronwall and Wrightson, 1974; Van Zomeren, 1981). It produces diffuse damage which affects how much and how rapidly information can be processed, in contrast to the specific and isolated deficits that result from penetrating brain injury.

This reduction of information processing capacity has therefore been used as a yardstick to measure the effects of mild head injury (MHI). In the majority of young healthy adults, normal scores on these measures are typically recorded within four weeks of injury (Gronwall and Sampson, 1974; Gronwall and Wrightson, 1974). However, there is now evidence that impairment may persist well beyond this time, at least on some measures of reaction time and attention (see Gentilini et al., Chapter 11, this volume). There is also evidence that return of test scores to a normal level does not necessarily imply full recovery from the trauma.

This chapter documents this evidence. To provide some background for the reader, the following section briefly describes the ways in which reduced processing capacity affects cognitive function, and some of the measures that have been used to chart recovery. The relationship between processing capacity and symptoms of the postconcussion syndrome is also outlined. Subsequent sections examine the factors that affect recovery after MHI, and evidence that MHI produces persistent and irreversible changes in CNS function.

## EFFECT OF REDUCED PROCESSING CAPACITY ON FUNCTION AFTER MHI

*Information processing capacity* is a term borrowed from communications theory (Hick, 1952). It can be broadly described as the number of operations the brain can carry out at the same time. For example, the normal 3-year old child can unwrap a toffee and can walk, but cannot do both at the same time. In contrast, an adult can walk and hold a conversation while unwrapping the sweet. However, if the demands on the adult's processing space are increased further—for example, should a companion ask a rather complex question—he or she will need to switch processing space from the locomotion and the unwrapping to deal with that question. He or she literally will have to stop and think.

After MHI, patients have difficulty in all areas that require them to analyze more items of information than they can handle simultaneously. They present as slow because it takes longer for smaller than normal chunks of information to be processed. They present as distractible because they do not have the spare capacity to monitor irrelevant stimuli at the same time as they are attending to the relevant stimulus. They present as forgetful because while they are concentrating on point A, they do not have the processing space to think about point B simultaneously. They present as inattentive because when the amount of information that they are given exceeds their capacities, they cannot take it all in.

These are all aspects of attention, and the relation between attention deficits and reduced information processing capacity after head injury has been fully documented elsewhere (Levin et al., 1987). However, historically, the most widely reported effects of MHI have been the subjective symptoms that make up the postconsussion syndrome (PCS). A brief discussion of the relation between reduced information processing capacity and PCS follows the outline of the types of tasks that have been used to measure recovery of function in MHI patients.

### Paced Auditory Serial Addition Task (PASAT)

PASAT samples information processing capacity by forcing the subject to carry out a series of simple operations at increasingly fast speeds. He or she is played a series of single digits and instructed to add them in pairs, so that the first number is added to the second, the second to the third, and so on, and to give his or her answer aloud. Four trials of this task are given, with increasingly fast pacing at each trial. The first trial is recorded with a 2.4-second interval from one number to the next, and normal adults score about 75% correct at this rate. The normal mean for the fourth and fastest trial (1.2-second pacing) is only 40%. Instructions for administration, as well as normative data for this test, are described in detail elsewhere (Gronwall, 1977).

PASAT data have been collected from MHI patients over a 15-year period, leading to the development of stable and reproducible recovery curves (Gronwall, 1986). These curves allow analysis of the effect of various factors on recovery. However, PASAT is obviously not the only measure of reduced information processing rate after MHI. Other aspects of attention that are also affected can be measured.

### Vigilance and Reaction Time

Vigilance tasks demand the ability to attend to an uninteresting task for an extended period of time. McCarthy (1977) used an auditory vigilance test, in which the subjects had to detect the infrequent times when the interval between a string of numbers was longer than the rest. She tested a group of young (<30 years) males who had been treated in an accident or emergency department after MHI, but had not been admitted to hospital. In addition to a control group of young non-head-injured males, she also tested a group (age >80 years) from a home for the aged. At the first test, the old group and the young MHI group did not differ significantly on any measure, and both groups performed significantly worse on this task than the young control group. However, when they were all tested again, some four to six weeks later, the MHI group no longer differed from the young controls, and both young groups performed significantly better than the 80-year olds.

The only other vigilance study of head-injury patients is that by Brouwer and van Wolffelar (1985). Although only one of their eight subjects had not had either a "severe" or a "very severe" head injury, these authors' conclusion—that this vigilance impairment is probably due to slower mental processing—may also apply after MHI.

The amount of information that can be processed concurrently also affects reaction times, especially on a complex task. The effect of MHI on reaction times is discussed fully by Gentilini et al. (Chapter 11, this volume).

### Relation to Postconcussion Symptoms

Postconcussion symptoms are described in detail elsewhere in this volume (see especially Chapters 14–18). A close relation between reduced processing capacity and some of these symptoms might be expected, since both effects typically follow MHI. By definition, problems with concentration would be predicted. Thus it is not surprising that poor concentration is the most commonly reported of all postconcussion symptoms (Binder, 1986). However, deficits in concentration and attention are not the only effects of reduced processing capacity. For example, operating at maximum capacity induces fatigue, as we know when we compare how we feel after sitting a three-hour examination with sitting for three hours of idle chatting. After MHI, activities (such as talking with visitors, for example) that do not normally demand full capacity may now use up all available processing space.

Apart from anecdotal accounts, there is other evidence that incidence of symptoms is related to information processing capacity, as measured by PASAT. In one study (Gronwall, 1976a), MHI patients were asked to rate the severity of ten common symptoms on a 5-point scale. This rating, and PASAT, were repeated at weekly intervals. Symptom ratings correlated significantly with PASAT scores in the MHI group. As PASAT scores improved, the number and severity of PCS symptoms decreased.

## FACTORS AFFECTING RECOVERY AFTER MHI

As noted above, most young MHI patients record normal PASAT scores about a month after injury. However, there is some variation, which is dependent on the degree of initial impairment. PASAT recovery curves have been generated from a consecutive series of 237 cases between 14 and 40 years of age. None had sufficiently severe injuries to warrant more than overnight observation in hospital. They had no neurological abnormalities nor skull fracture, and had no previous history of head injury. All had periods of posttraumatic amnesia (PTA) of less than seven days.

In spite of the apparent homogeneity imposed by the selection criteria, there was a wide variation in PASAT scores within this group, suggesting some shortcomings in the standard methods of defining severity of head injury. By any criteria (Glasgow Coma Scale, duration of PTA, etc.), all patients would be classified as MHI, yet reduction in information processing ability, as measured by PASAT, varied from minimal to very severe. The majority of cases (53%) fell within the middle range, with mean time scores between 4 and 5.5 seconds, and took from four to six weeks for normal scores to be recorded. Some 25% did better than this, and scored at a normal rate two weeks after injury. The remainder (more than 20%) showed more severe impairment initially, and also this impairment persisted for a longer period (Gronwall, 1986).

Recovery curves from the minimally to the moderately affected subgroups can be taken as the normal course of uncomplicated recovery. The next section examines some of the factors that alter this pattern.

### Effect of Age

The vigilance study described above showed how, in the first week after the accident, MHI patients in their 20s behaved in the same way as patients in their 80s. In practice, it is difficult to measure the extent of the aging effect in MHI in older groups. There is ample evidence that information processing capacity declines with age (Welford, 1958), and therefore, the PASAT is not useful for measuring MHI in people in their 50s or older, as the normal aging process alone is sufficient to depress scores. However, we would expect that older people would be more affected by head injury than younger people

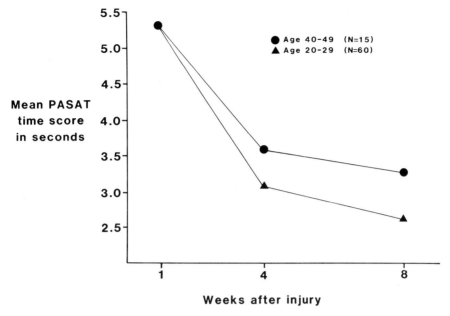

**Figure 10-1**  PASAT mean time scores from a young and an older group of MHI patients one, four, and eight weeks after injury.

because of the progressive loss of brain tissue with advancing age. When extra damage is suffered after MHI, the older person would be predicted to have less available reserves to cope with this insult.

Figure 10-1 compares PASAT recovery curves from MHI patients in their second and fourth decades 1, 4, and 8 weeks after injury. Sixty patients 20-29 years of age were compared with 15 patients 40-49 years of age. All met the criteria described at the beginning of this section, and all had first PASAT scores between 4.0 and 5.5 seconds. Because of this matching, there was no significant difference between the two groups at week 1 ($t = 0.5027$). By week 4, the younger group was performing more than half a second faster, on average, than the older (young: $M = 3.07$ seconds; old: $M = 3.595$ seconds). Eight weeks after injury, the group in their 40s were significantly slower than the group in their 20s ($t = 4.65$, $p < .001$).

### Effect of Previous Head Injury

When MHI is imposed on an older brain, the combined effect produces greater incapacity. The effect of repeated concussions is similar. Although full functional recovery is the norm, at least for young patients, CNS damage is not reversible. Thus when PASAT scores from patients who had no previous head injury are compared with those presenting after their second or third concussion, the latter are shown to be more severely affected, and to take longer to recover (Gronwall and Wrightson, 1975). The same effect, at the other end of the continuum, is the "punch-drunk" syndrome in boxers (Roberts, 1967).

Recently, there have been reports of cumulative MHI effects in amateur boxers, as well as in professionals (McLatchie et al., 1987).

## Extrainjury Factors

Although it is clear that older age and repeated head injury affect the time course of recovery, it is also clear that most MHI patients are young. Younger patients are more likely to present after a first injury. Therefore, extrainjury factors such as psychosocial and occupational status, which also affect recovery, are of obvious practical importance. A few examples will illustrate their importance.

### Patient and Family Expectations

How patients and their families cope with the effects of MHI plays a major role in how quickly these patients recover. If they are expected to carry on their normal activities while still functioning at a slower than normal rate, so that they are sleep-deprived as well as head-injured, then their PASAT scores will not improve at the expected rate. The problems relating to the management and rehabilitation of MHI patients, discussed more fully by Wrightson in Chapter 16, are perhaps one of the most common causes of plateaus in the recovery curves.

### High Achievers

Apparently faster than normal recovery is sometimes seen in patients who are highly motivated to show that they can do well. Such patients may achieve a normal PASAT score, but not in a normal manner. Normal subjects do not need two hours of sleep after the test session to recover from the effort, nor do they take two or three days to recover fully. Thus in the case of high achievers, the effect of the test, as well as the actual test results, needs to be taken into account.

### Intelligence Quotient (IQ)

The above-described "we try harder" effect is illustrated by the difference between PASAT recovery curves in high and low IQ groups. Although there is good evidence that, within the normal range, intelligence is not significantly correlated with PASAT performance (Gronwall and Sampson, 1974; Gronwall and Wrightson, 1974), it is one of the factors affecting the shape of PASAT recovery curves. A study comparing PASAT scores from a group of university students and a group of unskilled workers who had had similar head injuries, showed that although both groups performed at the same level at the first test, and both recovered to an identical level eventually, the recovery curves from the two groups differed in shape. Figure 10–2 shows this difference. Scores at the midpoint in the student group's curve were significantly higher than those of the unskilled workers (Gronwall, 1976b).

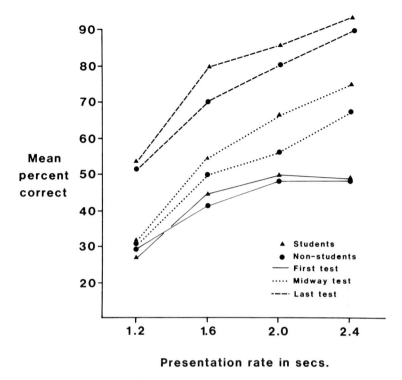

**Figure 10-2** PASAT scores from student and nonstudent groups after similar head injuries. (Reproduced from Gronwall, 1976b, by permission)

## EVIDENCE FOR PERSISTING EFFECTS OF MHI

Even where progress has been delayed or impeded, most young MHI patients appear to make a full functional recovery. Showing that these cognitive deficits may be temporary, however, does not mean that MHI is reversible. Indeed, for that to be the case would entail regeneration of CNS tissue. The cumulative effect of MHI, which has already been described, is evidence of a residual effect that is apparent in these cases only when the second head injury is imposed. There is other evidence of residual impairment, however: It is the persistent cognitive "fragility" to CNS stressors.

### Experimental Evidence

Ewing et al (1980) compared performance under mild hypoxia in a group of university students who had made a full "recovery" from MHI between one and three years before the study was done, with a matched group of control students who had never had a head injury. There was no group difference in PASAT scores, either at ground level or at a simulated altitude of 12,500 feet— a result that probably reflects the motivation factor already discussed. However, the MHI group was significantly poorer than controls on a memory and vigilance task performed where mildly hypoxic. Thus, although all the students who had had MHI more than a year before the study was carried out had returned to full-time university work, and were performing at the same level as before their accidents, the MHI had left a residual effect which impaired the ability to withstand another CNS stressor.

A similar effect may be responsible for the reports of reduced tolerance to alcohol shown by some MHI patients. However, an experiment documenting the effect of this stressor has yet to be done.

## Clinical Evidence

As clinicians working in a rehabilitation unit, we have learned that the fragility of MHI patients is not confined to CNS stressors such as hypoxia and alcohol. The following case history illustrates this.

*Case.* Mrs. B is a typical case. Her accident, which occurred in 1984, probably involved a multiple MHI: She was knocked unconscious when her car was hit by a truck reversing out of a driveway, and then there was another impact when the car was ricocheted into a brick wall on the other side of the street. She is a single parent in her 30s, with two young sons. Before the accident, she worked during school hours in a sole-charge office, where she was able to work at her own pace. She supplemented this income by working evenings in a bar.

Twelve months after the accident, she was coping reasonably well with the office job, although she could not return to her secondary employment because she still (i.e., three years postinjury) needs 10–12 hours of sleep. Until February of this year, we had not seen her since 1985. In September 1986, she changed jobs, and now works (the same hours) in a busy office that pays higher hourly rates. It is not sole charge. She now has to work under tight time constraints.

She had been coping well with a six-hour work day, but now she dreads anyone approaching her after lunch, by which time she, in her words, "can't even talk straight, let alone think straight." Headaches have returned, and the problem is compounded because she did not tell the firm about her accident when she applied for the job.

There are many Mrs. Bs. The factors that affect how quickly people recover from MHI also affect how well they do after they have "recovered." We are all vulnerable to stress and tension in our work and family lives, but MHI patients continue to have an extra vulnerability. There is no evidence to show that this vulnerability decreases over time since injury.

## PRACTICAL IMPLICATIONS

Ideally, all MHI patients should be screened, and also followed until they have recovered sufficiently to return to work. However, because of the numbers involved, such a program would be both expensive and impractical. We can, however, identify and provide assistance to those at risk for longer than normal periods of incapacity: (1) the older patient, (2) the patient who has a previous head injury, (3) the patient who is a high achiever or is in a demanding occupation, and (4) the patient who has family or social stressors. The importance of ensuring that support and counseling services are available for these groups is discussed fully by Wrightson (Chapter 16, this volume).

We also must make sure that all MHI patients are clearly informed about the importance of avoiding further injury. Caution is obviously most important in the early weeks after the accident because at this stage they are likely to be clumsy and uncoordinated, and have slowed reaction times. However, it is also important to let them know of the evidence that the effects of MHI can persist well beyond that time.

In summary, it has been shown that reduced information processing capacity is a reliable index of the effects of MHI on cognitive function, and that some of the clinical symptoms are related to this.

In most young adults, symptoms disappear, and information processing returns to a normal level in a matter of weeks, though the length of time before normal scores are recorded will depend on the measure that is used. Longer than normal recovery times have been shown to occur in two groups of patients: those who are older, and those who have had a second head injury. Before MHI, older people already have reduced information processing capacity, probably because of neuronal fallout. After injury, they recover more slowly, and sometimes incompletely. People who have a second head injury show a similar pattern, which may also be due to neuronal fallout.

Even those patients who appear to have made a full functional recovery, who record normal scores on all neuropsychological tests, and who have returned to their preinjury social and work life, may demonstrate persistent impairment when subjected to another stress. Experimentally such a stress may be metabolic (e.g., due to hypoxia) or cognitive (e.g., due to a second task's being added to the test). This persistent impairment is also demonstrated clinically, when situations of stress arise concerning work or family.

The conclusion is that MHI produces long-term damage, perhaps in the nature of neuronal fallout, which may not be apparent in normal circumstances, but which is evident when the system is stressed. These are the circumstances in which delayed or imperfect recovery from MHI can be expected.

## REFERENCES

Binder LM. Persisting symptoms after mild head injury: a review of the post-concussive syndrome. J Clin Exp Neuropsychol 8:323–346, 1986.

Brouwer WH, van Wolffelar PC. Sustained attention and sustained effort after closed head injury: detection and 0.10 Hz heart rate variability in a low event rate vigilance task. Cortex 21:111–119, 1985.

Ewing R, McCarthy D, Gronwall D, Wrightson P. Persisting effects of minor head injury observable during hypoxic stress. J. Clin Neuropsychol 2:147–155, 1980.

Gronwall D. Performance changes during recovery from closed head injury. Proc Aust Assoc Neurol 13:143–147, 1976a.

Gronwall D. Concussion: does intelligence help? NZ Psychologist 5:72–78, 1976b.

Gronwall D. Paced auditory serial addition task: a measure of recovery from concussion. Percept Mot Skills 44:367–373, 1977.

Gronwall D. Rehabilitation programs for patients with mild head injury: components, problems, and evaluation. J Head Trauma Rehab 1:53–62, 1986.

Gronwall D, Sampson H. The Psychological Effects of Concussion. Auckland: Oxford University Press, 1974.

Gronwall D, Wrightson P. Delayed recovery of intellectual function after minor head injury. Lancet 2:605–609, 1974.

Gronwall D, Wrightson P. Cumulative effects of concussion. Lancet 2:995–997, 1975.

Hick WE. On the rate of gain of information. QJ Exp Psychol 4:11–26, 1952.

Levin HS, Grafman J, Eisenberg HM (eds). Neurobehavioral Recovery from Head Injury. New York: Oxford University Press, 1987.

McCarthy D. Memory and Vigilance After Concussion. Unpublished MSc thesis, University of Auckland, 1977.

McLatchie G, Brooks N, Galbraith S, Hutchison JSF, Wilson L, Melville I, Teasdale E. Clinical neurological examination, neuropsychology, electroencephalography and computed tomographic head scanning in active amateur boxers. J Neurol Neurosurg Psychiatry 50:96–99, 1987.

Miller H. Accident neurosis. Br Med J 1:919–925, 1961.

Roberts AH. Brain Damage in Boxers. London: Pitman, 1967.

Van Zomeren AH. Reaction Time and Attention After Closed Head Injury. Lisse: Swets & Zeitlinger, 1981.

Welford AT. Aging and Human Skill. Oxford: Oxford University Press, 1958.

# 11

# Assessment of Attention in Mild Head Injury

MASSIMO GENTILINI,
PAOLO NICHELLI,
AND RUDOLF SCHOENHUBER

Impairment in attention has long been suggested as an explanation for the patterns of results from test batteries given to head-injured patients (Conkey, 1938; Ruesch, 1944). However, attention was rarely evaluated adequately, in part because of its virtual banishment from academic psychology by the dominant schools of Behaviorism and Gestalt psychology. With the development of modern cognitive psychology in the second half of this century, attention and its deficits have once again become a topic of empirical research.

Reference to the impairment of attention in head-injured patients is found even in the early literature. Meyer (1904) noted that some patients were "unable to concentrate their attention, even in occupations which serve for mere entertainment such as reading or playing cards . . . " During interviews, such patients are easily distracted and unusually tired when concentrating on a task. Some of them complain of difficulty in performing two tasks simultaneously. This finding supports the hypothesis that head-injured patients cannot divide their attention adequately.

This chapter focuses on attention deficits following head injury. We first present a general review of the literature concerning information processing in closed head injury and then discuss our studies, which are designed to evaluate the neuropsychological impairments that follow mild head injury—in particular, the problem of deficits in attention tasks.

## INFORMATION PROCESSING IN CLOSED HEAD INJURY: REVIEW OF THE LITERATURE

The reaction time (RT) technique in experimental psychology was first used by Obersteiner in 1874 to evaluate the mental capabilities of psychiatric patients. In 1922, two French studies reported prolonged RT in postencephalitic patients (see Blackburn and Benton, 1955). As early as 1938, Conkey noted that patients had difficulty in concentrating on tasks. Mental slowness was the outstanding feature of the head injury syndrome. RT therefore seemed an adequate method of investigation.

Ruesch (1944) was the first to use this technique with head-injured patients. He studied 25 patients with recent head injuries, 32 chronic patients suffering from prolonged posttraumatic syndromes, and 25 control subjects. Ruesch observed that both patient groups were slower than controls and concluded that visual RT could have a definite place in clinical evaluation. Unfortunately, his control group was significantly younger than the other patient groups; moreover, the severity of trauma and the interval between trauma and test were not specified.

Dencker and Lofving (1958) studied closed head injury with RT in 27 pairs of monozygotic twins. In each pair, one twin was afflicted and the other served as a control. Despite the rigorous methodological approach, test sessions were performed at an average interval of 10 years after trauma, by which time many of the mild injury cases had already recovered. These data illustrate both the recovery and relative mildness of the injuries. Both Norman and Svahn (1961) and Miller (1970) identified slowness in head-injured groups by using the technique of choice RT to a visual stimulus; however, significant differences were not revealed when simple RT was used. They concluded that head injury reduces decision-making and information-processing abilities. It is noteworthy, however, that these studies dealt with patients suffering from very severe cerebral concussion.

Klensch (1973) studied simple and choice RT in mildly injured patients. In simple RT sessions, subjects' responses to auditory and visual stimuli were tested, whereas in choice RT sessions, subjects were required to react solely to the combination of white light and a tone. There were no differences from controls in choice RT; only simple RT differentiated patients from controls. Gronwall and Sampson (1974) tested visual choice RT in 12 mildly concussed males having posttraumatic amnesia of less than one hour. The authors concluded that central processing time was significantly increased after trauma, a finding confirmed by Shiffrin and Schneider (1977).

Investigations of visual modality with the Stroop Color Test, the mirror-drawing task (Dencker and Lofving, 1958) and the card-sorting task with distracting stimuli (Miller and Cruzat, 1981), as well as auditory modality tests (Dencker and Lofving, 1958; Gronwall and Sampson, 1974), illustrate that speed of information processing is notably reduced in head-injured patients. Similar results were obtained by Gronwall and Sampson (1974) with the Paced Auditory Serial Addition Task (PASAT) for divided attention (Shiffrin and Schneider, 1977). This task involves dividing attention between stimuli, stored memory elements, mental transformations, and responding. They found that presentation had a significant influence on patients' performance and concluded that lower PASAT performance under time pressure is probably the result of slow execution of a qualitatively normal control strategy. Thomas (1981) did not find a deficit in PASAT performance with a slower presentation rate, a result which supports the importance of speed as a critical factor of information processing.

Van Zomeren and Deelman (1976) have studied speed of information processing in brain-injured patients with visual RT. In particular, they compared the sensitivity of different tasks, to determine whether simple or choice RT was most sensitive to brain damage. Comparison of simple visual RT with various types of choice RT revealed that both simple and four-choice RT can be used to differentiate head-injured patients. Their results agree with those of Norman and Svahn (1961), confirming the slowness of severe head injury patients in choice RT tasks. However, in their subgroup of mild head injury patients, they found a significant difference between patients and controls on the simple RT task only, as previously observed by Klensch (1973). The authors suggest that mildly injured patients might be slow in a basic stage of their information processing (e.g., delayed arousal or late response execution), and that the introduction of stages at higher cognitive levels, such as stimulus identification and response selection, may have similar effects as in normal subjects. In contrast, severely concussed patients could have a deficit especially at higher levels of information processing.

All these studies reveal that attention deficits following head injury are largely the result of a slowing down of information processing. Hence, the head-injured patient will experience more attention deficits than healthy subjects and will be confronted with his or her limited capabilities in situations demanding more global cognitive functions.

## ATTENTION DEFICITS FOLLOWING MILD HEAD INJURY: EXPERIMENT 1

The problem of evaluating neuropsychological functioning after mild head injury (MHI) is likely to be dependent on adequate selection not only of control subjects and statistical methods, but also of test procedures that tap those specific functional aspects more impaired after concussion. A general survey of neuropsychological abilities, as in test batteries aimed at examining different cognitive functions, may well be inefficient in isolating specific impairments.

In our first study (Gentilini et al., 1985), we evaluated neuropsychological deficits in a population of 50 patients whose head injuries were defined as mild according to precise criteria (i.e, loss of consciousness for less than 20 minutes, an initial score on the Glasgow Coma Scale of 13–15, hospitalization of less than three days, negative neurological examination upon admission and discharge, and no medical complications). MHI patient performances were compared to those of a control group closely matched for age, education level, and socioeconomic status (case–control approach). Patients younger than 13 or older than 75 years were excluded. Our neuropsychological battery consisted of six tests evaluating attention, memory, and intelligence. The patients were examined one month after the trauma.

## Testing Procedures

### Selective Attention Test
Each patient was presented with a matrix of 13 rows of 10 numbers (0–9). Patients were asked to mark each number indicated at the top of the matrix. The test was repeated three times. On the first matrix, there was a single-digit number; the second and third matrices had two and three single-digit numbers, respectively. Scores were calculated by the number of correct answers provided in the three matrices in a maximum time of 45 seconds per matrix.

### Digits Forward Test
The subject was asked to repeat progressively longer lists of digits. For each length, beginning with that of two numbers, two lists were administered; one point was given for the first list of each length correctly repeated, and an additional 0.5 point if the second list was also repeated correctly (De Renzi and Nichelli, 1975).

### Word Recognition Test
The subject was presented with 60 cards, each containing one word, which he or she read one at a time. There were 30 words with a high associative value and 30 with a low one. Immediately afterward, the same words were presented again one at a time in a random order, intermingled with an equal number of distractor items, and subjects were asked to say which words they had already seen (yes–no recognition procedure). Retention performance was measured by calculating the $d'$, an unbiased estimate of discriminability (Green and Swets, 1966), using the percentage of hits (correct "yes" responses) and false alarms (incorrect "yes" responses).

### Buschke's Test
This test is a verbal learning test on a list of 15 words, according to the technique of "selective reminding" proposed by Buschke (1973; Buschke and Fuld, 1974). The list was read at the speed of one word every two seconds, and the subject was asked for an initial partial recall. In each of the successive trials, the examiner repeated only those words not recalled from the previous trial. This procedure continued until the subject gave two consecutive recalls of the entire list or until a maximum of 10 trials was completed. For each subject, the learning curve, plotted as the number of words recalled on successive trials, was examined. These curves were found to be fitted by a linear regression of the type $y = a + bx$, where $y$ is the number of words correctly recalled, $x$ is the number of the trial, $b$ is the regression coefficient, and $a$ is the intercept on the ordinate at $x = 0$. This line being obtained, the theoretical number of trials required to recall the entire list ($N$) was calculated for each patient by the for-

mula $N = (15 - a)/b$. $N$ values constituted the score by which the performance of each single subject was evaluated.

### Working Memory Test
Four playing cards corresponding to the four suits (hearts, diamonds, clubs, and spades) were placed on a table. The subject was told to draw cards from the deck one by one as quickly as possible and to place them face up below the corresponding suit, while naming the number and suit of the card classified immediately before. The test was preceded by a warm-up trial with 10 cards. The number of cards correctly classified in one minute was scored.

### Raven Test
Raven Progressive Matrices (Raven, 1958) were used. The score was the number of correct answers within the time limit of 30 minutes.

### Results and Discussion

The multicovariance analysis performed on the standardized scores of the six neuropsychological tests by means of Hotelling's $t$-test was not significant ($F = 1.1809$; $d.f.$ 6/44, n.s.). Thus none of the multiple comparisons (Roy and Bose, 1953) proved to be significant. When the same comparisons were repeated by means of six univariate analyses, the performance of patients with MHI was found to be significantly lower than that of controls on the selective attention test ($F = 5.18$, $d.f.$ 1/49, $p < .05$). The study did not find a general neuropsychological impairment one month after MHI, but did provide some support for a specific attention deficit.

Van Zomeren and Deelman (1978) reported a follow-up study covering two years on a group of 57 young brain-injured males, divided into three subgroups according to the severity of injury. RT discriminated between subgroups, and a significant improvement during follow-up examination was shown. Choice RT discriminated severe from MHI patients better than simple RT and continued to do so throughout the entire follow-up period. Mac Flynn et al. (1984) examined 45 MHI patients on a four-choice RT test one day and six weeks after injury. In contrast to matched controls, the concussion cases displayed significantly poorer performance at both assessments. No differences, however, were detected between groups at six months. In contrast to these studies pointing to a specific and lasting attention deficit after MHI, McLean et al. (1983), using the Stroop Interference test, found that by one month after concussion, patients had recovered from deficits, even if they continued to report headaches, memory problems, and fatigue more than the controls, thus showing evidence of PCS.

### ATTENTION DEFICITS FOLLOWING MILD HEAD INJURY: EXPERIMENT 2

The contrasting results between the different studies may relate to the lack of a universally accepted definition of attention. We therefore devised a battery

**Table 11-1**  Means and Standard Deviations of
Demographic Features of the Experimental Groups

|          | Sex       | Age            | Education     |
|----------|-----------|----------------|---------------|
| Patients | 18 F, 30 M | 28.44 ± 14.08 | 9.00 ± 3.05  |
| Controls | 15 F, 33 M | 28.39 ± 13.95 | 9.10 ± 2.90  |

exploring different aspects of attention and administered it with the same methods described earlier in this chapter. Our aim was to determine whether MHI patients are specifically impaired at attention tasks and which tasks are more sensitive to damage. Forty-eight consecutive MHI cases, 15–65 years of age, were examined. All were right-handed, without left-handedness among relatives. The same inclusion criteria as in the previous experiment were followed. Patients on medications known to influence cerebral functions were excluded. Forty-eight right-handed subjects were chosen as controls (case-control approach). All patients were tested one month after the trauma; a subgroup of 28 subjects was retested with the same controls: 22 at three months, and 6 at five months after injury. Demographic features of the experimental groups are reported in Table 11–1.

The neuropsychological study consisted of three parts, each evaluating a different aspect of attention. Each patient was tested before his or her control subject was examined. Testing procedure and results are examined separately for each part of the study.

## Selective Attention

As in the previous experiment, each patient was presented with three matrices of 13 rows of 10 numbers. Patients were asked to mark as fast as possible the numbers corresponding to those indicated at the top of the matrices. All the subjects succeeded in completing the task in the given time (45 seconds per matrix); the precise execution time in seconds was therefore considered a further index of performance.

Table 11–2 shows scores and execution times by patients and controls tested one month after the trauma. Using a one-way analysis of variance (ANOVA) on the number of correct answers, there was no significant difference between the two groups tested one month after the trauma ($F = .64$, d.f. 1/47, n.s.). In contrast, execution time was significantly higher in MHI patients

**Table 11-2**  Means and Standard Deviations of Correct
Answers and of Execution Time at the Selective
Attention Test Obtained by Patients and Controls One
Month after MHI

|                      | Correct answers | Execution time |
|----------------------|-----------------|----------------|
| Patients ($N = 48$)  | 53.85 ± 4.82   | 81.88 ± 15.28 |
| Controls ($N = 48$)  | 53.19 ± 5.30   | 76.40 ± 13.03 |

**Table 11-3** Means and Standard Deviations of Execution Time at the Selective Attention Test Obtained by Patients and Controls Tested One and Three Months after Minor Head Injury

|  | One month | Three months |
| --- | --- | --- |
| Patients ($N = 22$) | 84.73 ± 16.50 | 81.55 ± 18.92 |
| Controls ($N = 22$) | 74.36 ± 12.37 | 72.82 ± 10.87 |

as compared with controls ($F = 3.64$, $d.f.$ 1/47, $p = .05$). The same was true also for 22 patients who were retested at three months post injury (Table 11-3):

At three months post injury, patients showed a significantly different speed of performance from controls ($F = 4.98$, $d.f.$ 1/42, $p = .029$). Interaction between experimental groups and repeated testing was not significant ($F = .307$, $d.f.$ 1/42, n.s.). In conclusion, as shown by Table 11-3, it seems that a significant impairment in selective attention is present as long as three months after a mild brain injury, but that the deficit is not manifested as an increased number of errors since a compensation for defective performance is found by slowing the execution of the task. We therefore suggest that execution time be used as an additional index of performance for selective attention tasks in MHI patients.

## Sustained and Divided Attention

### Sustained Attention
The ability to maintain sustained attention was evaluated by means of a simple RT task to stimuli appearing in the lateral visual fields. The subject sat with his/her head placed in a head-and-chin rest facing the screen of an Apple IIe personal computer located at a distance of 35 cm. The sequence of events started with the presentation of a fixation cross at the center of the screen. After a fixed interval of one second, an auditory warning signal lasting 25 msec preceded stimulus occurrence by a variable interval of 500-to 2500-msec. The stimulus was a bright square (0.5 × 0.5 degrees) presented for 100 msec at 10 degrees of eccentricity either to the left or the right of the central fixation point.

Each session consisted of two blocks of 25 test stimuli preceded by 10 practice trials. In the first block, subjects had to respond with the right hand to stimuli presented in the right visual field; in the second trial, left visual stimuli were responded to with the left hand. Half of the subjects began with the first block; half with the second. The subjects were instructed to fixate the central cross during the entire duration of each trial and to press a key with the right or left index finger as quickly as possible. The interstimulus interval between the end of each trial and the following was 500 msec. Eye movements were controlled by one of the examiners through a mirror attached to the PC monitor. In the rare cases when subjects shifted their gaze from central fixation, the trial was excluded and repeated at the end of the block. RT values greater than

**Sustained and Divided Att.**

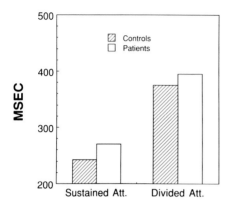

**Figure 11–1** RT of controls and patients on the Sustained and Divided Attention tests one month after the trauma.

1100 msec and shorter than 150 msec were eliminated and repeated at the end of the block.

### Divided Attention
The ability to divide attention between two concurrent tasks is a valid test procedure for deficits in control processing resources. Presentation of the stimulus and registration of RT were carried out as in the previous test, with the additional request to count backwards by 2s from 100 to 0 at a regular rate. When zero was reached before the end of the block, the subject started again from 100. Responses emitted during pauses in the subtracting task were eliminated and repeated at the end of the block.

Figure 11–1 shows RT of controls and patients on the Sustained and Divided Attention tests one month after the trauma. The median values of correct RT at Sustained and Divided Attention tests were taken into accont for statistical analysis of patients and controls' performances. An ANOVA on cor-

**Sustained and Divided Att.**

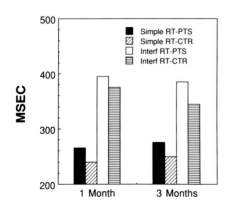

**Figure 11–2** RT of the limited sample retested after three months.

rect RT was performed. Visual field was included as a possible source of variability, but this was never the case.

Statistical analysis on the entire sample of patients tested one month after the trauma showed that, independently of the task (Sustained or Divided Attention), patients' responses were significantly slower than controls' ($F$ = 4.0, $d.f.$ 1/94, $p$ = .045). The analysis of data showed also that the concomitant task of counting backward by 2s, although very simple, was successful in interfering with the performance, since RTs on the Divided Attention paradigm were significantly slower than those recorded on the Sustained Attention Test ($F$ = 511.95, $d.f.$ 1/94, $p$ < .001). MHI patients and controls were equally impaired at Sustained and Divided Attention tests, as is shown by the lack of interaction between task and experimental group ($F$ = .21, $d.f.$ 1/94, n.s.). Patients tested one month after the trauma were not particularly sensitive to interference from the concomitant task, the impairment at both tasks being due rather to a general deficit in maintaining sustained attention.

RT values of the limited sample of 22 controls and patients retested after three months are shown in Figure 11–2. Statistical analysis once again showed a significant effect of the concomitant task ($F$ = 209.1, $d.f.$ 1/42, $p$ < .001). Furthermore, there was an interaction between time of test and type of task ($F$ = 14.01, $d.f.$ 1/42, $p$ < .001), which was due to a practice effect at the Divided Attention Test, independent from the experimental groups. The Sustained Attention Test, on the contrary, did not show any practice effect in either group, probably owing to the automatic nature of the task, which contrasted with a more controlled and effortful nature of the Divided Attention Test.

The effect of trauma was not a significant source of variability ($F$ = 2.57, $d.f.$ 1/42, n.s.), and the same was true for the interaction between trauma and time of test ($F$ = .69, $d.f.$ 1/42, n.s.) and for the third-order interaction between trauma, type of task, and time of test ($F$ = 3, $d.f.$ 1/42, n.s.).

Findings varied considerably in the two groups. In the entire group of 48 patients we found significant statistical differences in comparison to controls. In the subgroup of 22 patients examined at three months, no differences were found. Two explanations may account for these conflicting findings: either a leveling of performances after three months, or a higher power of the first analysis on the entire group. This latter hypothesis is supported by the fact that the subgroup of 22 patients did not show significant differences from control subjects even one month after the trauma.

## Distributed Attention

Subjects' ability to distribute attention across both visual fields was studied by having them respond to the simultaneous appearance of stimuli. Apparatus and experimental procedure were the same as for Sustained and Divided Attention tests, except that here the sequence of events was the following: A bright central cross and two squares (2.50 × 2.50 degrees) were presented on the screen at 13 degrees to the left and right of the fixation point. After a fixed interval of one second, an auditory warning signal was sounded for 25 msec, followed by the stimulus at a variable interval of 500–2500 msec. In 40% of

**Table 11–4**  Means and Standard
Deviations of RT to Target Stimuli on the
Distributed Attention Test of Patients and
Controls One Month after the Trauma

| | |
|---|---|
| Patients ($N = 48$) | 262.6 ± 49.7 |
| Controls ($N = 48$) | 241.0 ± 33.7 |

the trials, a bright spiral (2.25 × 2.25 degrees) was flashed for 20 msec in both
of the squares (target stimuli). In 40% of the trials, a single spiral (no-target
stimuli) was flashed in either the right or the left square, whereas in the remaining 20% no stimuli were presented (catch trials).

Subjects were instructed to fixate the central cross, to respond to target
stimuli by pressing a key with the right index finger as quickly as they could,
and to omit responding in the case of no-target stimuli. The response was followed by a visual feedback exposed for 500 msec, showing the speed of RT to
target stimuli and the accuracy of response in the case of no-target stimuli and
catch trials. The interstimulus interval between the end of each trial and the
following one was 500 msec.

Each test session consisted of two blocks of 50 trials, preceded by a practice session of 10 trials. Responses longer than 1,000 msec and shorter than
150 msec were eliminated. The median value of RT to target stimuli was taken
as the independent variable. The total number of errors did not exceed 10% of
trials and was not considered for statistical analysis.

Table 11–4 shows median RT to target stimuli obtained in the entire sample of 48 patients and their matched controls tested one month after the
trauma. The 48 patients tested after one month were, on the average, 21.6 msec
slower in responding to target stimuli than corresponding controls; this difference was highly significant ($F = 9.2$, $d.f.$ 1/47, $p = .004$).

Analysis of performance by the subgroup of 22 patients who were retested
after three months revealed an effect of trauma that was independent of time

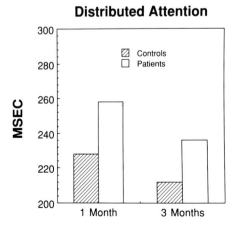

**Figure 11–3**  RT of controls and patients
on the Distributed Attention Test one and
three months after the minor head
trauma.

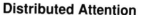

**Distributed Attention**

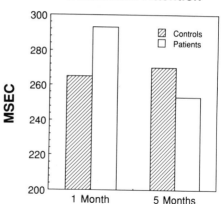

**Figure 11-4**   RT of patients and controls on the Distributed Attention Test five months after MHI.

of testing ($F = 7.3$, $d.f.$ 1/42, $p = .009$). A significant practice effect ($F = 24.7$, $d.f.$ 1/42, $p = .001$) was present in both patients and controls, as shown by Figure 11-3. Interaction between time of testing and brain trauma was not significant ($F = .49$, $d.f.$ 1/42, n.s.); there was no differential improvement of performance with time in the two experimental groups.

A small subgroup of six patients and their corresponding matched controls performed a second test five months after the trauma. Figure 11-4 shows their RT at the Distributed Attention Test. For this sample, ANOVA showed a significant effect of the interaction between trauma and time of testing ($F = 5.56$, $d.f.$ 1/10, $p = .38$). Only RT to target stimuli after one and five months reached significance, using the paired comparison according to the Newman–Keuls procedure (293.5 msec vs. 253.17 msec, diff. $= 40.3$ msec, $p < .05$).

The small size of this sample warrants careful interpretation of these results. However, note that the absolute value of mean RT of patients was slower than that obtained in control subjects one month after the trauma, whereas it was faster after five months. Available evidence therefore suggests an improvement of performance in the span of one to five months after MHI.

## DISCUSSION

The two studies on the neuropsychological performances of MHI patients at fixed intervals after the trauma gave quite different results. In the first study (Gentilini et al., 1985), concerning evaluation of patients' performance on a wide range of cognitive tasks, no significant difference was found between patients and controls except for a trend toward lower scores on a selective attention test, which was possibly obscured by the adoption of a multivariate statistical analysis. In contrast, significant differences between patients and controls were found in all of the tests from a battery devised specifically to explore different aspects of attention. Because sampling criteria of patients and controls were the same in the two studies, the different results can be due only to the fact that MHI patients are specifically impaired in those aspects of attention that were investigated by the latter study.

A specific impairment of attention after mild brain trauma has been shown by a number of studies (Gronwall and Sampson, 1974; Gronwall and Wrightson, 1974; Klensch, 1973; Mac Flynn et al., 1984; McLean et al., 1983; Van Zomeren and Deelman, 1976). However, in each of these, different criteria were adopted to define mild brain injury. Furthermore, each examined a single different aspect of attention, and none had a parallel study on the same group of patients to allow evaluation of the selectivity of the attentional impairment. Our two studies, therefore, present important evidence of the range of preserved and impaired abilities in a well-defined group of brain-injured patients.

A possible explanation for the selective impairment of attention in these patients can be related to mechanisms of concussional cerebral damage which, in patients clinically defined as mildly injured, tend to cause marginal axonal damage or only slight focal dysfunction. The most sensitive tasks for revealing cerebral dysfunction are therefore those that test functions involving the greatest number of cortical and subcortical areas simultaneously. This feature certainly applies to attentional tasks, especially those based on processing speed; in fact, RT values have been repeatedly shown to be more dependent on volume than on site of a cerebral lesion (Tartaglione et al., 1986).

The Distributed Attention Test seems to be the most sensitive among those we devised to investigate attention, as no improvement was detected in our sample as long as three months following the trauma. This finding has an important ecological validity, since distributing attention over space is crucial in many important activities of everyday life, such as driving a car or crossing the street in traffic. Further studies are necessary in order to evaluate the performance of single subjects on this task and also, more generally, to use the attentional test battery to define severity of impairment and degree of recovery.

## REFERENCES

Blackburn HL, Benton AL. Simple and choice reaction time in cerebral disease. Confin Neurol 15:327–338, 1955.

Buschke H. Selective reminding for analysis of memory and learning. J Verb Learn Verb Behav 12:543–550, 1973.

Buschke H, Fuld PA. Evaluating storage, retention, and retrieval in disordered memory and learning. Neurology, (Minn) 24:1019–1025, 1974.

Conkey RC. Psychological changes associated with head injuries. Arch Psychol 33:1–62, 1938.

Dencker SJ, Lofving BA. A psychometric study of identical twins discordant for closed head injury. Acta Psychiatr Neurol Scand 33(Suppl 122), 1958.

De Renzi E, Nichelli P. Verbal and non-verbal short-term memory impairment following hemispheric damage. Cortex 11:341–354, 1975.

Gentilini M, Nichelli P, Schoenhuber R, Bortolotti P, Tonelli L, Falasca A, Merli GA. Neuropsychological evaluation of mild head injury. J Neurol Neurosurg Psychiatry 48:137–140, 1985.

Green DM, Swets JA. Signal detection theory and psychophysics. New York: John Wiley, 1966.

Gronwall DMA, Sampson H. The Psychological Effects of Concussion. Auckland, NZ: Auckland University Press, 1974.

Gronwall D, Wrightson P. Delayed recovery after minor head injury. Lancet 2:605–609, 1974.

Klensch H. Die diagnostische Valenz der Reaktionszeitmessung bei verschiedenen zerebralen Erkrankungen. Fortschr Neurol Psychiatr 41:575, 1973.

MacFlynn G, Montgomery EA, Fenton GW, Rutherford W. Measurement of reaction time following minor head injury. J Neurol Neurosurg Psychiatry 47:1326–1331, 1984.

McLean A, Temkin NR, Dikmen S, Wyler AR. The behavorial sequelae of head injury. J Clin Neuropsychol 5:361–376, 1983.

Meyer A. The anatomical facts and clinical varieties of traumatic insanity. Am J Insanity 60:373–441, 1904.

Miller E. Simple and choice reaction time following severe head injury. Cortex 6:121–127, 1970.

Miller E, Cruzat A. A note on the effects of irrelevant information on task performance after mild and severe head injury. Br J Social Clin Psychol 20:69–70, 1981.

Norman B, Svahn EK. A follow-up study of severe brain injuries. Acta Psychiatr Scand 37:236–264, 1961.

Raven JC. Standard progressive matrices: sets ABCD and E. London: AK Lewis, 1958.

Roy SN, Bose RC. Simultaneous confidence interval estimation. Ann Math Statistics 24:513–536, 1953.

Ruesch J. Intellectual impairment in head injuries. Am J Psychiatry 100:480–496, 1944.

Shiffrin RM, Schneider W. Controlled and automatic human information processing: II. Perceptual learning, automatic attending and a general theory. Psychol Rev 84:127–190, 1977.

Tartaglione A, Bino G, Manzino M, Spadavecchia L, Favale E. Simple reaction-time changes in patients with unilateral brain damage. Neuropsychologia 24, 649–658, 1986.

Thomas C. Deficits of memory and attention following closed head injury. MSc thesis, Oxford University. Cited in Van Zomeren AH, Reaction time and attention after closed head injury. Lisse: Sweets & Zetlinger, 1981, p 93.

Van Zomeren AH, Deelman BG. Differential effects of simple and choice reaction after closed head injury. Clin Neurol Neurosurg 79:81–90, 1976.

Van Zomeren AH, Deelman BG. Long-term recovery of visual reaction time after closed head injury. J Neurol Neurosurg Psychiatry 41:452–457, 1978.

# 12

# Recovery of Memory After Mild Head Injury: A Three-Center Study

RONALD M. RUFF, HARVEY S. LEVIN,
STEVEN MATTIS, WALTER M. HIGH, JR.,
LAWRENCE F. MARSHALL, HOWARD M. EISENBERG,
AND KAMRAN TABADDOR

## REVIEW OF THE LITERATURE ON THE EFFECTS OF MILD HEAD INJURY ON MEMORY

Memory is commonly considered to encompass a number of separate but interacting systems that allow information about specific facts or events to become accessible to conscious awareness through recall or recognition (Luria, 1976; Norman, 1970; Pribram and Broadbent, 1970). These memory systems are often described by using a variety of biopolar distinctions, such as short term and long term (Wickelgren, 1975), episodic and semantic (Tulving, 1972), declarative and procedural (Cohen and Squire, 1980), or working and reference (Olton et al., 1979). No doubt there is overlap among the memory systems thus described since the distinctions among them are based more on experimental paradigm than on any generally accepted theory.

Historically, the loss of memory for events has been explained according to the "last in, first out" hypothesis. Evaluations of memory in patients with Korsakoff's syndrome or medial temporal lobe damage, for example, have documented a temporal gradient that demonstrates the greater susceptibility of more recent recollections to loss (Albert et al., 1979; Squire and Slater, 1979). However, conflicting findings have also been reported (Levin et al., 1985; Warrington and Sanders, 1971). Levin and colleagues, for example, did not find the same temporal gradient as that found in patients with Korsakoff's syndrome when they evaluated 20 closed head injury patients who were in various stages of recovery from posttraumatic amnesia. Furthermore, when the amnestic syn-

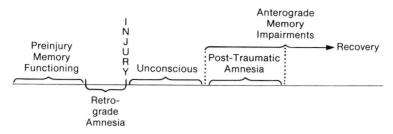

**Figure 12–1**  Schematic representation of the stages of recovery from closed head injury. Note that residual memory disturbance may persist beyond resolution of post-traumatic amnesia (i.e., gross anterograde amnesia characterized by inability to retain information about ongoing events and disorientation).

dromes of the head-injured patients are evaluated, another level of complexity is added; the time course preceding and following the injury may be evidence of different types of amnestic syndromes; and stages of recovery are common (see Figure 12–1).

In part, differences between head injury patients and other clinical populations can be attributed to the gradual onset of memory difficulties in the latter, particularly patients with Korsakoff's syndrome. Young head trauma victims are presumed to have normal long-term memory prior to injury. No available studies demonstrate significant retrograde amnesia in patients with minor head injury (MHI), and clinical observation suggests that extensive loss of memory for events preceding the trauma does not occur in these patients. Indeed, the classical studies by Russell and Nathan (1946) demonstrate that retrograde amnesia rarely extends for more than 30 minutes prior to the impact, except in those patients sustaining more severe closed head injury— that is, in those patients who experience more than one day of posttraumatic amnesia.

## Posttraumatic Amnesia

The term *posttraumatic amnesia* (PTA) refers to any disturbance of memory for events that occur in the period immediately following a head injury. This subacute form of anterograde amnesia is one of the most distinctive markers of closed head injury, and it is frequently encountered in patients with minor head injury. Clinically, the inability to store information into memory continuously causes the patient to be disoriented and confused. Once continuous memory has returned and the patient has become oriented to person, place, and time, other memory functions may still not have returned to their premorbid levels. These deficiencies are typically referred to as *anterograde memory deficits.*

In 1981, Gronwall and Wrightson evaluated the relationship between PTA and anterograde memory functioning in 71 patients from New Zealand who had simple head injuries (i.e., not requiring surgical evacuation of an intracranial lesion or repair of a depressed skull fracture). The patients were assessed between 4 and 27 days post injury. The results of the study indicate a relationship between the duration of PTA and the ability of a patient to consolidate information into long-term storage. However, the presence of PTA did not predict a patient's ability to retrieve information once it had been stored.

Barth et al. (1983) comprehensively assessed 71 minor head injury (MHI) patients three months after injury and found that a significant percentage suffered from cognitive impairments, primarily in the areas of attention and memory. However, this study had a number of methodological limitations, including the lack of exclusion for premorbid factors (multiple head injury, substance abuse, etc.) and the lack of matched controls.

Gentilini et al. (1985) compared 50 mildly head injured patients with 50 matched controls. All the patients were tested one month post injury. A multivariate analysis performed for six neuropsychological tests—three memory measures, two attention tests, and a test of intelligence—yielded no significant differences between the head-injured patients and the controls. The only major indication of poorer posttrauma performance among the head injury patients was documented on a measure of selective attention. In spite of a general trend toward impaired performance on this test, the investigators concluded that the MHI patients were not significantly impaired at one month post injury.

Dikmen et al. (1986) conducted a similar study of 20 patients suffering minor head injury who were compared to a group of matched controls. These investigators included memory measures in their extensive neuropsychological test battery. In general, they concluded that there were no major impairments in the MHI group. However, at one month post injury, the head-injured subjects did perform significantly below the controls on one memory test, specifically, the recall of a 12-word list after a lapse of four hours.

In summary, memory systems are frequently disturbed secondary to minor head injury in patients who may have suffered PTA lasting a few minutes to several hours. Moreover, such patients may also demonstrate anterograde memory loss. The extent and duration of such loss have not yet been fully studied. There are two key questions concerning the recovery of memory in patients who have suffered mild head injury: (1) What is the rate of recovery? and, (2) Do patients as a rule return to their premorbid levels of memory functioning?

## THREE-CENTER STUDY

From January 1982 through August 1984, a study was conducted at three medical centers to evaluate the degree of neurocognitive impairment following minor head injury and to ascertain the extent of recovery over a period of three months. The three medical centers were the University of California Medical Center at San Diego, California; John Sealy Hospital at the University of Texas

Medical Branch at Galveston, Texas; and the Jacoby Hospital of the Albert Einstein College of Medicine, Bronx, New York.

## Enrollment Criteria

Patients with minor head injury were enrolled in the study on the basis of the following diagnostic criteria:

1. A clinical history of cranial trauma. If this included a period of unconsciousness, the period must have been brief (20 minutes or less).
2. Upon admission, a Glasgow Coma Scale (GCS) score of 13–15, with no deterioration to a level below 13. At 48 hours, a GCS score of 15 was required, which is consistent with normal consciousness as reflected by spontaneous eye opening, comprehension of commands, and normal orientation.
3. No focal neurological deficits or evidence of intracranial mass lesion.
4. No hemiparesis or impaired eye movements.
5. Age 15–50 years at the time of injury.

Patients with extremity fractures or other injuries requiring general anesthesia were excluded from the study, as were patients with a premorbid history of neurological disease or injury or severe psychopathology.

## Conducting the Study

At the three medical centers, consecutively admitted patients who met all the diagnostic criteria were enrolled in the study. A baseline evaluation was completed on 155 patients within seven days following injury. A total of 57 patients received a follow-up examination 30 days post injury (±7 days). Halfway through the study, a three-month follow-up examination was added. A subgroup of 32 patients completed all three assessments. Each examination of the patients included the neuropsychological tests (see below) and an interview to assess post-concussional symptoms. Control subjects were given the neuropsychological tests only on a single occasion, and their examination did not include the interview that was given to patients to review their symptoms.

## Demographic Aspects

A major difference noted among the patients at three centers was in the mechanism of injury. Table 12–1 shows the etiology of injury for the patients studied at baseline. Motor vehicle accidents accounted for the highest percentage of patients in San Diego and Galveston, whereas 41% of the patients in the Bronx suffered minor head injuries secondary to an assault. This regional variation in the mechanism of injury raised questions as to sample differences among the three centers. Therefore, *local* control subjects were recruited and selected at each center to match the head-injured patients in age, education, race, and socioeconomic background. Table 12–2 shows the demographic char-

**Table 12-1**  Causes of Head Injury in Patients Studied at Baseline (Three Centers)

| Cause | Galveston (N = 62) | | Bronx (N = 51) | | San Diego (N = 42) | | Total (N = 155) | |
|---|---|---|---|---|---|---|---|---|
| | N | % | N | % | N | % | N | % |
| MVA | 27 | 43.5 | 7 | 13.7 | 25 | 59.5 | 59 | 38.1 |
| Assault | 10 | 16.1 | 21 | 41.2 | 3 | 7.1 | 34 | 21.9 |
| Fall | 9 | 14.5 | 9 | 17.6 | 6 | 14.3 | 24 | 15.5 |
| Sports | 5 | 8.1 | 0 | 0 | 2 | 4.8 | 7 | 4.5 |
| MVA/P. Ed. | 3 | 4.8 | 3 | 5.9 | 2 | 4.8 | 8 | 5.2 |
| Other | 8 | 12.9 | 11 | 21.6 | 4 | 9.5 | 23 | 14.8 |

*Abbreviations:* MVA, motor vehicle accident; P. Ed., physical education accident.

acteristics of those patients who returned for the one-month follow-up and corresponding characteristics for the control subjects.

### Testing Measures

The neuropsychological test battery used in the three-center study is described in detail in Levin et al. (1987). Here, we briefly describe those measures that pertain to memory.

1. *Galveston Orientation and Amnesia Test (GOAT)* (Levin et al., 1979). The initial portion of this test evaluates the subject's orientation to person, place, and time. A second portion of the test focuses on events that a patient is able to recall before and after injury; its purpose is to assess the extent and duration of retrograde and/or anterograde amnesia.

**Table 12-2**  Demographic Features of Head-Injured Patients Tested at One Month Post Injury and of Control Subjects at Three Centers (M ± SD)

| Center | Patients | Controls |
|---|---|---|
| *Galveston* | | |
| No. of subjects (sex) | 14 (9M, 5F) | 12 (8M, 4F) |
| Age | 21.9 ± 5.7 | 22.0 ± 4.2 |
| Education | 12.2 ± .9 | 12.0 ± 1.5 |
| Hollingshead | 53.6 ± 10.5 | 53.3 ± 14.0 |
| *Bronx* | | |
| No. of subjects (sex) | 26 (17M, 9F) | 26 (14M, 12F) |
| Age | 23.5 ± 8.1 | 25.8 ± 7.0 |
| Education | 12.8 ± 1.7 | 12.2 ± 2.3 |
| Hollingshead | 51.8 ± 15.8 | 52.6 ± 15.0 |
| *San Diego* | | |
| No. of subjects (sex) | 17 (9M, 8F) | 18 (11M, 7F) |
| Age | 23.9 ± 6.3 | 24.9 ± 8.3 |
| Education | 11.9 ± 2.3 | 12.4 ± .7 |
| Hollingshead | 53.2 ± 12.3 | 51.1 ± 12.5 |

2. *Mattis–Kovner Verbal Learning and Memory Test* (Mattis and Kovner, 1978). In this test, a list of 20 animal words is read to the subject, who is then asked to recall as many of the words as possible. Based on the subject's performance, a learning curve is established over a series of up to eight trials in which the examiner selectively reminds the subject of those words that were missed. Probes in the form of multiple-choice questions are used on trials 4 and 8 and again 20 minutes after presentation of the list.

3. *Benton Visual Retention Test* (Benton, 1974). In the first part of this test, the subject is asked to copy 10 different geometrical designs while looking at them. In the second part, a series of similar geometrical designs is presented for 10 seconds each. Once they have been removed, the subject is asked to draw the figures from memory.

4. *Digit Span of the Wechsler Adult Intelligence Scale (WAIS;* Wechsler, 1955). This measure assesses the subject's immediate recall of information (i.e., the subject's short-term memory). In the test, a series of digits is presented to the subject, who is then asked to repeat the series to the examiner, both foward and backward.

## Results

### Memory Performance Differences Among the Control Groups

Significant differences in memory performance were found among the regional control groups (see Table 12–3). On the verbal memory test, the controls from

**Table 12–3**  Performance on Memory Measures (Means $\pm$ SD) of Regional Control Groups

|  | Galveston ($N = 12$) | Bronx ($N = 26$) | San Diego ($N = 18$) |
|---|---|---|---|
| *Verbal memory* | | | |
| Percent correct, trial 4 | 83.1 $\pm$ 12.0 | 71.9 $\pm$ 7.9 | 82.7 $\pm$ 13.6 |
| Percent correct, trial 8 | 95.7 $\pm$ 5.5 | 84.3 $\pm$ 8.9 | 94.2 $\pm$ 6.6 |
| Total percent correct | 89.4 $\pm$ 8.8 | 78.1 $\pm$ 8.4 | 88.5 $\pm$ 10.1 |
| CLTR.[a], trial 4 | 42.1 $\pm$ 16.5 | 21.6 $\pm$ 8.3 | 38.7 $\pm$ 16.7 |
| CLTR.[a], trial 8 | 67.2 $\pm$ 10.4 | 47.0 $\pm$ 11.8 | 64.6 $\pm$ 15.6 |
| Total CLTR.[a] | [b]109.3 $\pm$ 26.9 | [b,c]68.6 $\pm$ 20.1 | [c]103.3 $\pm$ 32.3 |
| *Visual memory* | | | |
| No. correct, memory | 8.5 $\pm$ 1.1 | 7.0 $\pm$ 1.6 | 8.0 $\pm$ 1.5 |
| No. errors, memory | [d]1.8 $\pm$ 1.4 | [d]4.1 $\pm$ 2.6 | 2.7 $\pm$ 2.5 |
| No. correct, copy | 9.5 $\pm$ 0.8 | 9.7 $\pm$ 0.7 | 9.9 $\pm$ 0.3 |
| No. errors, copy | 0.5 $\pm$ 0.8 | 0.3 $\pm$ 0.7 | 0.1 $\pm$ 0.3 |
| *Digit span* | | | |
| Age-corrected scale score | 10.4 $\pm$ 2.6 | $\pm$ 12.1 $\pm$ 3.2 | $\pm$ 12.1 $\pm$ 2.7 |

[a]CLTR., consistent retrieval from long-term memory.

[b–d]A common superscript signifies a statistically significant ($p < .05$) difference according to The Wilcoxon Matched-Pairs Signed Ranks Test.

**Table 12–4**  Performances of Minor Head Injury Patients at Baseline at Three Centers (Means ± *SD*)

|  | Galveston (*N* = 62) | Bronx (*N* = 51) | San Diego (*N* = 42) |
|---|---|---|---|
| *Verbal memory* |  |  |  |
| Percent correct, trial 4 | 63.1 ± 19.5 | 54.8 ± 19.9 | 67.2 ± 17.5 |
| Percent correct, trial 8 | 74.4 ± 20.8 | 66.4 ± 21.5 | 79.6 ± 17.3 |
| Total percent correct | 68.8 ± 20.2 | 60.6 ± 20.7 | 73.4 ± 17.4 |
| CLTR.[a], trial 4 | 19.0 ± 16.9 | 11.1 ± 12.2 | 19.5 ± 13.5 |
| CLTR.[a], trial 8 | 39.8 ± 22.9 | 30.0 ± 20.6 | 43.7 ± 19.9 |
| Total CLTR.[a] | 58.8 ± 39.8 | 41.1 ± 32.8 | 63.2 ± 33.4 |
| *Visual memory* |  |  |  |
| No. correct, memory | 6.9 ± 1.8 | 5.4 ± 2.5 | 6.5 ± 2.1 |
| No. errors, memory | 4.5 ± 3.2 | 7.2 ± 5.2 | 4.5 ± 3.6 |
| No. correct, copy | 9.7 ± 0.9 | 8.8 ± 1.5 | 9.5 ± 0.9 |
| No. errors, copy | 0.4 ± 1.0 | 1.3 ± 1.7 | 0.5 ± 1.0 |
| *Digit span* |  |  |  |
| Age-corrected scale score | 9.2 ± 2.5 | 9.7 ± 3.0 | 10.5 ± 3.1 |

[a]CLTR., consistent retrieval from long-term memory.

the Bronx performed significantly below the controls from San Diego and Galveston. On the visual memory test (Table 12–3), significantly more errors were committed by the control subjects from the Bronx as compared to those from Galveston, without significant differences in the number of errors in copying the designs (i.e., while the material was held in view). In contrast, on a digit span measure of immediate retention, the performance of the Bronx group was comparable to that of the other two control groups.

### Baseline Evaluation
Table 12–4 shows the baseline (i.e., within one week of injury) performance of the patients at the three centers. On the verbal memory test, the patients' total recall of words (see Table 12–4) was approximately 40% below that of the control groups (see Table 12–3). Similarly, the patients had a significantly higher number of errors than the controls on the visual memory test.

Striking differences in memory performance were observed among the three centers. On both the verbal and visual memory measures, the control and patient groups from the Bronx scored significantly below the corresponding groups from Galveston and San Diego. In fact, the controls from the Bronx performed at a level comparable to that of the patients from the other two centers. For the digit span subtest, the scores of the patients were somewhat lower than the scores of the controls; however, no major differences among the centers were apparent.

### One Month Follow-Up
Although all three patient groups performed significantly below their respective control groups at baseline, all three groups showed significant gains at one month (see Table 12–5).

**Table 12–5** Performance of MHI Patients at Baseline vs. One Month at Three Centers

| | | Galveston (N = 14) | | Bronx (N = 26) | | San Diego (N = 17) | |
|---|---|---|---|---|---|---|---|
| | | Baseline | One month | Baseline | One month | Baseline | One month |
| *Verbal memory* | | | | | | | |
| Total CLTR.[a] | M | [b,]*68.7 | [b]98.8 | [c,]*43.3 | [c]61.9 | [d,]*67.6 | [d]96.9 |
| | | | | | ± | | |
| | ± SD | ± 45.7 | ± 41.8 | ± 32.3 | 34.0 | ± 28.5 | ± 25.7 |
| *Visual memory* | | | | | | | |
| No. errors, | | | | | | | |
| memory | M | *4.0 | 3.3 | [e,]*6.4 | [e]4.7 | [f,]*5.4 | [f]4.0 |
| | ± SD | ± 2.6 | ± 2.7 | ± 4.5 | ± 3.5 | ± 4.5 | ± 3.1 |
| *Digit Span* | | | | | | | |
| Age-corrected | | | | | | | |
| scale score | M | 9.2 | 9.6 | g*10.0 | [g]10.8 | *8.7 | *9.6 |
| | ± SD | ± 2.0 | ± 1.4 | ± 2.7 | ± 3.2 | ± 2.3 | ± 3.4 |

[a] CLTR., consistent retrieval from long-term memory.
[b-g] A common superscript signifies a statistically significant ($p < .05$) difference according to the Wilcoxon Matched-Pairs Signed Ranks Test.
*Differs significantly from respective control group.

### Three-Month Follow-Up

Patients at all three centers showed additional gains on the memory tests at the three-month follow-up. For the Galveston patients (Table 12–6), significant recovery was demonstrated on both the verbal and visual memory tests. In contrast, performance on the digit span test remained at about the same level on all three examinations.

The gains of the Bronx patients (Table 12–7) were similar to those of the patients in Galveston on both verbal and visual memory measures. Variation across time was noted on the digit span test; however, the significant gains in digit span were made between baseline and one month, but not between baseline and three months. This trend is atypical as compared with the changes in long-term memory.

Finally, for the San Diego patients (Table 12–8), there was clear improvement in verbal but not visual memory. With respect to the digit span test, the performance levels of the patients were consistently below those of the normals, but gains were minimal. In fact, the three-month digit span performance was the only significant deficit of the patients as compared to controls.

### Discussion

### Recovery of Memory Functioning

The three-center study demonstrated that a patient who has sustained a single, uncomplicated mild head injury generally shows compromised memory func-

**Table 12-6**  Galveston Patients: Baseline, One-Month, and Three-Month Evaluations (Means ± SD)

|                             | Baseline              | One month        | Three months           |
| --------------------------- | --------------------- | ---------------- | ---------------------- |
| *Verbal memory*             |                       |                  |                        |
| Percent correct, trial 4    | 80.7 ± 9.4            | 90.5 ± 7.5       | 95.3 ± 4.0             |
| Percent correct, trial 8    | 92.0 ± 9.1            | 94.5 ± 7.2       | 97.7 ± 1.9             |
| Total percent correct       | 86.4 ± 9.3            | 92.5 ± 7.4       | 96.5 ± 3.0             |
| CLTR.[a], trial 4           | 32.7 ± 18.5           | 51.3 ± 12.7      | 60.0 ± 17.1            |
| CLTR.[a], trial 8           | 60.5 ± 18.6           | 69.7 ± 9.8       | 71.0 ± 11.4            |
| Total CLTR.[a]              | [b]93.2 ± 37.1        | 121.0 ± 22.5     | [b]131.0 ± 28.5        |
|                             |                       |                  |                        |
| *Visual memory*             |                       |                  |                        |
| No. correct, memory         | 8.0 ± 1.2             | 7.3 ± 1.5        | 9.0 ± 0.8              |
| No. errors, memory          | [c]2.2 ± 1.3          | [d]3.3 ± 1.9     | [c,d]1.2 ± 1.1         |
| No. correct, copy           | 9.7 ± 0.7             | 9.7 ± 0.5        | 9.5 ± 0.5              |
| No. errors, copy            | 0.3 ± 0.7             | 0.3 ± 0.5        | 0.5 ± 0.5              |
|                             |                       |                  |                        |
| *Digit span*                |                       |                  |                        |
| Age corrected scale score   | 8.3 ± 2.4             | 8.7 ± 1.5        | 8.3 ± 3.9              |

[a]CLTR., consistent retrieval from long-term memory.

[b-d]A common superscript signifies a statistically significant ($p = .05$) difference according to the Wilcoxon Matched-Pairs Signed Ranks Test.

**Table 12-7**  Bronx Patients: Baseline, One-Month, and Three-Month Evaulations (Means ± SD)

|                             | Baseline               | One month         | Three months        |
| --------------------------- | ---------------------- | ----------------- | ------------------- |
| *Verbal memory*             |                        |                   |                     |
| Percent correct, trial 4    | 58.1 ± 21.5            | 66.3 ± 19.3       | 69.6 ± 15.1         |
| Percent correct, trial 8    | 67.8 ± 25.4            | 76.4 ± 16.9       | 76.8 ± 16.6         |
| Total percent correct       | 63.0 ± 23.5            | 71.4 ± 18.1       | 73.2 ± 15.9         |
| CLTR.[a], trial 4           | 12.9 ± 11.7            | 21.3 ± 18.4       | 25.3 ± 19.7         |
| CLTR.[a], trial 8           | 32.8 ± 22.4            | 42.6 ± 20.2       | 45.3 ± 20.2         |
| Total CLTR.[a]              | [b,c]*45.7 ± 34.1      | [b]63.9 ± 38.6    | [c]70.6 ± 39.9      |
|                             |                        |                   |                     |
| *Visual memory*             |                        |                   |                     |
| No. correct, memory         | 5.8 ± 2.4              | 6.3 ± 2.1         | 7.0 ± 1.5           |
| No. errors, memory          | [d,e]*6.6 ± 4.8        | [d]4.8 ± 3.2      | [e]3.8 ± 2.1        |
| No. correct, copy           | 9.3 ± 1.0              | 9.5 ± 0.7         | 9.3 ± 1.5           |
| No. errors, copy            | 0.8 ± 1.1              | 0.6 ± 0.9         | 0.8 ± 1.6           |
|                             |                        |                   |                     |
| *Digit span*                |                        |                   |                     |
| Age-corrected scale score   | [f]*9.9 ± 3.0          | [f]11.1 ± 3.7     | 10.9 ± 3.5          |

[a] CLTR., consistent retreival from long-term memory.

[b-f] A common superscript signifies a statistically significant ($p = .05$) difference according to the Wilcoxon Matched-Pairs Signed Ranks Test.

*Differs significantly from control group.

**Table 12–8** San Diego patients: baseline, one-month, and three-month evaulations (Means ± *SD*)

|  | Baseline | One month | Three months |
|---|---|---|---|
| *Verbal memory* | | | |
| Percent correct, trial 4 | 70.5 ± 11.7 | 80.0 ± 11.2 | 88.0 ± 6.0 |
| Percent correct, trial 8 | 88.7 ± 8.2 | 94.6 ± 4.6 | 96.3 ± 4.7 |
| Total percent correct | 79.6 ± 10.0 | 87.3 ± 7.9 | 92.2 ± 5.4 |
| CLTR.[a], trial 4 | 23.9 ± 12.3 | 36.9 ± 9.8 | 45.9 ± 10.9 |
| CLTR.[a], trial 8 | 53.4 ± 14.5 | 62.8 ± 8.6 | 70.4 ± 9.1 |
| Total CLTR.[a] | [b,c]*77.3 ± 26.8 | [b,d]99.7 ± 18.4 | [c,d]116.3 ± 20.0 |
| *Visual memory* | | | |
| No. correct, memory | 6.5 ± 2.5 | 6.9 ± 1.4 | 7.5 ± 2.2 |
| No. errors, memory | 4.9 ± 4.1 | 3.7 ± 1.8 | 3.4 ± 3.0 |
| No. correct, copy | 9.3 ± 0.9 | 9.5 ± 0.7 | 9.3 ± 1.0 |
| No. errors, copy | 0.9 ± 1.0 | 0.5 ± 0.7 | 0.7 ± 1.0 |
| *Digit span* | | | |
| Age-corrected scale score | *8.6 ± 2.2 | *8.1 ± 3.1 | *9.0 ± 1.8 |

[a]CLTR., consistent retrieval from long-term memory.

[b–d]A common superscript signifies a statistically significant ($p$ = .05) difference according to the Wilcoxon Matched-Pairs Signed Ranks Test.

*Differs from respective control group.

tioning when tested within one week of the trauma. Specifically, memory for verbal and visual information was found to be significantly below that of regional control subjects. In the period between baseline and one month, patients at all three centers recovered both verbal and visual memory functioning to a level that was no longer significantly below that of the controls.

Patients' performance on the digit span test followed a different pattern, however. Such a finding is not unexpected because the literature shows that performance on the digit span test often remains relatively intact in amnestic patients (Brooks, 1984). It is also known that immediate recall of numbers within an individual's span (i.e., when there is no interference or delay) primarily taps attention, which can be dissociated from short-term memory (i.e., the recall of a list of items after a brief delay). It is interesting to note that the performance of the Bronx patients on the digit span test was comparable to that of the patients at the other centers, whereas their performance on the two tests of memory was inferior. This supports the notion that the digit span test examines primarily attentional mechanisms rather than memory. Although this explanation is fairly well accepted for forward span, the capacity to reverse the sequence of digits on backward span may also engage short-term memory.

The patient groups who underwent all three assessments demonstrated significant gains in memory functioning between baseline and one month and more gradual recovery between one month and three months. However, the total number of subjects tested on all three occasions was small (Galveston, $N$ = 6; Bronx, $N$ = 16; San Diego, $N$ = 10), and hence these trends should be interpreted with caution.

*Postconcussion Symptoms*

The individual patients rated their physical, mental, and emotional symptoms following head injury in structured interviews. Subjective complaints were affirmed at baseline by all of the patients hospitalized in San Diego, by 93% of those from Galveston, and by 89% of those from the Bronx. With respect to cognitive dysfunctions, questions were asked during the interviews that required patients to assess their memory directly. An important finding of these interviews was the lack of correspondence between the patients' subjective complaints, which remained virtually unchanged at one month, and the significant gains that they showed on the neuropsychological tests. In other words, although the test performance of the patients improved, they continued to complain of postconcussional symptoms after one month. In fact, both the Galveston and the Bronx patient groups rated their cognitive symptoms as more severe at the one-month follow-up examination. At the three-month follow-up, however, fewer subjective symptoms were reported.

## IMPLICATIONS FOR THE CLINICAL MANAGEMENT OF DELAYED EFFECTS FOLLOWING MINOR HEAD INJURY

The three-center study found that when patients are evaluated within one week following a minor head injury, significant neurospychological deficits are present. This finding has now been supported by studies conducted in New Zealand, Europe and at other medical centers in the United States. Patients' complaints of postconcussional symptoms immediately following their injury do not appear to reflect the true extent of cognitive deficits as noted on the baseline examination. Moreover, measurable cognitive gains made during the first month are not reliably confirmed by the patients.

The patients' inaccurate assessments of their posttraumatic symptoms may be due to a variety of factors, such as premorbid personality characteristics, varying neuropathological substrate of injury, and primary and secondary psychological reactions to the trauma. However, the fact that patients' assessments tend to be inaccurate necessitates the inclusion of a thorough posttest consultation in each patient's clinical management. One purpose of this consultation should be to inform the patient of his or her neuropsychological condition. It is imperative that the patient be cautioned about participating in activities that would likely result in failures during the first month or so following injury. For example, a student preparing for finals, a carpenter preparing a bid on a major job, or an attorney facing a major court case who has sustained a minor head injury should be strongly advised to delay the activity or at least to obtain assistance. If patients suffer failure in complex activities following their injury, their postconcussional symptoms may be aggravated, resulting in confusion, depression, and self-doubt. This, in turn, can lead to bruised egos which then have to be dealt with not only in terms of the minor head injury itself but also in regard to subsequent failures.

One means of ameliorating secondary emotion problems is to initiate follow-up visits to provide a support system and to allow for the monitoring of the patient's improvement. It is also important to inform patients of gains they have made in their neurocognitive performance. Our data show that patients were often not aware of the improvement they had made during the three-month period over which they were tested. In the three-center study, the neuropsychological performance of the patients was found to have stabilized—if not to have improved—between the one-month and three-month testings. No significant drops were observed to have occurred during this interval, and a general trend toward improvement was found at all three centers.

In contrast, subjective postconcussional symptoms did not follow a similar recovery curve. Instead, some of the patients continued to complain of emotional, somatic, and cognitive problems at three months. These complaints were not homogeneous and varied considerably among the patients. It appears, therefore, that subjective complaints following minor head injury may increase over time. Clinically, one should expect such increases. The reason is that in the early phases of recovery, patients typically are not challenged by their environment; however, when they begin to resume those activities that they commonly engaged in, they have difficulty in accomplishing them, and it is at this time that subjective problems begin to surface.

In summary, it is possible for an individual who functions at the 90th percentile prior to injury to fall to the 60th percentile as a result of a minor head injury. Such a decline can significantly interfere with everyday or professional activities. Comparing these patients' data to an average population, using national norms or even regional norms, does not give us sufficient analytical power to make discriminations on an individual basis per se. In fact, it would be erroneous to conclude, on the basis of group comparisons, that patients recover from minor head injuries within three months. Because the three-center study was based on such comparisons, it is possible that the patients were suffering relative losses in a number of areas, and that these deficiencies were not detected. Furthermore, both compensation mechanisms and the effects of repeated testing could have played a role in the observed recovery of memory, and therefore, the existence of subtle neurological disturbances is not precluded (see Marshall and Ruff, Chapter 18, this volume).

## ACKNOWLEDGMENTS

This work was suported by National Institute of Neurological and Communicative Disorders and Stroke Contract NO1 NS9 2312.

## REFERENCES

Albert MS, Butters N, Levin J. Temporal gradients in the retrograde amnesia of patients with alcholic Korsakoff's disease. Arch Neurol 36:211–216, 1979.
Barth JT, Macciocchi SN, Giordani B, et al. Neuropsychological sequelae of minor head injury. Neurosurgery 13:529–533, 1983.

Benton AL. The Revised Visual Retention Test: Clinical and Experimental Applications, 4th ed. New York: The Psychological Corporation, 1974.

Brooks N. Cognitive deficits after head injury. *In* Brook N (ed), Closed Head Injury: Psychological, Social, and Family Consequences. New York: Oxford University Press, 1984.

Cohen NJ, Squire LR. Preserved learning and retention of pattern-analyzing skill in amnesia: dissociation of knowing how and knowning that. Science 210:207–210, 1980.

Dikmen S, McLean A, Temkin N. Neuropsychological and psychosocial consequences of minor head injury. J Neurol Neurosurg Psychiatry 49:1227–1232, 1986.

Gentilini M, Nichelli P, Schoenhuber T, el al. Neuropsychological evaluation of mild head injury. J Neurol Neurosurg Psychiatry 48:137–140, 1985.

Gronwall D, Wrightson P. Memory and information processing capacity after closed head injury. J Neurol Neurosurg Psychiatry 44:889–895, 1981.

Levin HS, O'Donnell VM, Grossman RG. The Galveston Orientation and Amnesia Test: a practical scale to assess cognition after head injury. J Nerv Ment Dis 167:675–684, 1979.

Levin HS, High WM, Meyers CA, von Laufen A, Hayden ME, Eisenberg HM. Impairment of remote memory after closed head injury. J Neurol Neurosurg Psychiatry 48:556–563, 1985.

Levin HS, Mattis S, Ruff RM, Eisenberg HM, et al. Neurobehavioral outcome following minor head injury: a three-case center study. J Neurosurg 66:234–243, 1987.

Luria AR. The Neuropsychology of Memory. New York: John Wiley, 1976.

Mattis S, Kovner R. Different patterns of mnemonic deficits in two organic amnestic syndromes. Brain Lang 6:179–191, 1978.

Norman DA (ed). Models of Human Memory. New York: Academic Press, 1970.

Olton DS, Becker JT, Handelmann GE. Hippocampus, space, and memory. Behav Brain Sci 2:313–365, 1979.

Pribram KH, Broadbent DE (eds). Biology of Memory. New York: Academic Press, 1970.

Russell WR, Nathan PW. Traumatic amnesia. Brain 69:183–187, 1946.

Squire LR, Slater PC. Anterograde and retrograde memory impairment in chronic amnesia. Neuropsychologia 16:313–322, 1978.

Tulving E. Episodic and semantic memory. *In* Tulving E, Donaldson W (eds), Organization of Memory. New York: Academic Press, 1972.

Warrington EK, Sanders HI. The fate of old memories. Q J Exp Psychol 23:432–442, 1971.

Wechsler D. Wechsler Adult Intelligence Scale Manual. New York: Psychological Corporation, 1955.

Wickelgren WA. The long and the short of memory. *In* Deutsch D, Deutsch JA (eds), Short-Term Memory. New York: Academic Press, 1975.

# 13

# Neurobehavioral Outcome of Mild Head Injury in Children

HARVEY S. LEVIN
LINDA EWING-COBBS,
AND JACK M. FLETCHER

The literature on the neurobehavioral outcome of head trauma in children consists primarily of (1) studies confined to patients who were hospitalized in a comatose condition or who suffered moderate injuries, and (2) studies in which patients were markedly heterogeneous with respect to severity of injury. Although children with mild head trauma have occasionally been included as a comparison group, the focus has been on the outcome of severe head trauma. Clinicians and investigators have only recently recognized the importance of specifically studying the outcome of mild head injury defined according to research diagnostic criteria.

In this chapter, we review various facets of mild head injury in children (see Goldstein and Levin, 1985 for a review which focuses on severe pediatric head trauma). The first section is devoted to the epidemiology of mild head injury in children and the evidence for predisposing factors. Next we discuss developmental issues, including distinctive pathophysiological features of head injury in children and the vulnerability of emerging cognitive and linguistic skills at various ages. Third, we review early and long-term effects of mild head injury on neurobehavioral functioning in children, and finally we conclude by pointing out gaps in our current understanding of mild head injury in children and indicate directions for future research.

## EPIDEMIOLOGY

This section summarizes findings concerning the epidemiology of head injury in children with an emphasis on mild head trauma. The reader is referred to

Kraus and Nourjah (Chapter 12) to gain a perspective on the epidemiology of mild head injury in all age ranges.

A recent epidemiological investigation of pediatric head injury by Kraus et al. (1986) based on prospective evaluation of injury severity yielded an estimate of incidence that closely approximated the figures reported earlier by Annegers (1983), who reviewed medical and public health records for Olmsted County, Minnesota. In a study of new occurrences of brain injury in 1981 among residents under 15 years old of San Diego County, California, Kraus and colleagues (1986) found an overall incidence per 100,000 population of 185 for boys and 132 for girls. The incidence of head injury in children was similar to that in adults. Kraus et al. classified the severity of head injury according to the Glasgow Coma Scale (GCS) of Teasdale and Jennett (1974), which was used throughout the trauma system of San Diego County during the period of data collection. Of the 688 children with brain injury who were admitted to a hospital, 606 (88%) had a *mild* brain injury (i.e., GCS score 9–15, duration of hospitalization < 48 hours, no intracranial surgery, and no abnormal CT findings), 46 (7%) had a *moderate* head injury (i.e., GCS score 9–12, hospitalization longer than 48 hours, intracranial surgery, and/or abnormal CT), and 36 (5%) had a *severe* brain injury (GCS score ≤ 8). Note that the criteria used by Kraus et al. for mild injury encompassed a more impaired level of consciousness as compared with other studies (cf. Levin et al., 1988). Kraus and colleagues assumed that most of the injuries that did not result in hospitalization were also mild (not included in incidence). Extrapolation of these figures to the U.S. population under 15 years suggests that nearly 95,000 children suffered traumatic brain injury in 1981, including 83,000 cases of mild injury.

Figure 13–1 shows that the total percentage of brain injury accounted for by mild cases increased as a function of age until age 14, when there was a rise in the percentage of severe cases. Overall, falls predominated as the cause of injury in children 4 years and under, whereas recreational activities (especially bicycle-related injuries) and motor vehicle accidents accounted for most of the injuries in older children and adolescents. Of interest, three-fourths of the mildly injured children were transported to the hospital by private vehicles as compared with one-fourth of mildly injured adults. Consistent with previous findings (Klonoff, 1971), Kraus and co-workers reported that the incidence of head injury in children reached a peak during the spring and summer months, particularly for bicycle-related injuries.

### Predisposing Factors and Risk of Second Head Injury

Fabian and Bender (1947) identified predisposing factors in 21 of 86 pediatric admissions (24%) for head injury to the Bellevue Hospital in New York City during the period 1934–44. These factors included mental deficiency (8 cases), epilepsy (5 cases), brain disease (6 cases), and psychosis (2 cases). Of the 65 head-injured children with no previous disability, 33 (51%) had been involved in two or more major accidents. This finding led the authors to infer "accident proneness" as a contributing factor. They also implicated the role of alcohol-

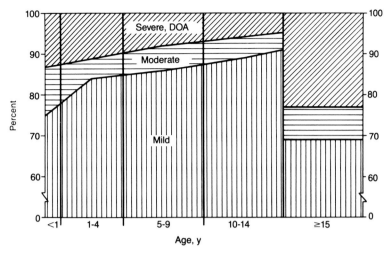

**Figure 13-1**  Distribution of severity of brain injury in 1981 as a function of age among residents under 15 years old of San Diego County, California. (Reproduced from Kraus et al., 1986, by permission)

ism and personality disorders in the parents. However, interpretation of the Fabian and Bender study is hampered by their lack of a comparison group of children without head injury.

Klonoff (1977) found no excess of developmental anomalies or previous trauma (including head injury) in children who sustained head injury in Vancouver as compared to a control group of school children matched on demographic variables. However, congested residential areas, lower income housing, marital instability, and lower socioeconomic status of fathers were overly represented in the head injury group.

Perhaps the most impressive evidence for a risk factor related to head trauma is the increased likelihood of a second head injury. In an analysis of pediatric head injury in Olmsted County, Minnesota for the period 1935–1974, Annegers (1983) found that boys with head trauma had a twofold risk of subsequent head injury. Increased risk of a second injury was nearly as great in head-injured girls. Although the investigators compared the risk of subsequent head trauma to the risk in uninjured children during the same time period, it is still unclear whether the increased risk is a nonspecific accident proneness or a consequence of the initial head injury (e.g., related to cognitive changes, slowed reaction time, or alteration of personality). A comparison group of children sustaining orthopedic injuries could potentially resolve this issue.

## DEVELOPMENTAL ISSUES IN EVALUATING THE CLINICAL COURSE AND OUTCOME OF MILD HEAD INJURY IN CHILDREN

In comparison with closed head injury (CHI) in adults, children differ with respect to the etiology and pathophysiology of brain injury (Kraus et al., 1986).

As discussed by Kraus and his colleagues (1986, and in Chapter 2 of this volume), falls (i.e., relatively low-velocity injuries) contribute immensely to head injury in young children, whereas motor vehicle accidents (which presumably impart greater acceleration to the head) predominate in adolescents, particularly in suburban and rural areas. Apart from age-related differences in injury input variables, investigators have suggested that there are distinctive pathophysiological features of CHI in children. Snoek, Minderhoud, and Wilmink (1984) reported that delayed deterioration of consciousness after a lucid or symptom-free period occurred in about 4% of patients aged 2 months to 17 years who sustained apparently mild head injuries. The reader is referred to Dacey (Chapter 6, this volume) for a discussion of deterioration after apparently mild injury in adults. Assessment of conscious level must be modified for infants and young children in whom "flexes and extends" represent the ceiling of the motor component rather than "obeys" commands (Raimondi and Hirschauer, 1984). Similarly, vocalizations (i.e., cries) constitute the ceiling of the verbal portion of the Children's Coma Scale for infants (Raimondi and Hirschauer, 1984). Diffuse brain swelling occurs more frequently in pediatric head injury (including noncomatose cases) as compared with CHI in adults (Bruce et al., 1978, 1979). Although the reports by Bruce suggested a lower frequency of hemispheric mass lesions in pediatric head trauma than in adult head injuries, a more recent study (Berger et al., 1985) based on a centralized system of trauma care has questioned this distinction. Finally, the full implications of mild to moderate head injury during infancy or early childhood may not be appreciated until complex behavior and cognitive processes can be assessed several years later.

### Diffuse Axonal Injury

In view of evidence implicating diffuse axonal injury after mild head trauma in adults (Oppenheimer, 1968) and in nonhuman primates subjected to experimental acceleration/deceleration injury (Jane et al., 1985), it is plausible that similar effects can be demonstrated microscopically in children sustaining mild head injury. Whether the occurrence of mild head injury during a phase of rapid myelination such as the first decade of life (Yakovlev and Lecours, 1967) is related to increased vulnerability to developmental delays and possibly later cerebral insult is unknown. However, the finding that recovery of cognitive functioning after a mild head injury is more prolonged for adults suffering a second mild head injury as compared to adults sustaining their first head trauma has implicated a subtle, residual reduction in "cerebral reserve" (Gronwall and Wrightson, 1975).

### Focal Brain Lesions

Evidence in support of greater potential for recovery from brain injury in children as compared with adults has emanated primarily from studies of unilateral focal lesions (Basser, 1962). Infantile right hemiplegia and left hemispherectomy have been compatible with acquisition of language of variable quality

(Basser, 1962). Most clinicians and investigators agree that the resolution of aphasia is more rapid and more complete in children as compared to adults, while acknowledging that the manifestations of language disorder are different in the two groups (Hecaen, 1976). Greater potential for participation of homologous regions of the right hemisphere and/or reorganization of function in adjacent areas of the language-dominant hemisphere may subserve the observed recovery in children (Lenneberg, 1967).

However, these conclusions regarding developmental issues in recovery from focal brain lesions have been questioned because of methodological problems such as the contribution of diffuse cerebral insult to the sequelae of head trauma. Etiology (as opposed to age) may also be an important variable in recovery from aphasia. Although stroke is uncommon in children, it is a leading cause of aphasia in adults. The observed rapid improvement of language in children rendered aphasic by head injury may reflect the recovery characteristics of this etiology rather than a feature intrinsic to children per se as compared with adults. Dennis (1980) reported persistent aphasia in a child who sustained a left temporoparietal vascular insult; this aphasia resembled the language problems typically found in adults with comparable vascular lesions. Finally, the upper age range compatible with displacement of language to the right hemisphere in children sustaining left hemisphere insult may be as early as 12–14 months (Satz and Bullard-Bates, 1981). How do these findings impinge on the outcome of mild head injury? Recent evidence suggests that focal parenchymal abnormalities are frequently visualized by magnetic resonance imaging in adults admitted for mild CHI (Levin et al., 1987). Consequently, it is conceivable that focal lesions may be more common in children with mild impairment of consciousness than hitherto thought. Application of advanced neuroimaging technologies may elucidate the presence and localization of intracranial lesions after mild head injury in children.

### Methodological Issues in Studies of Neuropsychological Sequelae of Mild Head Injury

Methodological concerns include selection of sufficiently narrow age ranges to permit analysis of differences in outcome that might be obscured by recruiting children with a wide disparity of age for a single group. Other issues include the selection of an appropriate comparison group. Although normative data are available for many neuropsychological tests, the samples of children on which published data are collected may differ along pertinent socioeconomic variables from the CHI children under investigation. A recent study of neurobehavioral outcome of minor head injury in adults (see Ruff et al., Chapter 12, this volume) disclosed marked differences in neuropsychological performance across both the samples of patients and the normal comparison subjects who were recruited at three geographically diverse centers. Children sustaining orthopedic injuries could to some extent control for nonspecific stress related to trauma and hospitalization, but occult mild head injury and the effects of both pain and analgesics potentially contaminate this comparison group. Approaches to recruiting normal children for control groups have included classmates selected by their teacher for scholastic ability similar to the head-injured patients (Gulbrandsen, 1984) and identical twins (Lyons and Matheny, 1984).

Collection of normative data at a single point in time is of limited usefulness for comparison with serial findings in head-injured children. Changes in performance related to maturation and repeated exposure to the test materials can be partially assessed by serially studying the comparison group at intervals corresponding to the assessment schedule of the head-injured children. The time course and scheduling of follow-up examinations are of particular importance in studying outcome of head-injured in children who are undergoing marked maturational changes. Test–retest intervals as brief as six months may normally be associated with improved performance on cognitive and memory tests, owing to maturational changes (apart from the practice effects, which accrue from repeated testing in adults) in children, whereas a relatively stable cognitive level may be assumed in neurologically normal adults. The issues surrounding practice effects and appropriate comparison groups are complex. Serially studying normal children at intervals corresponding to the intertest periods used in a head-injured cohort does not ensure equivalent practice effects. The initial experience with a test is presumably better retained by an uninjured child than equivalent exposure to the procedure in a child studied within several days of sustaining even a mild head injury. An alternative to serially testing normal children in order to assess the effects of repeated exposure is to study head-injured patients repeatedly over a short period of time (e.g., one month). This relatively brief follow-up interval would provide an estimate of maximal practice effects which could be used to adjust the results of serial assessment for repeated exposure to the test materials in head-injured cohorts. The residuals after such an adjustment could be interpreted as reflecting recovery.

## EARLY EFFECTS OF MILD CLOSED HEAD INJURY

The term "early" here refers to findings obtained during the initial hospitalization or shortly after discharge. As will be seen, the temporal relationship between the initial assessment and resolution of posttraumatic amnesia (i.e., confusion, disorientation, and gross impairment of memory for ongoing events) is a pertinent issue. Moreover, procedures to assess posttraumatic amnesia (PTA) in children have only recently been developed and require refinement pending studies of orientation in normal children. Levin and Eisenberg (1979a) studied children following closed head injury (CHI) of varying severity, including 14 children 6–12 years of age and 24 adolescents 13–18 years of age, who had brief or no loss of consciousness and were following commands on admission to the hospital. Although the brief duration of unconsciousness was consistent with mild CHI, all three of the younger patients who underwent computed tomography (CT) had abnormal findings (small ventricles, focal lesion of the right hemisphere), whereas three of the 11 adolescents who were referred for CT had abnormal scans (focal lesion of the right hemisphere, small ventricles). While performing CT on all pediatric cases of mild CHI has to be weighed against cost, radiation burden, and necessity for sedation in young children, these preliminary data suggest that cerebral swelling (as reflected by small ventricles) or focal hemispheric lesions may be present in about one-third of the cases. Further study utilizing magnetic resonance imaging could pursue this point.

Levin and Eisenberg (1979a,b) administered neuropsychological tests that encompassed the domains of language (e.g., naming), visuospatial function (e.g., block construction), memory (e.g., learning and retention of a list of words), somatosensory function (e.g., stereognosis for geometrical shapes), and motor speed (e.g., reaction time). The presence of a neuropsychological deficit was inferred from a score that fell two or more standard deviations below the mean for normal children of the same age. Within the group 6–12 years old, there were deficits in all areas, including language (29% of children), visuospatial function (21%), memory (13%), somatosensory function (33%), and motor speed (21%). The low percentage of deficits for memory might reflect the fewer cases who were given the relevant tests. Among the mildly injured adolescents, the corresponding findings included deficits in language (17%), visuospatial function (4%), memory (25%), somatosensory function (20%), and motor speed (13%). In contrast to these findings, memory deficit was the most frequent neuropsychological residual in severely injured children and adolescents. In the absence of follow-up assessment and evaluation of an appropriate comparison group of children and adolescents without brain injury, the long-range implications of this investigation for sequelae of mild CHI are uncertain.

In a study concerning the early effects of CHI on language, Ewing-Cobbs, Levin, Eisenberg, and Fletcher (1987) included 14 children and 21 adolescents who had sustained mild head trauma according to an admission GCS score of 13–15. The Neurosensory Center Comprehensive Examination for Aphasia (Spreen and Benton, 1969), a series of expressive and receptive language tests, was administered. To examine the effects of CHI on various language functions, the subtests were grouped into categories of naming, expressive language (other than naming), receptive skills, and graphic ability (e.g., writing to dictation). Percentile scores on each subtest were derived from normative data and averaged within a category to yield an overall percentile for the domain. As shown in Table 13–1, the mean percentile scores on the language tests were generally within the average range for both the children and adolescents who sustained a mild head injury. However, the relatively low graphical percentile score in children led the investigators to postulate that a skill in a rapid phase of development such as writing was more vulnerable to the effects of injury than was a more firmly established capacity (e.g., receptive language). The most common writing errors were omission of words (and occasionally letters), capitalization errors, and misspellings, a pattern which the investigators attributed to attentional and organizational difficulties as opposed to primary semantic, syntactic, or apraxic deficits. The finding of greater vulnerability of written language is compatible with the previous results by Hécaen, Perenin, and Jeannerod (1984), who reported more frequent dysgraphia in children sustaining left hemisphere lesions (secondary to trauma, tumor, or hematoma)

**Table 13-1**   Mean Composite Language Percentiles (Corrected for
Age) Obtained on Baseline Examination of Children and Adolescents
Sustaining a Mild Head Injury

|  | Children (5–10 years) | Adolescents (11–15 years) |
|---|---|---|
| Naming |  |  |
| *n* | 10 | 11 |
| *M* | 63.6 | 69.8 |
| *SD* | 28.2 | 4.9 |
| Expressive |  |  |
| *n* | 11 | 11 |
| *M* | 53.8 | 47.7 |
| *SD* | 16.7 | 16.6 |
| Receptive |  |  |
| *n* | 11 | 8 |
| *M* | 46.9 | 58.9 |
| *SD* | 10.5 | 14.4 |
| Graphical |  |  |
| *n* | 8 | 10 |
| *M* | 37.5 | 54.8 |
| *SD* | 14.6 | 16.5 |

*Source:* Adapted from Ewing-Cobbs et al. (1987), by permission.

who were younger than 10 years, as compared with adolescents. Moreover,
disproportionate impairment of written language in head-injured children is
consistent with normative data indicating that this capacity develops most rapidly between the ages of 6 and 8 years (Gibson and Levin, 1975).

## LONG-TERM NEUROPSYCHOLOGICAL SEQUELAE

This review is confined to studies that included a group of children with mild
head injury, or at least a combined group with mild and moderate injuries.
Consequently, investigations that were based on heterogeneous (or unspecified) injuries ranging from mild to severe were excluded. The results of the
studies are summarized in Table 13–2. In general, the neuropsychological outcome of mild head injury in children has been studied for comparison with
severe pediatric head injury rather than as the focus of inquiry. This constraint
is illustrated in the series of seminal papers by Rutter and his associates
(Brown, et al., 1981; Chadwick et al., 1981; Rutter, 1982; Rutter et al., 1980),
who matched orthopedic injury controls on pertinent demographic variables
and preinjury history to children with severe head injury (i.e., duration of PTA
of one to four weeks). However, a mild injury group had more frequent preexisting school adjustment problems (28% of patients) and below average school
achievement (35% of patients) in comparison with 14% of the children in the
control and severe injury groups. Moreover, boys comprised three-fourths of
the mild head injury group as compared with 57% of the controls and severe

injuries. A socially disadvantaged background was also more common in the mild injury group. Notwithstanding the disparities in preinjury adjustment and socioeconomic background, mean age at injury was about 10 years in all three groups, Rutter and co-workers defined a mild injury according to PTA duration (i.e., the postinjury interval for which the patient has no recollection) which ranged from one hour to less than seven days. This relatively long interval of amnesia exceeds the duration of PTA typically used to define a mild injury (cf. Jennett and Teasdale, 1981).

Follow-up assessment at 2¼ years after injury revealed that two children in the mild injury group had been placed in schools for the educationally subnormal, but this transfer had been initiated prior to the trauma in both cases (Chadwick et al., 1981). Two mildly injured children (8%) were referred for psychiatric treatment during the follow-up period, as compared with 11 of the 28 (39%) severely injured cases. Given the preexisting behavioral problems in the mild injury group, this finding provides no convincing evidence of increased psychiatric morbidity following their head trauma. Administration of the Wechsler Intelligence Scale for Children–Revised (WISC-R) to the mildly injured children disclosed that their Verbal and Performance IQs were about 8–10 points below the scores of the orthopedic group on the initial assessment and at one year post injury, with a trend toward lower Performance IQ (mean = 107) at two and one-quarter years after injury as compared with controls (mean = 116). As depicted in Figure 13–2, the mild injury group failed to exhibit gains comparable to the other two groups over the the follow-up period. This is especially evident in the marked increment from baseline to 1 year in the controls and the severely injured children. In contrast to the unequivocal deficit in Performance IQ of the severe CHI patients (Figure 13–2), their initial Verbal IQ (mean = 96) was similar to that of the mild injury group (mean = 97).

Chadwick et al. inferred from the recovery patterns depicted in Figure 13–2 that the impaired Performance IQ was due to brain damage in the severe injury group but not in children who sustained mild head trauma. Persistent intellectual impairment, which the investigators defined as an initial deficit in Performance IQ that was still below 70 at follow-up, was present in about one-third of the severely injured children but in none of the patients with mild head trauma. The investigators contended that mild head injury produced no impairment on the Verbal or Performance portions of the Wechsler Intelligence Scale. Although more than 40% of the mildly injured children had a reading level below expectation for age at follow-up (vs. 18% of the controls), the authors surmised that this finding reflected a premorbid condition.

An implication of the Chadwick et al. study is the importance of serially assessing control subjects at intervals that correspond to the follow-up assessments of the head-injured patients. Although the findings provide evidence for intellectual deficit in severely injured children, the comparison between mildly injured patients and controls is equivocal because of disparities in demographic background, preinjury scholastic achievement, and psychosocial adjustment.

More recently, Levin and Benton (1986) reported scholastic achievement

**Table 13-2** Summary of Studies Concerning Long-Term Neuropsychological Sequelae of Mild Head Injury in Children

| Authors | Study sample and age | Indices of severity | Neuropsychological measures (injury–test interval) | Findings | Comments |
|---|---|---|---|---|---|
| Chadwick et al., 1980 | mild head injury ($n$ = 29), $M$ age = 9.6 yr; severe head injury ($n$ = 31), $M$ age = 10.1 yr; orthopedic controls ($n$ = 28), $M$ age = 10.0 yr | PTA duration >1 hr, <1 week in mild injury; ≥1 week in severe injury | WISC (baseline 1 yr, 2¼ yr) | 1. Performance IQ of mildly injured cases improved (nonsignificant) ($M$ = 98) over 2¼ yr ($M$ = 107) as compared with Performance IQ of 107 initially in controls who improved to 116. Verbal IQ was initially 97 in milds, 106 in controls. 2. Slight change in Performance IQ after mild head injury was interpreted as evidence for the low premorbid level rather than for the effects of injury. | 1. Mildly injured children were drawn from lower SES and had more premorbid problems in school than controls. 2. PTA duration was longer than specified by most definitions of mild injury and of questionable reliability. |
| Gulbrandsen, 1984 | Mild head injury ($n$ = 56), age = 9–13 yr; classmates matched on age, sex, and academic level ($n$ = 56) | Unconscious ≤15 min; ≥2 Sx: LOC, amnesia, nausea or vomiting | WISC, Reitan–Indiana Battery (4–8 mo post injury) | 1. Injured children performed below controls on tests of complex sensorimotor integration (Tactual Performance Test, Grooved Pegboard), problem solving (Category Test), and the Picture Completion and Comprehension subtests of the WISC. | 1. Preliminary 2-yr follow-up data show resolution of group differences. |

| Study | Subjects | Classification | Tests | Results | Comments |
|---|---|---|---|---|---|
| Bawden et al., 1985 | Mild head injury (n = 47), M age = 9.4 yr; moderate head injury (n = 23), M age = 9.5 yr; severe injury (n = 17), M age = 9.6 yr | GCS score 8–14; unconscious ≤20 min in mild, >20 min in moderate; GCS score ≤7 in severe injuries | WISC-R, motor tests (1 yr post injury) | 1. MHI patients obtained average-level IQs (Verbal = 92, Performance = 99) which exceeded scores in severely injured (Verbal IQ = 87, Performance = 80), but not moderately injured (Verbal IQ = 93, Performance = 95). 2. Mild patients consistently performed at the average level on psychomotor (e.g., mazes) and motor (e.g., finger tapping) tests and exceeded the scores of severely injured children. 2. Pattern of greater group differences in young children (9–10 yr) was shown. 3. Teachers reported no increase in scholastic problems of injured children. | 1. Retrospective GCS scores. 2. No control group. 3. Assumes that normative data were obtained from children of similar background. |
| Lyons and Matheny, 1984 | Mild head injury in MZ twins, 12–36 mo (n = 5), 36–48 mo (n = 8) | Retrospective estimate of duration of unconsciousness by parents, noncompound skull fracture | WPPSI (all children tested at age 6 yr) | 1. Injury at 12–36 mo resulted in average IQs (Verbal = 101, Performance = 106) vs. cotwin (Verbal = 104, Performance = 102). 2. Injury at 36–48 mo resulted in lower Performance IQ (Verbal | 1. Two of the children injured at 36–48 mo had durations of unconsciousness that were long for a mild injury. |

**Table 13-2** *Continued*

| Authors | Study sample and age | Indices of severity | Neuropsychological measures (injury–test interval) | Findings | Comments |
|---|---|---|---|---|---|
| Levin et al., 1988 | Mild injury (*n* = 14), moderate injury (*n* = 16), severe injury (*n* = 28); children studied in 3 age ranges at injury: 6–8, 9–12, 13–15 yr | Mild: GCS score 13–15, unconscious ≤ 20 min; moderate: GCS score 9–12 or higher, with depressed fx or abnormal CT; severe: GCS score ≤8 | Selective reminding (verbal, memory); continuous recognition memory (tested after clearing of PTA and 1 yr post injury) | 1. Combined group of mild/moderate injuries (9–12 yr) were impaired on baseline recognition memory as compared with controls, but no other differences were significant initially or 1 yr later. = 95, Performance = 92) vs. cotwins (Verbal = 98, Performance = 101). | 1. Controls tested on only one occasion, leaving open the possibility that adverse effects on the patients are underestimated owing to practice effects. |

*Abbreviations:*
LOC, loss of consciousness; MZ, monozygous; PTA, posttraumatic amnesia; SES, socioeconomic status; WISC, Wechsler Intelligence Scale for Children; WISC-R, Wechsler Intelligence Scale for Children–Revised; WPPSI, Wechsler Preschool and Primary Scale of Intelligence.

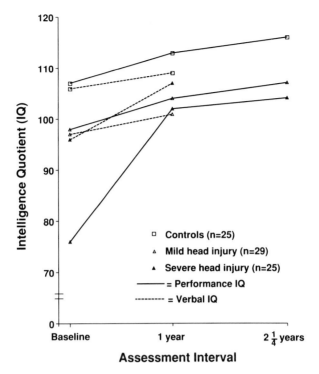

**Figure 13–2** Verbal and Performance IQ of orthopedic control and head-injured groups plotted against the assessment interval. Note that Verbal IQ was obtained on the initial examination and at the one-year follow-up assessment, but not at the 2¼-year evaluation. (Adapted from Chadwick et al., 1981, by permission)

data for children and adolescents (median age at injury = 10.3 years) who were tested at least six months after CHI of varying severity. In contrast to the longitudinal investigation completed in London, Levin and Benton excluded children with a preinjury history of neuropsychiatric disorder or learning disability that was documented in the school records. As indicated in Table 13–3, age-percentile reading scores on the Wide-Range Achievement Test were at the average level in both mild to moderate and severe CHI groups (defined according to the postresuscitation or lowest GCS scores). However, mathematics scores fell below reading in both groups of pediatric head-injured patients, a finding which Levin and Benton attributed to the demands of timed calculation on attention and information processing speed as compared with the more automatized, unspeeded test of reading. It is seen in Table 13–3 that spelling was also performed at a higher level than mathematics in the severely injured group.

In a study of neuropsychological functioning of children (mean age, 9.5 years at injury; range, 2.5–17) one year after CHI of varying severity, Bawden, Knights, and Winogron (1985) defined an injury as mild according to an admission GCS score of 8–14 and loss of consciousness ≤ 20 minutes (with or without a linear skull fracture) based on medical records which the inves-

**Table 13-3**  Comparison of Achievement Test Percentile Scores for Age Within the Head-Injured Group (N = 34)

|  | *Reading %tile for age | | Mathematics %tile for age | | Spelling %tile for age | |
| --- | --- | --- | --- | --- | --- | --- |
|  | Median | Range | Median | Range | Median | Range |
| Total series (N = 34) | 64[a] | 3–97 | 26[a,b] | 2–92 | 46[b] | 2–99 |
| GCS score ≤ 8 (n = 17) | 75[a] | 5–94 | 34[a,b] | 2–92 | 47[b] | 5–94 |
| GCS score > 8 (n = 17) | 56[a] | 5–93 | 15[a] | 2–75 | 31 | 2–81 |

[a,b]A common superscript signifies a statistically significant ($p < .05$) difference according to the Wilcoxon Matched-Pairs Signed Ranks Test.
*Source:* Levin and Benton (1986), by permission.

tigators assessed retrospectively. These patients were distinguished from moderate head injuries primarily by the duration of unconsciousness (> vs. ≤ 20 minutes), whereas severe head injury was defined by a GCS score ≤ 7. Bawden et al. administered the WISC-R and a series of neuropsychological tests which they grouped according to the demand for speeded performance (e.g., finger tapping was considered highly speeded, whereas solving a maze was moderately speeded). Raw scores on the neuropsychological tests were transformed to standard scores based on normative data which were previously collected, but no control group was evaluated. Although the three groups were matched on age and sex, there was no mention of socioeconomic variables. However, children with preexisting, neuropsychiatric disorders were excluded from the study.

As depicted in Table 13-2, the mildly injured children had scores within the average range on the WISC-R (mean Verbal IQ = 92.3, $SD$ = 14.5; mean Performance IQ = 99.4, $SD$ = 19.2), findings which were similar to the moderate CHI group, but clearly above the results obtained in severely injured patients. The Performance IQ of severly injured patients was significantly below that of the mild group. The impression that mildly injured patients recovered to within the average range of intellectual functioning was supported by their consistently normal scores on a series of neuropsychological tests including highly speeded (e.g., finger and foot tapping, pegboard assembly) and moderately speeded (e.g., mazes) procedures on which they performed significantly better than the severely injured patients. While acknowledging the constraint imposed by the lack of a control group, Bawden and co-workers inferred from the test scores that it was unlikely that the mildly injured children suffered "any major intellectual impairment" (Bawden et al., 1985, p. 49).

Contrary to the impression of essentially full recovery (or at least full resolution of measurable sequelae) after mild CHI in the pediatric age range, Gulbrandsen (1984) reported that children (9–13 years at injury) tested four to eight months after head trauma producing less than 15 minutes of uncon-

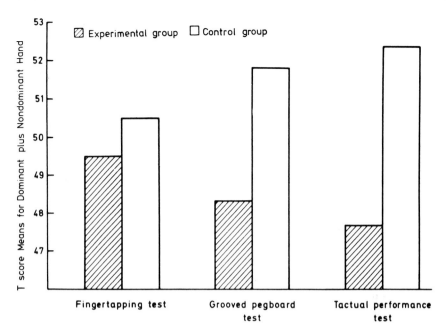

**Figure 13-3** Comparison of performance on neuropsychological tests as a function of task complexity in children evaluated four to eight months following mild head injury and in uninjured classmate controls. (Reproduced from Gulbrandsen, 1984, by permission)

sciousness exhibited impairment on several neuropsychological tests comprising the Reitan–Indiana Battery as compared with classmates who were matched on age and sex but not socioeconomic background (children with preexisting neuropsychiatric disorder were excluded). Teachers of the head-injured children had selected the classmates for comparability in scholastic performance. In contrast to the results of Bawden et al. which implicated impaired performance on speeded tests following severe head injury, Gulbrandsen found that procedures involving complex sensorimotor integration accounted for most of the significant differences (Figure 13–3). Exceptions to the pattern were the Picture Completion and Comprehension subtests of the WISC, which involved no motor response. Although Gulbrandsen's controlled study implicates sequelae of mild head injury, she subsequently found that the observed neuropsychological deficits had resolved on a two-year follow-up assessment (Gulbrandsen, personal communication, 1987). Moreover, at the time of the four- to eight-month follow-up examination, the teachers reported no excess of scholastic problems in the head-injured children, and they were frequently unaware that an injury had occurred.

In a study of monozygotic male twins in whom one twin of each pair sustained a noncompound skull fracture within the age range of 12–36 months ($n$ = 5) or 36–48 months ($n$ = 8), Lyons and Matheny (1984) compared Wechsler Preschool and Primary School Intelligence test scores obtained in the injured twins tested at age six years with findings of the cotwins. Retrospective reports of the injuries obtained from the parents disclosed that all but two injured infants had lost consciousness for periods less than one hour and that 10 of the patients had been hospitalized for periods of one day or less. However, the estimated durations of unconsciousness of two hours and 48 hours in two of the infants were hardly compatible with a mild head injury. Separate analyses of the intellectual test findings for the two age ranges disclosed no difference in cognitive function between the twins injured at 12–36 months and their cotwins, whereas the infants injured between 36 and 48 months had lower scores on several subtests (e.g., Animal House, Picture Completion, Block Design) of the Performance scale as compared with the cotwins. These differences, which were marginally significant, included the infants who had been unconscious for two hours and 48 hours. Consequently, it is questionable whether the differences in cognitive performance between the injured twins and their cotwins would have been significant with deletion of the two cases who had persistent impairment of consciousness. Prospective study of monozygotic twins offers the opportunity to control for genetic (and usually psychosocial) determinants of intellectual performance.

## Memory Functiong After Mild to Moderate Head Injury in Children

Despite the frequent finding of memory deficit during the early stages of recovery from mild head injury in adults (see Ruff et al., Chapter 12, this volume) and after severe CHI in the pediatric age range (Levin et al., 1982), relatively few studies have focused on this problem in mild head-injured children. Levin, High, Ewing-Cobbs, et al. (1988) studied three age ranges of pediatric head-injured patients (6–8 years, 9–12 years, and 13–15 years) following resolution of PTA and one year after injury. Because of the relatively small number of patients, the investigators combined the mild (i.e., GCS score 13–15, with loss of consciousness less than 20 minutes) and moderate (GCS score 9–12 or 13–15, with unconsciousness persisting longer than 20 minutes) injuries within each age range into a single group for comparison with a severe head injury and control groups. Levin and colleagues administered the Selective Reminding Test (Buschke, 1973) to assess verbal learning and memory, and the Continuous Recognition Memory Test (Hannay et al., 1979) which evaluated the capacity to differentiate recurring pictures of familiar living things from distractors that appeared on only a single trial. In view of the relative immaturity of mnemonic strategies in children as compared with adolescents, the investigators had postulated that verbal learning and memory would be relatively unaffected in the younger age groups whereas recognition memory would be similarly impaired in the children and adolescents.

Figure 13–4A shows that the mildly to moderate injured children in the group 6–8 years of age exhibited no impairment of verbal learning and memory at baseline, and their performance tended to exceed the level of a severely injured group one year later. Although Figure 13–5A depicts a decrement in recognition memory at baseline as compared with the control group, this difference was nonsignificant. It is seen that recognition memory in the children

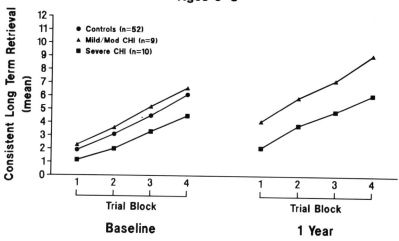

**Figure 13–4(A)**  Mean consistent long-term retrieval of a word list plotted against trial blocks of the Selective Reminding Test for children 6–8 years old who sustained mild to moderate or severe closed head injury and completed baseline and one-year follow-up examinations. Data are also shown for a control group of normal school children of similar age who were tested on a single occasion. (Reproduced from Levin et al., 1988, by permission)

**Figure 13–4(B)**  Mean consistent long-term retrieval of a word list plotted against trial blocks of the Selective Reminding Test for children 9–12 years old who sustained mild to moderate or severe closed head injury and completed baseline and one-year follow-up examinations. Data are also shown for a control group of normal school children of similar age who were tested on a single occasion. (Reproduced from Levin et al., 1988, with permission)

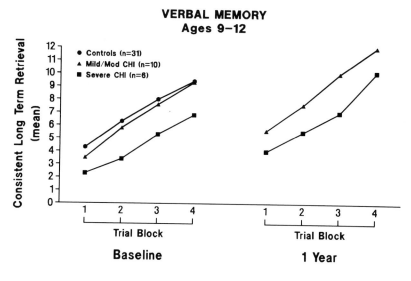

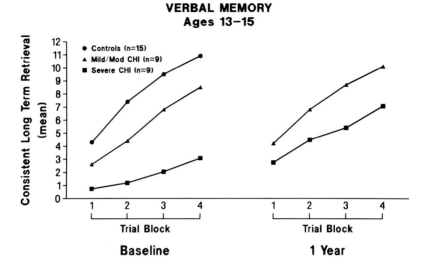

**Figure 13–4(C)** Mean consistent long-term retrieval of a word list plotted against trial blocks of the Selective Reminding Test for adolescents 13–15 years old, who sustained mild to moderate or severe closed head injury and completed baseline and one-year follow-up examinations. Data are also plotted for a control group of normal adolescents who completed the test on a single occasion. (Reproduced from Levin et al., 1988 by permission)

**Figure 13–5(A)** Mean $d'$ (an index of memory sensitivity) on the Continuous Recognition Memory test plotted for children ages 6–8 years who sustained mild to moderate or severe closed head injury and a control group of uninjured, normal children of similar age. The results for the head-injured patients are shown for baseline and one year postinjury. (Reproduced from Levin et al., 1988, by permission)

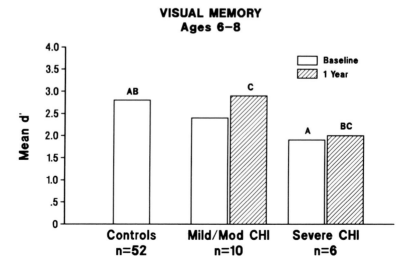

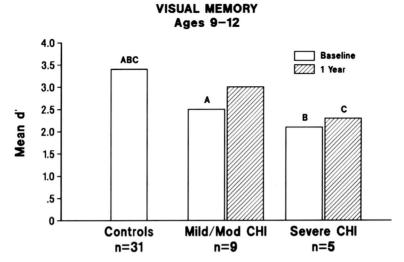

**Figure 13–5(B)** Mean $d'$ (an index of memory sensitivity) on the Continuous Recognition Memory Test plotted for children ages 9–12 years who sustained mild to moderate or severe closed head injury and a control group of children of uninjured, normal children of similar age. The results for the head-injured patients are shown for baseline and one year postinjury. (Reproduced from Levin et al., 1988, by permission)

**Figure 13–5(C)** Mean $d'$ (an index of memory sensitivity) on the Continuous Recognition Memory test plotted for adolescents ages 13–15 years who sustained mild to moderate or severe closed head injury and a control group of uninjured, normal children of similar age. The results for the head injured patients are shown for baseline and one year post injury. (Reproduced from Levin et al., 1988, by permission)

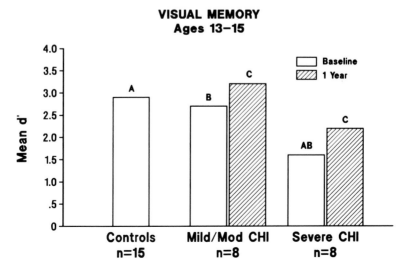

sustaining mild to moderate injuries recovered one year later to a level significantly above that of the severely injured group (Figure 13–5A). Similar to the youngest groups, the 9- to 12-year-old children sustaining mild/moderate head injuries showed no evidence of impaired verbal learning and memory (Figure 13–4B). However, Continuous Recognition Memory was initially impaired in the children who sustained mild/moderate injury during the age range of 9–12 years (Figure 13–5B), but this capacity later recovered to a level which approximated that of the control group.

Despite the apparent deficit in verbal learning and memory in the adolescents sustaining mild to moderate injuries (Figure 13–4C), their scores did not differ significantly from the findings of controls (but exceeded the level of the severely injured adolescents). Similarly, adolescents sustaining mild to moderate head injury did not differ from controls in recognition memory (Figure 13–5C), but they performed above the level of the severely injured group on both the baseline and follow-up examinations.

Taken together, the results obtained by Levin and co-workers provide no convincing evidence of persistent memory deficit after mild to moderate head injury. However, serial assessment of controls is needed to equate for the concurrent effects of maturation and repeated exposure to the test materials.

## Posttraumatic Behavioral Changes

Early studies depicting sequelae of pediatric head injury emphasized the debilitating effects of behavioral changes (e.g., irritability, anger control problems) rather than postconcussional symptoms such as headache which resolved and had relatively minor effects on overall adjustment (Black et al., 1969; Dillon and Leopold, 1961). However, there was no specific analysis of mild head injury in these studies nor were control groups of uninjured children or orthopedic injuries included for comparison. The presence of physical symptoms and psychosocial changes one month after minor head injury were recently reported for a series of 204 children (mean age, 4.4 years) treated in the emergency room at the Children's Hospital of Philadelphia (Casey et al., 1986). In contrast to the studies of neuropsychological outcome after mild head injury summarized in Table 13–2, the Philadelphia series selected cases who had no loss of consciousness, skull fracture, or neurological symptoms at the time of their initial evaluation. By comparison with children rendered unconscious (however briefly), the injuries studied by Casey and co-workers could be considered "minimal." Findings obtained one month after injury disclosed that physical symptoms were infrequently reported by the children. Headache, the most common symptom, was reported by less than 7% of the children, whereas other symptoms typically found in head-injured adults were present in 1% or less of the series. Although Casey et al. found that absenteeism from school and diminished social activities were present during the month after "minimal" head injury, the study lacked a comparison group of children matched on psychosocial background and medical history (e.g., parental occupation, previous head injury). It is conceivable that emergency room treatment for extracranial injuries might have resulted in a comparable reduction of

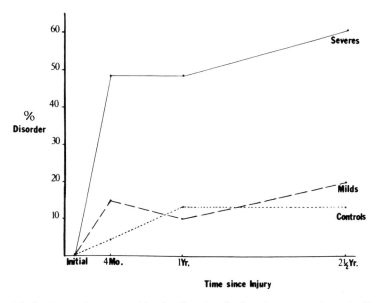

**Figure 13–6** Rate of new psychiatric disorder during the two and one-half years following injury depicted for mild head injury, severe head injury, and orthopedic injury in children. (Reproduced from Rutter, 1982, by permission)

activities over the one-month period. In any case, there is evidence that head-injured children are not representative of the pediatric population with respect to psychosocial variables (Rutter et al., 1980). Be as it may, the study by Casey and co-workers confirms earlier work showing that children consecutively treated for minimal head injury have relatively few postconcussional complaints.

The presence of adverse psychosocial and ecological conditions associated with lower income housing and marital instability which could predispose to behavioral problems was noted in the foregoing section on Epidemiology. This point is illustrated by a prospective study of psychiatric sequelae of head-injured children in London, which disclosed that school adjustment problems antedated mild head injury in nearly 28% of the sample as compared with 14% of orthopedic controls (Brown et al., 1981; Rutter et al., 1980). The investigators identified preexisting behavioral problems by interviewing the parent shortly after injury before the emergence of posttraumatic changes which could have substantially influenced the results. By determining the rate of behavioral disorder that arose after the injury and comparing the results over time to findings in orthopedic injury controls, Brown and co-workers (1981) controlled for nonspecific effects of trauma and hospitalization. As depicted in Figure 13–6, there was no significant difference in the development of new psychiatric disorders (i.e., which were not present before injury) in children sustaining mild head trauma as compared with children who had orthopedic injuries. In contrast, the rate of new psychiatric disorder was markedly elevated following severe head injury as compared with the other two groups. As was the case for acquired cognitive deficit, the findings of the London study implicated brain injury in the genesis of behavioral disorder after severe, but not mild head trauma. These conclusions are in accord with incidental observations of normal behavior in a recent study concerning sequelae of mild head injury (Gulbrandsen, 1984).

### Influence of Parental Reactions

The possibility that parental anxiety at the time of injury and acute treatment might influence the child's residual complaints and morbidity during the following month was studied by Casey, Ludwig, and McCormick (1987). These investigators found that physical complaints, absenteeism from school (after initially returning to class), and reduced activities were essentially confined to children of parents who were highly anxious at the time of emergency room treatment for minimal head trauma (i.e., no loss of consciousness, no neurological deficit, no complications or surgery). Moreover, 85% of the parents were considered to be moderately or severely anxious at the time their children were treated in the emergency room. In contrast, an intervention consisting of supplementary information provided by a nurse concerning the injury and its clinical course proved to have no effect on the outcome reported by the parents one month after trauma as compared with a control group of parents who were given on additional instructions. In summary, the Philadelphia study implicates the impact of the parental reaction on sequelae of minimal head injury in children. Further research is necessary to examine the influence of parental response on postconcussion symptoms in children who sustain mild to moderate head injury.

### DIRECTIONS FOR FUTURE RESEARCH

Gaps in our current knowledge of mild head injury in children include the implications of heterogeneity in the pathophysiology of injury (including maturational variables, differences in etiology, and susceptibility to complications such as brain swelling) for neuropsychological outcome. Preliminary CT findings indicate that focal hemispheric lesions and brain swelling are present more often in children with minimally impaired consciousness than previously thought. Would MRI yield findings of additional focal lesions? What is the time course for resolution of these focal lesions? Is there a relationship between the presence of focal lesions and neuropsychological sequelae? The outcome of mild head injury occurring in infancy has been pursued in only a single study to date (Lyons and Matheny, 1984), which was based on retrospective documentation of the trauma without assessment of neuropsychological capacities apart from intellectual functioning.

In general, controlled studies are needed to assess the long-term effects of mild head injury on a wide range of neuropsychological abilities including memory and attention. Skills that are relatively undeveloped at the time of injury may appear initially to be spared with evidence of impairment emerging when the injured area of the brain normally becomes functionally mature. Consequently, follow-up periods of one to two years may be insufficient to demonstrate long-term sequelae, depending on the age at injury. To this end, assessment of appropriately matched control children is necessary to appreciate persisting effects of mild head injury in children and to evaluate critically the possibility of chronic impairment (Boll, 1983). This point is underscored by the progressive demands on learning and retention imposed by the educational system in children who are injured during the first five or six years of life. Depending on the results of the proposed longitudinal studies, the educational implications should be considered. What special procedures (if any) should be followed in counseling the child, the family, and school personnel following a mild head injury?

The markedly increased risk of a second head injury in children sustaining head trauma merits further study. Is this a nonspecific indication of accident proneness or secondary effect of diminished attention and psychomotor retardation? Are the neurobehavioral effects of mild head injury in children cumulative, similar to the findings reported for adults? In view of the high incidence of mild head injury in children, the answers to these questions and others warrant further research.

## ACKNOWLEDGMENTS

Research completed by the authors was supported by the Javits Neuroscience Investigator Award, NS-21889. The authors are grateful to Liz Zindler for manuscript preparation.

## REFERENCES

Annegers JF. The epidemiology of head trauma in children. *In* Shapiro K (ed), Pediatric Head Trauma. Mount Kisco, NY: Futura Publishing, 1983, pp. 1–10.

Basser LS. Hemiplegia of early onset and the faculty of speech with special reference to the effects of hemispherectomy. Brain 85:427–460, 1962.

Bawden HN, Knights RM, Winogron HW. Speeded performance following head injury in children. J Clin Exp Neuropsychol 7:39–54, 1985.

Berger MS, Pitts LH, Lovely M, Edwards MSB, Bartkowski HM. Outcome from severe head injury in children and adolescents. J Neurosurg 62:194–199, 1985.

Black P, Jeffries JJ, Blumer D, Wellner A, Walker AE. The posttraumatic syndrome in children. *In* Walker AE, Caveness WF, Critchley M (eds), The Late Effects of Head Injury. Springfield, IL: Charles C Thomas, 1969, pp 142–149.

Boll TJ. Minor head injury in children—out of sight but not out of mind. J Clin Child Psychol 12:74–80, 1983.

Brown G, Chadwick O, Shaffer D, Rutter M, Traub M. A prospective study of children with head injuries: III. Psychiatric sequelae. Psychol Med 11:63–78, 1981.

Bruce DA, Schut L, Bruno LA, Wood JH, Sutton LN. Outcome following severe head injuries in children. J Neurosurg 48:679–688, 1978.

Bruce DA, Raphaely RC, Goldberg AI, Zimmerman RA, Bilaniuk LT, Shut L, Kuhl,

DE. Pathophysiology, treatment, and outcome following severe head injury in children. Child's Brain 5:174–191, 1979.

Buschke H. Selective reminding for analysis of memory and learning. J Verb Learn Verb Behav 12:543–550, 1973.

Casey R, Ludwig S, McCormick MC. Morbidity following minor head trauma in children. Pediatrics 78:497–502, 1986.

Casey R, Ludwig S, McCormick MC. Minor head trauma in children: an intervention to decrease functional morbidity. Pediatrics 80:159–164, 1987.

Chadwick O, Rutter M, Brown G, Shaffer D, Traub M. A prospective study of children with head injuries: II. Cognitive sequelae. Psychol Med 11:49–61, 1981.

Dennis M. Stroke in childhood. I. Communicative intent, expression, and comprehension after left hemisphere arteriopathy in a right-handed 9 year old. In Reiber RW (ed), Language Development and Aphasia in Children. New York: Academic Press, 1980, pp 45–67.

Dillon H, Leopold RL. Children and the post-concussion syndrome. JAMA 175:110–116, 1961.

Ewing-Cobbs L, Levin HS, Eisenberg HM, Fletcher JM. Language functions following closed head injury in children and adolescents. J Clin Exp Neuropsychol 9:575–592, 1987.

Fabian AA, Bender L. Head injury in children: predisposing factors. Am J Orthopsychiatry 17:68–79, 1947.

Gibson, EJ, Levin H. The Psychology of Reading. Cambridge: MIT Press, 1975.

Goldstein FC, Levin HS. Intellectual and academic outcome following closed head injury in children and adolescents: research strategies and empirical findings. Dev Neuropsychol 1:395–214, 1985.

Gronwall D, Wrightson P. Cumulative effect of concussion. Lancet 2:995–997, 1975.

Gulbrandsen GB. Neuropsychological sequelae of light head injuries in older children 6 months after trauma. J Clin Neuropsychol 6:257–268, 1984.

Hannay HJ, Levin HS, Grossman RG. Impaired recognition memory after head injury. Cortex 15:269–283, 1979.

Hécaen H. Acquired aphasia in children and the ontogenesis of hemispheric functional specialization. Brain Lang 3:114–134, 1976.

Hécaen H, Perenin MT, Jeannerod M. The effects of cortical lesions in children: Language and visual functions. In Almli CR, Finger S (eds), Early Brain Damage, Vol 1: Research Orientations and Clinical Observations. New York: Academic Press, 1984, pp 277–298.

Jane JA, Steward O, Gennarelli, T. Axonal degeneration induced by experimental noninvasive minor head injury. J Neurosurg 62:96–100, 1985.

Jennett, B, Teasdale, G. Management of Head Injuries. Philadelphia: F.A. Davis Company, 1981.

Klonoff H. Head injuries in children: predisposing factors, accident conditions, accident proneness and sequelae. Am J Public Health 61:2405–2417, 1971.

Kraus JF, Fife D, Cox P, Ramstein K, Conroy C. Incidence, severity, and external causes of pediatric brain injury. Am J Dis Child 140:687–693, 1986.

Lenneberg E. Biological Foundations of Language. New York: John Wiley, 1967.

Levin HS, Amparo E, Eisenberg HM, Williams DH, High WM Jr, McArdle CB, Weiner, RL. Magnetic resonance imaging and computed tomography in relation to the neurobehavioral sequelae of mild and moderate head injuries. J Neurosurg 66:706–713, 1987.

Levin HS, Benton AL. Developmental and acquired dyscalculia in children. In Flehmig

I, Stern L (eds), Child Development and Learning Behavior. Stuttgart: Gustav Fisher, 1986, pp 317–322.

Levin HS, Eisenberg HM. Neuropsychological impairment after closed head injury in children and adolescents. J Pediatr Psychol 4:389–402, 1979a.

Levin HS, Eisenberg HM. Neuropsychological outcome of closed head injury in children and adolescents. Child's Brain 5:281–292, 1979b.

Levin HS, Eisenberg HM, Wigg NR, Kobayashi K. Memory and intellectual ability after head injury in children and adolescents. Neurosurgery 11:668–673, 1982.

Levin HS High WM Jr, Ewing-Cobbs L, Fletcher JM, Eisenberg HM, Miner ME, Goldstein, FC. Memory functioning during the first year after closed head injury in children and adolescents. Neurosurgery 22:1043–1052, 1988.

Lyons MJ, Matheny AP. Cognitive and personality differences between identical twins following skull fractures. J Pediatr Psychol 4:485–494, 1984.

Oppenheimer DR. Microscopic lesions in the brain following head injury. J Neurol Neurosurg Psychiatry 31:299–306, 1968.

Raimondi AJ, Hirschauer J. Head injury in the infant and toddler: coma scoring and outcome scale. Child's Brain 11:12–35, 1984.

Rutter M. Developmental neuropsychiatry: concepts, issues, and prospects. J Clin Neuropsychol 4:91–115, 1982.

Rutter M, Chadwick O, Shaffer D, Brown G. A prospective study of children with head injuries: I. Design and methods. Psychol Med 10:633–646, 1980.

Satz P, Bullard-Bates C. Acquired aphasia in children. In Sarno MT (ed), Acquired Aphasia. New York: Academic Press, 1981, pp 399–426.

Snoek JW, Minderhoud JM, Wilmink JT. Delayed deterioration following mild head injury in children. Brain 107:15–36, 1984.

Spreen O, Benton AL. Neurosensory Center Comprehensive Examination for Aphasia: Manual of Directions. Victoria, B.C.: Neuropsychology Laboratory, University of Victoria, 1969.

Teasdale G, Jennett B. Assessment of coma and impaired consciousness: a practical scale. Lancet 2:81–84, 1974.

Yakovlev PI, Lecours, A-R. The myelogenetic cycles of regional maturation of the brain. In Minkowski A (ed), Regional Development of the Brain in Early Life, Proceedings of a symposium organized by the Council for International Organizations of Medical Sciences. Philadelphia: FA Davis, 1967.

# V
# Postconcussion Symptoms

# 14

# Postconcussion Symptoms: Relationship to Acute Neurological Indices, Individual Differences, and Circumstances of Injury

WILLIAM H. RUTHERFORD

## NOMENCLATURE

The term *minor head injury* is so widely accepted that it is almost impossible to avoid using it. However, it is not an ideal name, for "minor head injury" is not simply a minor injury to the head. Such injuries as a facial wound, a dislocated jaw, a tear in the conjunctiva, or a bite of the pinna of the ear are all minor injuries of the head, yet clearly different from what is meant by "minor head injury." The term *minor brain injury* would be less open to confusion.

Another term that is used in connection with these cases is *concussion*. This is clear and succinct, and to my mind preferable to "minor head injury." However, it is also a term to which different meanings have been given, and if it is to be more widely used in this connection, it is well that it should be clearly defined. My suggestion would be:

*Concussion is an acceleration/deceleration injury to the head almost always associated with a period of amnesia, and followed by a characteristic group of symptoms such as headache, poor memory, and vertigo.*

In the past, it was understood that concussion was a transient state where no organic damage resulted. It was the term used by pathologists to describe a condition in which the appearance of the brain was normal yet the clinical history indicated a period of unconsciousness. It was contrasted with conditions like contusion, laceration, or hemorrhage, where the lesion could be clearly seen (Tan and Kakular, 1981). From the studies of Oppenheimer (1968), it is clear that with careful examination of the concussed brain, microscopic damage can be found. It has also been understood in the past that concussion was a minor head injury. Although minor head injury is the subject of

**Table 14-1**  Early and Late Concussion Symptoms

| Early symptoms | Late symptoms |
| --- | --- |
| Headache | Headache |
| Dizziness | Dizziness |
| | |
| Vomiting | Irritability |
| Nausea | Anxiety |
| Drowsiness | Depression |
| Blurred vision | Poor memory |
| | Poor concentration |
| | Insomnia |
| | Fatigue |
| | Poor hearing |
| | Poor vision |

this particular book, the definition of concussion given above does not impose any limit in terms of severity. All acceleration/deceleration head injuries, no matter how severe, result in the same type of brain damage, and all the symptoms seen following the mild cases are seen in the major cases also. Should hemorrhage occur, an urgent and often life-threatening situation may result. Should a patient survive, he or she will be left with the aftereffects of concussion, not of brain hemorrhage.

Concussion or minor head injury is sometimes defined in relation to unconsciousness rather than amnesia. Ambulancemen (paramedics) are trained observers, but will be able to give an opinion about the patient's condition only after their arrival, which is usually 15–20 minutes after the accident. Relatives and friends may or may not be able to give a clear description of what happened. In every case there is a patient, and only very occasionally does it prove difficult to establish whether or not there is a gap in the patient's memory exactly corresponding to the trauma to the head. There are rare cases where the patient never experiences a total loss of memory and yet develops the characteristic symptoms after an acceleration/deceleration head injury. The definition as worded above is wide enough to accept these as being genuine cases of concussion.

If one accepts this definition of concussion, which is essentially a clinical rather than a pathological definition, then one would expect the symptoms that characterize it to be spoken of as *concussion* symptoms rather than *postconcussion* symptoms. The pain of fractured ribs may continue for some weeks, yet nobody refers to such pain as "post rib fracture" pain.

## EARLY AND LATE SYMPTOMS

Table 14–1 lists what may be considered the common early and late symptoms. The *early* symptoms are what the patient complains of immediately after regaining full consciousness, and are the typical complaints on the following morning. The *late* symptoms are those that are reported at clinical visits a few weeks later. In different studies a certain amount of variation is found in the late symptom list because it is possible to subdivide some of the symptoms. For instance, some studies will mention sensitivity to noise as a distinct symptom, whereas others report the same complaint under the general heading of irritability.

It is interesting to note that vomiting, nausea, drowsiness, and blurred vision are short-lived complaints. It is extremely uncommon to hear patients complaining of these at a late stage, except for a few of the patients involved in litigation. In these instances it is reasonable to have reservations about the reality of the complaints. It is equally interesting to note the symptoms complained of under the "late" heading which are not mentioned in the early stage. Why do these symptoms appear only "late" and when did they appear? The answer may be that the underlying dysfunction of the brain is present from the moment of impact, but that it takes time and the stresses and strains of daily life to make the patient realize what has happened. Thus while lying quietly in a hospital bed, the patient is unaware of any irritability or sensitivity to noise. However, a fond father may have two or three young children at home. After his head injury, he may discover that he cannot tolerate the noise they make, and he is disconcerted by the way he keeps losing his temper with them. It is at this stage that he will complain to his doctor of irritability.

Not all the stresses and strains of life may be evident in the first few days. It is evident, for example, that a patient may be able to cope with life while on leave from work, yet when normal working is resumed, the added responsibilities may tax the brain function beyond what it is yet able to perform. This does not prove that the only factor in late symptoms is the reduced ability of the brain, but it does suggest that the appearance of a symptom for the first time some weeks or months after the injury is not in itself proof that that symptom is neurotic rather than organic.

## INCIDENCE OF LATE SYMPTOMS

Table 14–2 sets out the results of a number of studies reporting estimates of the incidence of symptoms at various times after a head injury is sustained.

**Table 14–2**  Incidence of Late Concussion-Symptoms

| Reference | Six weeks | Three months | One year | One to two years | Three years |
|---|---|---|---|---|---|
| Rutherford et al., 1977 | 51% | | | | |
| Rimel et al., 1981 | | 84% | | | |
| Wrightson and Gronwall, 1981 | | 60% | | | |
| Lidvall et al., 1974 | | 24% | | | |
| Rutherford et al., 1978 | | | 14.5% | | |
| Amphoux et al., 1977 | | | | 49% | |
| Fee and Rutherford, 1987 | | | | | 34% |

There is considerable variation between different authors and different studies. For example, the incidence of symptoms at three months varies between 24% and 84%. The differences may be due in part to differences in methodology. It is very important to ascertain whether the data relate to symptoms spontaneously volunteered, or whether patients were questioned against a previously agreed-upon list of symptoms. In our own studies at six weeks and one year (Rutherford et al., 1977, 1978), we were very aware of the possibility of suggesting symptoms to patients. However, in patients who were sure they had no symptoms, we did take them through a checklist. In some studies it is not clear how the questioning was carried out, and in these the significance of the estimate is uncertain.

Another reason for different estimates is that the cases have been selected differently. The most obvious example here is the study by Fee and Rutherford (1987), in which all the patients had been involved in litigation. In contrast, the series by Rutherford et al. (1977, 1978) was a general prospective series of patients with concussion in whom only 6% were so involved.

Kelly (1975) has put forward the view that the symptoms rate is related to the quality of medical care received by the patients. It is plausible that the relatively low incidence of symptoms shown in our studies is associated with the efforts to prevent the occurrence of a secondary neurosis.

Finally, the study of Amphoux et al. (1977) was a retrospective study, and one would expect in such a study that a number of patients who had head injuries and rapidly recovered might forget about the incident, whereas those with continuing symptoms would be less inclined to do so. This would result in a distortedly high estimate of the percentage of head-injured patients with symptoms.

## DURATION OF SYMPTOMS

Table 14–3 is taken from the article by Amphoux et al. (1977), working as physicians in the French construction industry. These authors had been impressed by frequent complaints of head injury symptoms in the annual med-

**Table 14–3**  Head Injuries and Concussion Symptoms Among French Construction Workers

| Time since injury | No. of patients reporting head injury | No. of patients recovering from Sx | Patients with persisting Sx | |
|---|---|---|---|---|
| | | | Number | Percent |
| <1 yr | 165 | 6 | 72 | 43.6 |
| 1–2 yr | 149 | 10 | 73 | 49.0 |
| 3–4 yr | 123 | 12 | 63 | 51.2 |
| 5–8 yr | 144 | 21 | 64 | 44.4 |
| 9–15 yr | 142 | 15 | 65 | 45.8 |
| 16+ yr | 85 | 4 | 22 | 25.9 |

*Source:* Amphoux et al. (1977), by permission.

**Table 14–4** Sex by Symptoms at Six Weeks

|  | No symptoms | One symptom | More than one symptom | $\chi^2$, $p$ |
|---|---|---|---|---|
| Male | 55 (59.8%) | 10 (10.9%) | 27 (29.3%) | $\chi^2$ (2 $df$) = 12.85 |
| Female | 16 (30.2%) | 14 (26.4%) | 23 (43.4%) | .01 > $p$ > .001 |

ical checkup of their work force, and undertook this investigation to quantify the effect. The results refer to head injuries for any reason and not just work-related accidents. The number involved in litigation was low. It is surprising to find so little variation in the reported percentage of head-injured patients continuing to complain of symptoms at any time between one year and 15 years. It is also interesting that some patients were still complaining more than 16 years after their accident. Merskey and Woodford (1972) also reported a patient with symptoms 14 years after minor head injury.

## FACTORS ASSOCIATED WITH THE PRESENCE OF LATE SYMPTOMS

These associations are based on our earlier follow-up studies at six weeks and one year (Rutherford et al., 1977, 1978).

### Sex

Table 14–4 shows the positive relationship between the female sex and late symptoms. (In all our work we have accepted a value of $p < .05$ as being statistically significant.) This association was confirmed in the study by Lidvall et al. (1974).

### Age

Table 14–5 shows that in our one-year follow-up study, the figure for symptoms in people aged 40 years and over just fell short of the significant value. I would be surprised if a larger study did not confirm this association.

### Posttraumatic Amnesia

Table 14–6 is based on those patients in our six-week study who had a negative blood alcohol. Although the results do not approach significance, there does

**Table 14–5** Age by Symptoms at One Year

|  | No symptom | Symptoms | $p$ |
|---|---|---|---|
| <20 yr | 37 (86.8%) | 6 (13.2%) |  |
| 20–39 yr | 44 (93.6%) | 3 (6.4%) | $\chi^2$ = 5.74, .07 > $p$ > .05 |
| >40 yr | 31 (75.6%) | 10 (24.3%) |  |

**Table 14-6** Posttraumatic Amnesia in Patients with Negative Blood Alcohol by Symptoms at Six Weeks

|  | No symptoms | Symptoms | $\chi^2$, $p$ |
|---|---|---|---|
| <15 min | 11 (45%) | 13 (55%) | $\chi^2$ (2 d.f.) = 0.278 |
| 15–59 min | 10 (42%) | 14 (58%) |  |
| >60 min | 6 (38%) | 10 (62%) | .7 > p > .5 |

appear to be a clear association of lower symptoms rates with shorter posttraumatic amnesia (PTA), and higher symptom rates with longer PTA. This trend awaits confirmation in a larger study, in which cases with positive blood alcohols would be excluded. However, in a study of personality and behavioral change after severe blunt head injury, Brooks and McKinlay (1983) did not find any correlation with postraumatic amnesia.

## Headache

Table 14–7 shows that the presence of a headache within 24 hours of recovery of consciousness is associated with a higher symptom rate at six weeks. Few would believe that this headache was the result of neurosis, but if it is an organically caused symptom then there would appear to be some organic factor involved with the symptoms at six weeks.

## Diplopia, Anosmia, or any Positive CNS Finding on the Second Morning

All of these complaints are associated with a higher symptom rate at six weeks (Table 14–8, 14–9, and 14–10), and all are clearly evidence of organic factors involved.

## Whose Fault?

At the six-week follow-up appointment in our study, patients were asked to give their opinion as to who was to blame for their injury. We then separated those who blamed either their employer or a large impersonal body—such as the Belfast Corporation or the British Army—from the rest (Table 14–11). The association of a high symptom rate among the selected group was not unexpected, and was also clear evidence of nervous and emotional factors at work in the production of symptoms.

**Table 14-7** Headache at 24 Hours by Symptoms at Six Weeks

|  | No symptoms | 1 symptom | >1 symptom | $\chi^2$, $p$ |
|---|---|---|---|---|
| Absent | 25 (67.6%) | 6 (16.2%) | 6 (16.2%) | $\chi^2$ (2 d.f.) = 8.32 |
| Present | 46 (42.6%) | 18 (16.7%) | 44 (40.7%) | .02 > p > .01 |

**Table 14–8** Diplopia at 24 Hours by Symptoms at Six Weeks

|  | No symptoms | 1 symptom | >1 symptom | $p$ |
|---|---|---|---|---|
| Absent | 69 (51.9%) | 21 (15.8%) | 43 (30.3%) | .0324 |
| Present | 2 (16.7%) | 3 (25.)% | 7 (58.3%) | |

**Table 14–9** Anosmia at 24 Hours by Symptoms at Six Weeks

|  | No symptoms | 1 symptom | > 1 symptom | $\chi^2, p$ |
|---|---|---|---|---|
| Absent | 63 (51.6%) | 22 (18.0%) | 37 (30.3%) | $\chi^2$ (2 $d.f.$) = 5.99 |
| Present | 8 (34.8%) | 2 (8.7%) | 13 (56.5%) | $.05 > p > .02$ |

## Significance of These Studies

In the United Kingdom, the article by Miller (1961) was very influential. His central interest was accident neurosis, but many of the cases in his series were cases of minor head injury. He was convinced that the severity of the symptoms was inversely proportional to the severity of the primary injury. His cases were all involved in litigation, and the symptoms persisted until settlement and then disappeared. The effect of this article was to give wide credence to the view that the symptoms of concussion were essentially neurotic or even due to malingering. Our studies in 1977 and 1978 were valuable in producing good evidence that organic factors were implicated. This view is confirmed not only by the pathological studies of Oppenheimer (1968), but by the many studies that, with the use of psychometric testing, showed alterations following minor head injuries (Gronwall and Wrightson, 1974; MacFlynn et al., 1984; McMillan and Glucksman, 1987; Montgomery et al., 1984; Stuss et al., 1985).

**Table 14–10** Any Positive CNS Sign at 24 Hours by Symptoms at Six Weeks

|  | No symptom | 1 symptom | >1 symptom | $\chi^2, p$ |
|---|---|---|---|---|
| Absent | 54 (54.5%) | 22 (18.2%) | 27 (27.3%) | $\chi^2$ (2 $d.f.$) = 11.3 |
| Present | 13 (32.5%) | 4 (10.0%) | 23 (57.5%) | $.005 > p > .001$ |

**Table 14–11** Whose Fault, by Symptoms at Six Weeks

|  | No symptom | 1 symptom | > 1 symptom | $\chi^2, p$ |
|---|---|---|---|---|
| Employer/Impersonal Organization | 7 (31.8%) | 1 (4.5%) | 14 (63.6%) | $\chi^2$ (2 $d.f.$) = 10.1 |
| Self, Other Person, "Act of God" | 61 (48.2%) | 23 (17.0%) | 35 (34.8%) | $.01 > p > .001$ |

However, we did not conclude that the late symptoms were solely organic, for we were able to demonstrate also the correlation with motivation.

## THE EFFECT OF LITIGATION UPON LATE SYMPTOMS OF MINOR HEAD INJURIES

The question of whether the late effects of concussion of the spine were organic as advocated by Ericksen (1882) or neurotic as Page (1885) believed started over 100 years ago. The closely related debate regarding concussion of the brain has flourished to an even greater extent, and one gathers from recent correspondence in the *Journal of the Royal Society of Medicine* (Kelly; Field; Trimble; Guthkelch, 1981) that the controversy is still alive and well.

For some years now solicitors in Belfast have sought medicolegal reports on virtually all the cases of minor head injury that have been admitted to the Observation Ward of the Royal Victoria Hospital in Belfast under the author's charge. In our previous studies (Rutherford et al., 1977, 1978), we had already documented symptom rates for such patients at six weeks and at one year after injury; therefore, we decided to examine the symptom rate of a consecutive series of patients for whom medicolegal reports had been written for comparison. The full details of the study will be published shortly in the *Archives of Emergency Medicine,* and the methodology will be fully described there.

In comparing symptom rates among our general series and our litigation series, we wanted to establish whether there was any obvious bias in the selection of the litigation series that might account for the differences. It can be seen (Table 14–12) that as far as posttraumatic amnesia and sex are concerned, there is no difference between the two groups. The age distributions are different, but it will be noticed that the main difference is that those below 20 years of age are underrepresented in the litigation group. Our previous work did not suggest that this group had significantly different symptom rates from the group 20–40 years of age. The group over 40 years of age is slightly but not significantly overrepresented in the litigation group. As regards headaches and abnormal CNS signs at 24 hours, there is no significant difference. In our previous study, falls from a height appeared to be associated with higher symptom rates at six weeks, though not at one year. In this respect, the litigation series is significantly underrepresented in accidents from such falls, so that such bias as may exist is toward a lower late symptom rate in this series.

The early series on which we reported the symptom rates at six weeks and one year (Rutherford et al., 1977, 1978) did contain at least 6% of patients involved in litigation. Because it is possible that some cases so involved escaped our attention, we felt it safer to call this first series the "general" series. It is likely that a comparison between a litigation series with a series in which none of the patients was involved in litigation would show even more marked contrasts than are seen in this study.

In the litigation series we have documented symptom rates at three stages: (1) at the time of writing the medicolegal reports (mean 12.9 months post accident), (2) at the time of settlement (mean 22.1 months post accident), and (3)

**Table 14–12** Distribution of Posttraumatic Amnesia, Age, Sex, Headaches, and Abnormal CNS Signs at 24 Hours, and External Cause of Accident in Litigation Series and General Series

| | | Litigation series | General series | $\chi^2$, $p$ |
|---|---|---|---|---|
| Posttraumatic amnesia | 15 min | 21 (49%) | 41 (31%) | $\chi^2 = 4.350$ |
| | 15–59 min | 11 (26%) | 46 (35%) | d.f. 2 |
| | 60 min | 11 (26%) | 44 (34%) | $.2 > p > .1$ |
| | 20 yr | 4 (9.3%) | 43 (33%) | $\chi^2 = 9.198$ |
| Age | 20–40 yr | 22 (52%) | 47 (36%) | d.f. 2 |
| | 17 yr | 17 (40%) | 41 (31%) | $.02 > p > .01$ |
| Sex | M | 33 (75%) | 83 (63%) | $\chi^2 = 1.510$ |
| | | | | d.f. 2 |
| | F | 11 (25%) | 48 (37%) | $.3 > p > ./2$ |
| Headaches at 24 hr | Yes | 24 (69%) | 108 (74%) | $\chi^2 = 0.274$ |
| | No | 11 (31%) | 37 (26%) | $.7 > p > .6$ |
| | | | | d.f. 2 |
| Positive CNS signs at 24 hr | Yes | 5 (14%) | 40 (29%) | $\chi^2 = 2.353$ |
| | | | | d.f. 1 |
| | No | 30 (86%) | 99 (71%) | $.3 > p > .1$ |
| Caused by falls | Yes | 3 (6.8%) | 33 (23%) | $\chi^2 = 4.58$ |
| | | | | d.f. 2 |
| | No | 41 (93%) | 112 (77%) | $.05 > p > .02$ |

*Note:* In the litigation series, PTA was unknown in one case, and headaches and CNS signs were unknown in nine cases. In the general series, CNS signs were unknown in six cases.

one year later (mean 34.1 months post accident). Eighty-two percent of the patients had contacted their solicitor within two months of their accident.

At the time of writing the report, 57% of patients had symptoms; at the time of settlement, 39%; and one year later, 34% (Table 14–13). We were surprised to find that such a high percentage had already become symptom free before their report was written. Equally interesting was that a certain improvement was seen in the 9.2 months between report and settlement. We had frequently heard the view expressed that once the settlement was over, there would be a spectacular improvement. In our series a few cases did improve at this stage, but the improvement was relatively small.

On comparing the incidence of symptoms at the time of the report (57%) with that at six weeks in our general series (51%), there was virtually no difference (Table 14–13). The real difference was in the time interval from accident. A similar comparison between the symptom rate one year after settlement in the legal series (34%) with the symptom rate one year after accident in the general series (14.5%) shows the rate to be 2.3 times higher in the legal group, a finding confirmed as being highly significant.

It is clear that the symptom rates in the two series are different. The question remains, do patients with worse symptoms engage in litigation, or is the different outcome due to the strains and stresses generated by the experience of litigation? It was only at the end of our study that we realized how central

**Table 14–13** Distribution of Symptom Rates at Intervals after Injury in Litigation Series and General Series

| Litigation series | Sx | No Sx | General series | | $\chi^2, p$ |
|---|---|---|---|---|---|
| | | | *Sx | No Sx | |
| Litig. series at report (mean, 12.9 mo) | 25 | 19 | 74 | 71 | $\chi^2 = 0.251$ |
| General series at six weeks | (57%) | (43%) | (51%) | (49%) | d.f. 1 $.7 > p > .8$ |
| Litig. series at settlement (mean, 22.1 mo) | 16 | 25 | | | |
| | (39%) | (61%) | | | |
| Litig. series 1 yr after settlement | 14 | 27 | 19 | 112 | $\chi^2 = 7.17$ |
| General series at 1 yr | (34%) | (66%) | (14.5%) | (85.5%) | d.f. 1 $.01 > p > .001$ |

*Note:* Three cases are unsettled at the time of writing.

this question was. In our comparisons between the two series (Table 14–13), it can be seen that in the litigation series there are nine missing cases in the sections relating to headaches and abnormal CNS signs. The reason is that documentation of these aspects was not made compulsory at the start of the series. However, our previous work did identify several factors that were clearly associated with higher late symptom rates: These were (1) female sex, (2) headaches or abnormal CNS signs at 24 hours, and (3) falls from a height. The only one of these with a significantly different distribution between the two series is the falls, and in this case it should be associated with a lower incidence of symptoms in the litigation series. It is still conceivable that there is some other factor of which we are so far unaware, and that the litigation series suffers its higher symptom rates because of this bias. All that we can say at this point is that we have been unable to identify any such factor. Over 80% of our litigation patients had contacted their solicitors within two months. They presumably had been discussing the possibility of taking such action with friends and relatives from an even earlier stage. At this point, the majority of patients would be experiencing symptoms, yet they would not be able to predict whether their symptoms were likely to resolve quickly or not. Admittedly, those patients who are already symptom free in the very early period may be somewhat less likely to proceed with litigation, and this may result in some bias. However, we can see that having no concussion symptoms at the time of writing a report does not make patients pull out of litigation, and it is likely that those patients who feel that they have a just claim will not be deferred, even by having no concussion symptoms from the first day or two after injury. As well as questions of pain and suffering and loss of earnings, the decision to embark on litigation might be taken because of symptoms from coexisting injuries or damage to property.

Our earlier work (Rutherford et al., 1977, 1978) showed that psychological factors could influence late symptoms. There seems little doubt that being the object of litigation is an experience that causes considerable emotional strain. Even patients not involved in litigation find it difficult and embarrassing to try to explain to others the exact nature of their complaint. The embarrassment is increased for litigation patients if they feel that they are under suspicion of magnifying their conditions for the sake of their claims.

Tarsh and Royson (1985) have shown that such reactions are not limited to the patient, but extend to the family circle. Whereas outsiders are inclined to treat avowed symptoms with deep suspicion, the family reacts with total belief. As a result, roles inside a family are often reversed. The patient is now carried by the rest of the family, and a less dominant spouse will take over the leading role previously exercised by the patient. Once this pattern is established, it is difficult to reverse.

## CONCLUSIONS

1. Minor head injuries may give rise to morbidity which sometimes lasts for many years if not for life.
2. Late symptoms are caused by an interplay of organic and neurotic factors.
3. Treatment is mainly directed toward the prevention of a secondary neurosis, and this is best done by a physician who will care for the patient throughout the whole of his or her illness.
4. If litigation results in more than doubling the long-term symptom rate, then its justice is questionable.
5. The organic damage is irreversible. Doctors who treat patients with head injuries of any degree of severity should be deeply involved in preventive measures.

## REFERENCES

Amphoux M, Gagey P-M, Le Flem A, Pavy F. The development of the postconcussion syndrome. Rev Med Travail 5:53–75, 1977.

Brooks DN, McKinlay W. Personality and behavioural change after severe blunt head injury—a relative's view. J Neurol Neurosurg Psychiatry 46:336–344, 1983.

Ericksen JE. On Concussion of the Spine. London: Longmans Green, 1882.

Fee CRA, Rutherford WH. A study of the effect of legal settlement on postconcussion symptoms. Arch Emerg Med 4:159, 1987.

Field H. Correspondence on post-traumatic syndrome. J R Soc Med 74:630, 1981a.

Field H. Correspondence on post-traumatic syndrome. J R Soc Med 74:941–942, 1981b.

Gronwall D, Wrightson P. Delayed recovery of intellectual function after minor head injury. Lancet 2:605–609, 1974.

Guthkelch AN. Correspondence on post-traumatic syndrome. J R Soc Med 74:940, 1981.

Kelly R. The posttraumatic syndrome, an iatrogenic disease. Forensic Sci 6:17–24, 1975.

Kelly R. Correspondence on post-traumatic syndrome. J R Soc Med 74:630–631, 1981.

Lidvall HF, Linderoth B, Norlin B. Causes of the post concussional syndrome. Acta Neurol Scand 50:1–143, 1974.

MacFlynn G, Montgomery EA, Fenton GW, Rutherford WH. Measurement of reaction time following minor head injury. J Neurol Neurosurg Psychiatry 47:1326–1331, 1984.

McMillan TM, Glucksman EE. The neuropsychology of moderate head injury. J Neurol Neurosurg Psychiatry 50:393–397, 1987.

Merskey H, Woodforde, JM. Psychiatric sequelae of minor head injury. Brain 95:521–528, 1972.

Miller H. Accident neurosis. Br Med J 1:991–998, 1961.

Montgomery A, Fenton GW, McClelland RJ. The post-concussional syndrome. Lancet 1:1011, 1984.

Oppenheimer DR. Microscopic lesions in the brain following head injury. J Neurol Neurosurg Psychiatry 31:299–306, 1968.

Page HW. Injuries of the Spine and Spinal Cord. London: Churchill, 1885.

Rimel RW, Giordani B, Barth JT, Bell TJ, et al. Disability caused by minor head injury. Neurosurgery 9:221–228, 1981.

Rutherford WH, Merrett JD, McDonald JR. Sequelae of concussion caused by minor head injuries. Lancet 1:1–4, 1977.

Rutherford, WH, Merrett JD, McDonald JR. Symptoms at one year following concussion from minor head injuries. Injury 10:225–230, 1978.

Stuss DT, Ely P, Hugenholtz H, Richard MT, et al. Subtle neuropsychological deficits in patients with good recovery after closed head injury. Neurosurgery 17:411–447, 1985.

Tan N, Kakular BA. Pathology of head injuries. In Dinning TAR, Connelley TJ (eds), Head Injuries. Brisbane: John Wiley, 1981.

Tarsh MJ, Royston, C. A follow-up study of accident neurosis. Br J Psychol 146:18–25, 1985.

Trimble MR. Correspondence on post-traumatic syndrome. J R Soc Med 74:940–941, 1981.

Wrightson P, Gronwall D. Time off work and symptoms after minor head injury. Injury 12:445–454, 1981.

# 15

# Neuropsychological Recovery: Relationship to Psychosocial Functioning and Postconcussional Complaints

## SUREYYA S. DIKMEN, NANCY TEMKIN, AND GAY ARMSDEN

Patients with minor head injury commonly report problems with headache, dizziness, fatigue, irritability, and concentration soon after injury. By our definition of minor head injury, such patients show no objective neurological deficits. Consistent with the severity of the head injury, the majority of the patients (including those with early symptoms) recover satisfactorily. The fact that a sizable minority of patients complain of persisting and disabling problems—postconcussional syndrome (PCS)—has raised questions concerning the etiology of their symptoms.

For some time, the view was generally accepted that very few minor head injury patients reported postconcussional symptoms (PCS) beyond one month post injury. This view has been contradicted by studies of consecutive cases which indicate that PCS are indeed reported for one year or longer after injury (Cartlidge, 1977; Rutherford et al., 1979). Various avenues of investigation have been undertaken to explain the persistence of PCS. Possible psychological and motivational factors, especially litigation, have been cited as causes of continued PCS in the absence of neurological deficits (Miller, 1961). This lack of correspondence between severity of injury and persistence of symptoms has been cited to support a psychogenic etiology of PCS.

Contrary to the view that emotional disturbance and/or motivation for compensation primarily contribute to the morbidity of minor head trauma, there is evidence of neuropathological and neurophysiological alterations after these injuries, including neuronal damage, reduced cerebral blood flow, altered brainstem evoked potentials, and reduced speed of information processing (Gronwall, 1976; Gronwall and Wrightson, 1975, 1981; Jane et al., 1985; Noseworthy et al., 1981; Oppenheimer, 1968; Schoenhuber and Gentilini, 1986, and Chapter 9, this volume; Taylor and Bell, 1966). Gronwall (1976) demonstrated an association between improved information-processing speed on the Paced Auditory Serial Addition Test (PASAT) and reduction in postconcussional symptoms in patients whom she serially studied after minor head injury. This finding, together with evidence of a broad spectrum of neuropsychological and psychosocial problems as late as three months post injury (Barth et al., 1983; Rimel et al., 1981), have bolstered arguments for an organic etiology of PCS. However, recent neuropsychological studies that have included control groups and head-injured samples without preexisting conditions have concluded that by one to three months after minor head injury there is little evidence of cognitive impairment (Gentilini et al., 1985; Levin et al., 1987).

Given these inconsistencies in the literature on neurobehavioral sequelae of minor head injury, methodological differences among the studies need to be evaluated as a contributing source. At the same time, more systematic efforts need to be made in the direction of identifying deficits due to head injury, the natural history of recovery, and factors contributing to the persistence of problems in some individuals.

The remaining sections of this chapter are focused on our work concerning minor head injury. The chapter is organized to address the following questions: (1) What are the neuropsychological and psychosocial consequences of minor head injury and are these time contingent? (2) What are some of the factors that contribute to psychosocial consequences and to reporting of postconcussional symptoms? and (3) How do these results relate to the broader issues of conceptualizing disability and postacute treatment following minor head injury?

## NEUROPSYCHOLOGICAL AND PSYCHOSOCIAL CONSEQUENCES

### Neuropsychological Consequences

The Behavioral Outcome in Head Injury Project at the University of Washington, funded by the National Center for Health Services Research, has produced two studies dealing with minor head injury (Dikmen et al., 1986a; McLean et al., 1983). The subjects for both minor head injury studies (which involved partial overlap in samples) were drawn from the larger sample of 102 head injury cases studied and described elsewhere (Dikmen et al., 1986b; McLean et al., 1984). The larger sample was drawn from consecutive head-injured patients who were hospitalized at Harborview Medical Center. In terms of severity, the selection criteria included any period of coma or post-traumatic amnesia of at least one hour, or objective evidence of cerebral trauma (e.g., positive neurological signs). Case selection was limited to subjects without preexisting neurological and neuropsychiatric conditions. A comparison group, also screened for preexisting conditions, was selected from friends of the controls. The age range was between 15 and 60 years for both groups. All subjects were English speaking.

The study by McLean et al. (1983) included 20 head-injured patients and 52 controls who were uninjured friends of head trauma patients studied at our center. The 20 head-injured persons were selected from the total series of 102 patients on the basis that they had to be sufficiently neurologically intact to undergo testing three days post injury. In a strict definitional sense, some patients in this group sustained more severe trauma than minor head injuries; however, their injuries were mild enough to be testable at three days post injury. (Details of the injury severity are reported by McLean et al.) The mean age and education of the head-injured group were 23.25 and 12.20 years, respectively. The corresponding values for the controls were 22.83 and 12.51 years. A brief battery of cognitive tasks that included the Selective Reminding Test of verbal memory (Buschke, 1973) and the Stroop Color Test (Dyer, 1973; Stroop, 1935) was administered to the 20 head-injured subjects at three and at 30 days post injury. The control subjects were tested once.

Neuropsychological scores obtained at three and at 30 days post injury were compared with the scores of the control group (Table 15–1). The results on the Stroop Test indicated significant difficulties at three days post injury on the more difficult portion of the test (Part II) which requires the ability to inhibit responding to competing stimuli, but not on Part I which simply requires reading printed words. However, no significant differences were found at one month post injury. The results on the Selective Reminding Test indicated impaired memory in the head-injured patients at three days, but not at one month post injury. Although the one-month comparisons were not statis-

**Table 15–1**  Mean Test Scores at Three-Day and One-Month Testings

|  | | Head injured | |
| --- | --- | --- | --- |
| *Tests* | Controls at one month ($N = 52$)[a] | At three days ($N = 20$) | At one month ($N = 20$) |
| *Stroop Color Test* | | | |
| Part I | 39.48 | 50.82 | 42.36 |
| Part II | 91.58 | 124.54* | 99.43 |
| *Selective Reminding Test* | | | |
| Sum recall | 87.33 | 71.45‡ | 84.30 |
| Sum, long-term retrieval | 82.85 | 58.30‡ | 76.20 |
| Sum, long-term storage | 85.69 | 66.40‡ | 78.75 |
| Sum, consistent long-  term retrieval | 73.90 | 40.65† | 68.65 |
| Immediate recall | 9.46 | 6.95‡ | 9.15 |
| Immediate recognition | 9.98 | 9.45† | 9.95 |
| Delayed recall[b] | 8.48 | 6.77 | 7.40 |
| Delayed recognition | 9.94 | 9.71 | 10.00 |

[a]The sample size for the Stroop Color Test was smaller than for the other measures. The test was administered to 42 control subjects, 11 head-injured patients at three days after injury and to 14 head-injured patients at one month after injury.

[b]The length of the delay for the Selective Reminding Test was different for the two examination periods. For the three-day examination the delay was 10 minutes, whereas for the one-month examination the delay was 30 minutes.

*$p < .01$, †$p < .001$, ‡$p < .0001$; significance levels of Wilcoxon Rank Sum Test comparing controls with head-injured patients at three-day and one-month testings.

*Source:* McLean et al. (1983).

tically significant, there was an obvious trend for the head injury cases to perform slightly worse than the controls.

The second study (Dikmen et al., 1986a) included 20 cases who fulfilled the following selection criteria for severity of head injury: (1) any period of coma not exceeding one hour, or, if no coma, posttraumatic amnesia of at least one hour; (2) a Glasgow Coma Scale (GCS) score greater than 12 on admission; and (3) no clinical evidence of cortical or brainstem contusion. Seven of the 20 subjects were also subjects in the McLean et al. (1983) study. The 1986 study employed an extensive battery of neuropsychologial and psychosocial measures given at one month and at 12 months post injury. Of the 20 cases examined at one month, one was lost to follow-up at one year. In this study, uninjured friends serving as controls were individually matched to the head-injured patients on sex, age, and education, and were given an identical battery of measures with the same test–retest interval.

Table 15–2 presents the median neuropsychological test scores of the head injured at one month post injury and of the uninjured subjects. The measures

**Table 15–2**   Median Scores on the Neuropsychological Measures. One-Month Evaluations

|  | Score refers to | HI | Uninjured |
|---|---|---|---|
| *Motor and psychomotor* | | | |
| Finger tapping speed D | No. of taps in 10 sec | 51 | 50 |
| Finger tapping speed ND | No. of taps in 10 sec | 45 | 48 |
| TPT[a] total time | time per block (sec) | .36 | .33 |
| | | | |
| *Attention, flexibility, and quickness* | | | |
| Speech Sounds Perception | No. errors | 5 | 4 |
| Seashore Rhythm | No. correct | 26 | 28* |
| Trail Making Test A | time to complete (sec) | 20 | 20 |
| Trail Making Test B | time to complete (sec) | 58 | 51 |
| | | | |
| *Memory and learning* | | | |
| Wechsler Memory Scale (WMS) | | | |
| Logical Memory—Immed. | verbal units recalled | 11 | 11 |
| Log. Mem.—Delay 30 min | the same 30 min later | 9 | 9 |
| Visual Reproduction Immed. | spatial units recalled | 13 | 13 |
| Vis. Reprod.—Delay 30 min | the same 30 min later | 11 | 12 |
| Associate Learning—Easy | No. pairs recalled | 18 | 18 |
| Associate Learning—Hard | No. pairs recalled | 8 | 10 |
| Selective Reminding Test | | | |
| Total recall | No. words recalled (max 100) | 84 | 85 |
| Consistent long-term retrieval | No. words recalled (max 100) | 68 | 65 |
| Delayed recall—30 min | No. words recalled (max 10) | 8 | 9 |
| Delayed recall—4 hr | No. words recalled (max 10) | 7 | 9* |
| | | | |
| *Reasoning* | | | |
| Category Test | No. errors | 26 | 24 |

[a]Tactual Performance Test
*P < .05.
*Source:* Dikmen et al. (1986a).

cover a broad spectrum of functions including attention, memory, motor skills, and reasoning.

The results indicate that the performances of both the head-injured and control groups are quite intact by any standard. There is, however, a trend for the head injured to perform slightly less adequately than the uninjured controls. Group differences on Seashore Rhythm, a measure of sustained attention, and the four-hour delayed recall trial of the Selective Reminding Test reached statistical significance. All group differences were nonsignificant at one year post injury.

These neuropsychological findings are in general agreement with the results of other controlled studies, such as those by Gentilini et al. (1985) and Levin et al. (1987), and the data summarized by Ruff et al. (Chapter 12, this volume). All three studies either have found no difference or, when differences were reported, have indicated only mild and selective impairments by one to three months post minor head injury.

## Psychosocial Consequences and Postconcussional Complaints

The subjects in the Dikmen et al. (1986a) study were also given a battery of behavioral/psychosocial measures. This battery included the Sickness Impact Profile (Bergner et al., 1976), a Head Injury Symptom Checklist, and a Modified Function Status Index (Patrick et al., 1973; Reynolds et al., 1974). These

**Figure 15–1** Mean percent dysfunction on the Sickness Impact Profile (SIP). (Reproduced from Dikmen et al., 1986a, by permission)

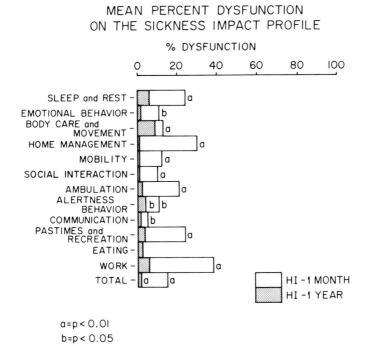

MEAN PERCENT DYSFUNCTION
ON THE SICKNESS IMPACT PROFILE

% DYSFUNCTION

a=p< 0.01
b=p< 0.05

measures rely on the subjects' report of changes in functioning or performance due to head injury and health.

Figure 15–1 presents the mean percent dysfunction of the head-injured subjects at one month and 12 months post injury on the Sickness Impact Profile. The mean percent dysfunction scores for the controls were zeros, and therefore are not presented. The results indicate considerable dysfunction at one month across different categories of functioning, ranging from basic physical abilities to higher-level performance such as major role activities and social interactions. Definite improvements are noted in all areas of psychosocial functioning among the head injured over the one year postinjury period. Also noteworthy is the finding that at both one month and 12 months, cognitive and emotional difficulties were among the less frequently endorsed problem areas.

With respect to resumption of work and leisure activities (as represented on portions of the Function Status Index), most patients were limited in both of these areas at one month post injury (Table 15–3). By one year, however, most minor head injury patients had resumed both work and leisure activities. Although a 10% unemployment rate among the head injured at one year may seem high, it is the same rate as that for the controls who were working at the one-month examination but not at 12 months.

Figure 15–2 shows the percentage of head-injured subjects endorsing various posttraumatic symptoms at one month post injury, compared with controls. These results indicate that head-injured patients endorse a substantial number of symptoms. Equally interesting is the finding that these symptoms are also reported by uninjured controls, although to a lesser extent.

## CONTRIBUTORS OF PSYCHOSOCIAL DISRUPTION AND POSTCONCUSSIONAL SYMPTOMS

The results of our psychosocial assessments suggest that HI patients at one month post injury display significant and major disruption of their everyday

**Table 15–3**   Resumption of Major and Other Activities

| Modified function status index | One month | One year |
|---|---|---|
| *Return to major activity* | | |
| With no limitations | 4 | 15 |
| With limitations | 4 | 2 |
| No return | 9 | 2[a] |
| Could not determine—summer | 2 | 0 |
| | | |
| *Resumption of leisure/recreational activity* | | |
| With no limitations | 3 | 12 |
| With limitations | 15 | 6 |
| No resumption | 1 | 0 |
| No resumption, not injury related | 0 | 1 |

[a]One of the two HI patients who had not returned at one year, had problems that were not head injury related.

*Source:* Dikmen et al. (1986a).

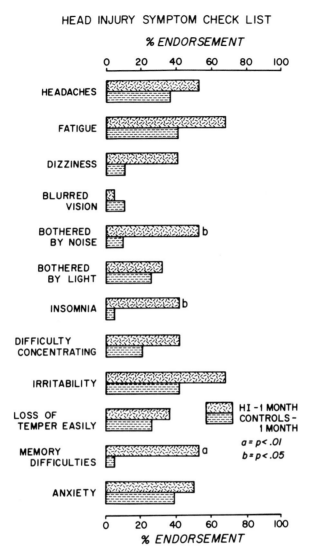

**Figure 15–2**  Median percent endorsement on the Head Injury Symptom Checklist. (Reproduced from Dikmen et al., 1986a, by permission)

life in numerous areas including work and leisure, and they also endorse many postconcussional symptoms. The magnitude of the psychosocial difficulties and postconcussional symptoms exceed what would be anticipated on the basis of the neuropsychological impairments presented earlier on the same subjects.

In light of this unexpected disability, factors contributing to psychosocial disruptions in three areas were also examined: work, leisure, and postconcussional symptoms. With respect to disruption of work and leisure, at one month post injury there appears to be a strong detrimental effect of other system injuries sustained in the same accident (Table 15–4). For instance, 1 of the 8 patients with isolated head injury had not returned to work or school, and 9

**Table 15-4**  Contribution of Other System Injuries (e.g., Orthopedic and Soft Tissue Injuries) at One Month Post Injury

|                        | HI only | HI + other injuries |
|------------------------|---------|---------------------|
| *Work/School*          | (8)     | (11)                |
| Not applicable         | 0       | 1                   |
| Without limitations    | 3       | 1                   |
| With limitations       | 4       | 0                   |
| Not doing              | 1       | 9                   |
| *Leisure activity*     | (8)     | (11)                |
| Without limitations    | 3       | 0                   |
| With limitations       | 5       | 10                  |
| Not doing              | 0       | 1                   |

*Source:* Dikmen et al. (1986a).

of the 11 patients who sustained head injury concomitantly with other system injuries had not resumed their prior major activity. Neuropsychological functioning, however, did not appear to differentiate those who did and those who did not return to work.

Also examined was the contribution of several different sets of variables to the occurrence of postconcussional symptoms reported by patients as newly occurring or worse than baseline. High (6+) and low (≤5) symptom reporters, based on one-month data, were compared on preinjury, injury, and postinjury characteristics. Given the small sample size and the number of variables examined, the results need to be interpreted very cautiously. Several *trends* are noteworthy, however, and have some support from other reports in the literature based on research or clinical impressions.

No significant differences between the high versus low symptom reporters were found on preinjury characteristics that included age, education, sex, job stability, and job skill level. However, a trend was evident for the high symptom reporters to be somewhat older and less educated, and to have lower job skill levels. The severity of the head injury, as assessed by posttraumatic amnesia, was not significantly different in high versus low symptom reporters. Although the high endorsers had fewer other system injuries (38% vs. 70% for the low symptom endorsers), this disparity also fell short of statistical significance. A trend for high symptom endorsers to have returned to work earlier and to be emotionally more distressed was nonsignificant.

Although severity of head injury did not distinguish the high symptom reporters, they consistently performed below the low symptom reporters on neuropsychological tests. Statistically significant differences between the high and low symptom endorsers were found on several measures at both one month and 12 months post injury. The less adequate neuropsychological functioning of the high symptom endorsers is important and warrants further investigation. The critical question, of course, is whether or not the lower neuropsychological performance of patients reporting substantial symptoms was caused by or preceded the injury. Given the small sample size and lack of *ade-*

*quate* premorbid information, no firm conclusions could be drawn from these results. However, there are several findings (e.g., lower educational and job skill levels) that would support the contention that a lower level of functioning may have preceded the injury in patients who subsequently reported high levels of symptoms. Furthermore, the similar curves of improvement in neuropsychological functioning for the high and low symptom groups over the one-year postinjury period is consistent with a comparable severity of head trauma.

## DISCUSSION

There is growing evidence for neuropathological, neurophysiological, and neuropsychological changes in patients with minor head injury. However, these changes (at least the neuropsychological sequelae) appear to be time contingent. Our results indicate that minor head injury is associated with neuropsychological difficulties within days of injury. By one to three months post injury, the neuropsychological effects of a single, uncomplicated minor head injury in previously healthy young people are selective and subtle. This generalization probably applies to the majority, but not to all cases. These early changes represent the *subacute* effects of minor head injury. The results of our studies and those of other controlled investigations support this contention (Gentilini et al., 1985; Gronwall and Wrightson, 1974; Levin et al., 1987). Overinterpretation of results and methodological artifacts (e.g., high attrition, with those followed constituting the nonrecovered cases; no comparison group) need to be considered as potential explanations for claims of major and continued neuropsychological deficits beyond three months in consecutive, unselected cases. Major disruptions in psychosocial functioning such as work and leisure are seen, but these types of activities appear to be strongly influenced by the presence of other system injuries.

Information regarding the natural history of recovery from PCS is less conclusive. There is no doubt that PCS are common, and although these symptoms decline with time, they appear to persist in a number of cases beyond one month post injury (as indicated by our results and those of others). A small number of patients fail to recover within the time frame common to the majority of the cases and go on to present persistent *chronic* effects of minor head injury. These are the cases difficult for clinicians to understand and treat, and not the majority of minor head injury patients who may show acute, time-limited effects. Patients with chronic sequelae have also been the source of much controversy regarding an organic versus psychogenic etiology for persistent complaints.

The major research and clinical emphasis in minor head injury has been on neuropathological, neurophysiological, and neuropsychological changes. The implied model of causation in these investigations is a medical one, which assumes that physical or objective signs underlie the problems reported by or observed in patients with minor head injury. The results of such investigations have shown that there are indeed objective/physical changes. Although these findings have helped us to understand possible mechanisms responsible for the acute effects, they have made only limited contributions toward elucidating or resolving the dilemma of patients with chronic effects. The problem is that the injury model is overly simplistic when applied to patients with chronic sequelae. Whereas early PCS may be caused by subtle effects of brain damage or disruptions of brain functions, persistent symptoms probably have as their origins multiple factors including preexisting individual vulnerabilities, head injury-related losses, reactions of others to those losses, litigation, etc. In this vein, Rutherford et al. (1979) have suggested that PCS are caused and maintained by the interaction of organic and psychological factors; psychological factors may prevent the resolution of originally organically based symptoms or produce new symptoms. Other investigators have supported the view that psychological factors are important in contributing to PCS (Binder, 1986; Levin et al., 1982; Lishman, 1973), but this conclusion appears to be drawn from eliminating the contributions of other variables rather than through direct evidence from research studies.

The reason for the emphasis on "objective" findings in research or clinical endeavors likely derives from the problems of measurement of personality and emotional factors. In determining the effects of head injury, the task confronting the clinician and the researcher alike is to ascertain whether or not the functioning of the individual is impaired and, if so, whether the head injury caused it. The emphasis on objective neuropsychological or neurological measures reflects the fact that these types of measures are more face valid, widely acceptable, and easier to obtain and communicate than indices of psychosocial adjustment. Neuropsychological measures are relatively straightforward and have guidelines for determining which patients are impaired and which are nonimpaired; the cause of the impairments, if present, is usually assumed to be central nervous system related.

In contrast, measurement of personality and emotional factors is more complex. The available measures are sufficiently transparent that patients can feign difficulty; there is no general agreement on what constitutes "impaired" functioning; there is even less willingness to attribute emotional or personality styles to the head injury. Despite the advantages of studying neuropsychological or neurological factors rather than personality or emotional ones, there are several shortcomings of this line of inquiry. First, there is no close correspondence between objective (e.g., head injury severity) neurological or neuropsychological findings and persistent PCS or distress. Second, even if neuropsychological or neurological impairments are established, it does not necessarily mean that the head injury produced them or caused the PCS. Our findings relating to neuropsychological performance in high versus low symptom reporters raise a cautionary note regarding attribution of cause. The mildly injured patient with long-persisting PCS and disabilities, despite negative neurological and neuropsychological findings, presents a formidable clinical challenge. In some of these cases, the most prominent and disabling difficulties are emotional in nature. Although this is not an unusual observation, and although personality and emotional factors have been implicated in the genesis of posttraumatic syndrome, this line of inquiry has not been pursued sufficiently. Despite the difficulties, further exploration of emotional factors is necessary.

## FUTURE DIRECTIONS

First and foremost, concerted efforts should be directed to educate the patients to prevent the development of persisting and secondary complications. More research is needed to identify persons at high risk for persistent PCS, emotional distress, and disability, as these persons should receive more intensive preventive work. Our preliminary findings and those of Rutherford et al. (1979) suggest certain characteristics that may predispose certain individuals to excessive or persistent PCS. It is important to note that these preliminary findings are not idiosyncratic to head injury. In examining the literature of other disciplines, certain characteristics of the high symptom reporter emerge. Those characteristics include older age, female gender, low socioeconomic class, ineffective coping style, poor social suport network, low social competence, low self-esteem, and negative labeling of stressful or ambiguous events (Pennebaker, 1982).

Second, even though the problem is complex, more concerted effort is needed to separate the truly distressed from those few that are malingering. Furthermore, the negative connotations that have come to be associated with "psychological," "psychogenic," or "neurotic" factors need to be dispelled. Attempting to better understand why certain patients are at high risk and the process by which they become disabled may guide efforts to prevent disabilities from developing and to treat those patients who have developed them. Constructs such as coping skills and social support are more positive than global psychiatric classifications (e.g., neurotic) and lend themselves to more specific intervention strategies.

Third, from a treatment perspective, perhaps we need to borrow some ideas or models used by other disciplines. The treatment approach taken by pain clinics around the country offers an excellent example. The problems of pain patients are quite analogous to those of minor head injury patients. Both types of patients endure pain, suffering, and disability in the face of oftentimes negative physical/neurological findings. The strategy of pain clinics has been not to focus on the legitimacy of the patients' complaints, but rather to approach the problem of suffering, pain, and disability from a broader rehabilitation perspective. More effective pain programs recognize the difference between pain and suffering. Such a perspective involves identifying factors contributing to the suffering and disability and applying behavioral methods to increase activities and reduce excessive disability (Fordyce et al., 1985).

## ACKNOWLEDGMENTS

This work was supported by Grant Nos. HS 04146 and HS 05304 from the National Center for Health Services Research, Office of the Assistant Secretary of Health. We thank Joan Machamer for her invaluable assistance in various aspects of our studies including careful review of the manuscript.

## REFERENCES

Barth JT, Macciocchi SN, Giordlani B, Rimel R, Jane JA, Boll TJ. Neuropsychological sequelae of minor head injury. Neurosurgery 13:529–533, 1983.

Bergner M, Bobbitt RA, Pollard WE, Gilson BE. The Sickness Impact Profile: validation of a health status measure. Med Care 14:57–67, 1976.

Binder LM. Persisting symptoms after mild head injury: a review of the postconcussive syndrome. J Clin Exp Neuropsychol 8:323–346, 1986.

Buschke H. Selective reminding for analysis of memory and learning. J Verb Learn Verb Behav 12:543–550, 1973.

Cartlidge NEF. Post-concussional syndrome. Scott Med J 23:103, 1977.

Dikmen S, McLean A, Temkin N. Neuropsychological and psychosocial consequences of minor head injury. J Neurol Neurosurg Psychiatry 49:1227–1232, 1986a.

Dikmen S, McLean A, Temkin N, Wyler A. Neuropsychologic outcome at one-month post injury. Arch Phys Med Rehab 67:507–513, 1986b.

Dyer FN. The Stroop phenomenon and its use in the study of perceptual cognitive, and response processes. Mem Cognit 1:106–120, 1973.

Fordyce WE, Roberts AH, Sternbach RA. The behavioral management of chronic pain: a response to critics. Pain 22:113–125, 1985.

Gentilini M, Nichelli P, Schoenhuber R, Bortolotti P, Tonelli L, Falasca A, Merli G. Neuropsychological evaluation of mild head injury. J Neurol Neurosurg Psychiatry 48:137–140, 1985.

Gronwall D. Performance changes during recovery from closed head injury. Proc Aust Assoc Neurol 13:143–147, 1976.

Gronwall D, Wrightson, P. Delayed recovery of intellectual function after minor head injury. Lancet 2:605–609, 1974.

Gronwall D, Wrightson P. Cumulative effect of concussion. Lancet 2:995–997, 1975.

Gronwall D, Wrightson P. Memory and information processing capacity after closed head injury. J Neurol Neurosurg Psychiatry 44:889–895, 1981.

Jane JA, Steward O, Gennarelli T. Axonal degeneration induced by experimental non-invasive minor head injury. J Neurosurg 62:96–100, 1985.

Levin HS, Benton AL, Grossman RG. Neurobehavioral consequences of closed head injury. New York: Oxford University Press, 1982.

Levin HS, Mattis S, Ruff RM, Eisenberg HM, Marshall LF, Tabaddor K, High WM Jr., Frankowski RF. Neurobehavioral outcome following minor head injury: a three-center study. J Neurosurg 66:234–243, 1987.

Lishman, WA. The psychiatric sequelae of head injury: a review. Psychol Med 3:304–318, 1973.

McLean A, Jr. Temkin NR, Dikmen S, Wyler AR. The behavioral sequelae of head injury. J Clin Neuropsychol 5:361–376, 1983.

McLean A, Jr., Dikmen S, Temkin N, Wyler AR, Gale JL. Psychosocial functioning at 1 month after head injury. Neurosurgery 14:393–399, 1984.

Miller, H. Accident neurosis. Br Med J 1:919–925; 992–998, 1961.

Noseworthy JH, Miller J, Murray TJ, Regan, D. Auditory brainstem responses in postconcussion syndrome. Arch Neurol 38:275–278, 1981.

Oppenheimer DR. Microscopic lesions in the brain following head injury. J Neurol Neurosurg Psychiatry 31:299–306, 1968.

Patrick DL, Bush JW, Chen MM. Toward an operational definition of health. J Health Soc Behav 14:6–23, 1973.

Pennebaker JW. The Psychology of Physical Symptoms. New York: Springer-Verlag, 1982.

Reynolds W, Rushing W, Miles D. The validation of a Function Status Index. J Health Soc Behav 15:271–288, 1974.

Rimel RW, Giordani B, Barth JT, Boll TJ, Jane JA. Disability caused by minor head injury. Neurosurgery 9:221–228, 1981.

Rutherford WH, Merrett JD, McDonald JR. Symptoms at one year following concussion from minor head injuries. Injury 10:225–230, 1979.

Schoenhuber R, Gentilini M. Auditory brain stem responses in the prognosis of late postconcussional symptoms and neuropsychological dysfunction after minor head injury. Neurosurgery 19:532–534, 1986.

Stroop JR. Studies of interference in serial verbal reactions. J Exp Psychol 18:643–662, 1935.

Taylor AR, Bell TK. Slowing of cerebral circulation after concussional head injury. Lancet 2:178–180, 1966.

# VI
**Disability and Rehabilitation**

# 16

# Management of Disability and Rehabilitation Services After Mild Head Injury

PHILIP WRIGHTSON

The development of current views on the nature of the symptoms that can follow mild head injury are described earlier in this book (e.g., see Benton, Chapter 1). Previous concepts are epitomized by the monograph of Lindval, Linderoth, and Norlin (1974). They concluded that there was no evidence of an organic defect of brain function and that the symptoms were psychogenic, owing to the stress and insult of the accident. The situation changed when it was recognized that the psychometry that had been used up to that time was only marginally sensitive to the effects of head injury. When appropriate tests were used, particularly those that measured the rate at which information could be processed, consistent changes were found, even in minor injuries, which related well to symptoms and clinical progress. This provided a convincing explanation for some of the symptoms and an expectation that others were similarly based.

The relation of the behavioral symptoms to the cognitive defects was clarified over the next few years. Studies of an unselected population with mild head injury (Rimel et al. 1981) and of a subsection of young physically fit men (Wrightson and Gronwall, 1981) showed that there was a group of symptoms that were common to the great majority of people after mild head injury. They were present at all ages, whether there were claims for compensation or not, and sportsmen were not exempt, as some had claimed. The reaction to these symptoms varied according to their severity and to the personality and circumstances of the victim, as would the response to any threat. The patient's state depended on the sum of the direct effect of injury and the reaction to it, and recovery on the separate resolution of each of these two factors.

A third factor of great clinical importance emerged as the effect of stress on cognitive performance. This had been shown in laboratory experiments

(Wrightsman, 1962) and was obvious in the clinical situation. The stress of being unable to cope diminished cognitive capacity, which made coping more difficult, and resulted in a spiral of deterioration.

On this basis, a philosophy of treatment could be developed. Activity was reduced to a level that cognitive capacity could manage, and increased only as function could be shown to improve. The reactions to incapacity were managed by counseling and support. No measure seemed to have a major effect on the rate at which cognitive capacity increased (Gronwall, 1986), and it seemed necessary to wait for recovery and to prevent complications while this occurred.

As these concepts developed, and the extent and cost of mild head injury became clear, it was apparent that traditional management had been ineffective medically and economically, and that is was worth setting up special facilities for treatment. Physicians and other health professionals, people injured, and the community at large needed to be educated, to recognize the symptoms, to know that help was available, and to treat the victim with understanding and compassion.

## CLINICAL PRESENTATION

Patients who have had a mild head injury present for help, suffering from symptoms that fall into three main groups:

### Acute Group

These symptoms are present immediately after the injury and continue for some days at least in about half of all people who have been concussed. Unless they are particularly severe or continue for more than two or three weeks, specialist advice is not usually sought. They are:

1. Headache, nausea, and general malaise
2. Dizziness, which may be true vertigo related to movement, but is often a term used by the patient to describe a sense of detachment and unreality
3. Irritability, and sensitivity to light and noise
4. Inability to concentrate, memory impairment, and lack of insight
5. Rapid fatiguability and a need for long hours of sleep

In addition there may be such neurological findings as anosmia, blurred vision, diplopia, or ataxia. These constitute a different aspect of the problem and will not be referred to again.

### Middle Group

These symptoms occur in a small proportion of people who have been concussed. Such patients commonly come for help one to several months after the injury. There is usually a history of symptoms of the acute group, but they may not have been severe. Groups of symptoms can be distinguished by the nature of the problems they present:

1. Change in behavior, shown by bad temper, irritability, and sensitivity to light and noise. Family and social relations deteriorate. Insight may be poor. There may be impotence.
2. Impairment of cognitive function, shown by poor concentration and memory, slow responses, and failure to cope with work.
3. Fatigue, which comes on after a predictable period of activity, and which cumulates rapidly if the activity continues. With its onset, the other symptoms increase in severity. Paradoxical insomnia may coexist with the fatigue.
4. Headache, due to scalp and neck injury, and also stress.
5. Reaction to these symptoms, in the form of depression, anger, or stress effects such as headache.

### Late Group

These symptoms are seen in a yet smaller group of people who have been living at a disadvantage for months or years after a mild head injury. They may present because they cannot cope with their work, owing to a specific cognitive deficit or fatigue, or because of family or social problems. There may be other symptoms of the middle group, but often the complaints are limited. The connection with injury may not have been realized; or, sometimes it has been endorsed by the patient but denied by physicians or insurers.

### DIAGNOSIS AND ASSESSMENT

The history of injury and the subsequent symptoms, which constitute a syndrome as constant as any in clinical medicine, will usually leave the diagnosis in little doubt. Formal neuropsychological testing will confirm it, will quantitate the general depression of cognitive function, and will reveal any areas of particularly marked deficit which may need special attention in management.

The common occasion of uncertainty is an excessive or atypical reaction to an undoubted injury, suggesting either preexisting emotional instability or malingering. The doubt can usually be resolved by the neuropsychological tests, which will show a disproportion between the deficits and the symptoms. Obvious inconsistencies within the tests will suggest frank malingering.

Patients with symptoms of the late group present the most difficulty in diagnosis. The connection with injury may be uncertain. The reaction to a long and puzzling disability may suggest that the symptoms were of psychiatric origin from the outset. In the negotiation for compensation, it may appear that the symptoms are being exaggerated. In coming to a decision, most weight will be placed on the result of neuropsychological testing. A clear deficit in one or more cognitive functions will support an organic origin. Well-documented evidence of a change in capacity at work or in home-making clearly related to an accident will be valuable. When the problem is predominantly one of family and social relations, or of fatigue alone, diagnosis may depend on the consistency of the history, and be difficult to demonstrate to someone not familiar with the syndrome.

## MANAGEMENT

### Principles

We postulate that the basis of the symptoms is that the primary neuronal damage disturbs cognition and emotion and, by a means as yet not understood, results in fatigue and an abnormal sleep pattern. Secondary to this incapacity follow anxiety, depression, and frustration, as would occur with any illness or threat to being. The third factor is the stress that results from the other two; stress increases the effect of the primary damage on function and creates a spiral of deterioration.

### Acute Stage

The general malaise requires relief of headache, nausea, and the pain of associated injuries. Demands on brain function are kept to a minimum. The circumstances of the accident and its consequences may need business or legal management, and it may not be appreciated that the patient is not able to cope with this properly, so that he or she may need both support and protection; impaired insight may add to the difficulties. Counseling about symptoms is needed but may not be tolerated.

### Middle Stage

The middle stage forms the major workload of mild head injury management. A full clinical diagnosis and certainly a complete neuropsychological assessment are not possible until the acute symptoms have receded. Counseling then becomes practical, for patients are then able to accept the reason for their symptoms and can begin to accept reassurance that they will improve. Group sessions with patients at all stages become important: Patients learn much more from each other than the professionals can teach them. When anxiety is a prominent feature, relaxation techniques are used.

Progress is followed by formal interview and observation in group sessions. Simpler tests, such as choice reaction times, are repeated regularly. The patient is kept well informed of the results. As capacity increases, physical and cognitive activities are stepped up, but symptoms are monitored carefully and tests are given to prevent overload, which is evidenced by fatigue, diminished performance, and falling test scores.

Eventually, activity related to normal work can be considered. Depending on its nature and the facilities available, this activity can be attempted either in the rehabilitation facility or at the normal workplace. It is vital that the hours of work be carefully controlled, and it may be necessary to begin with very limited periods, such as two hours three times a week (see below under Fatigue).

## The Patient and the Community

As the patient improves, a major problem emerges. He or she looks normal, and there is nothing apparent to family, friends, or employer as to why the patient cannot return to a normal life. Accusations of softness or malingering are in the air, even if not explicitly stated. This is very difficult for the patient to bear, and the stress it causes can be destructive. As patients commonly say, if their leg was in a cast, people would understand. It is useful to invite the family—and even the employer—to a group session, so that they can better understand what the problems really are.

## Specific Cognitive Rehabilitation

If the neuropsychological assessment demonstrates specific defects of memory or perception that are disproportionate to the general effects of MHI, the patient should attend special sessions directed to these problems.

## Fatigue

Probably the most important single factor that patients must deal with in returning to work is fatigue. At each stage, it is essential for the patient to work within the limits that fatigue imposes. As soon as fatigue exceeds a critical level, function deteriorates, stress accumulates, and symptoms such as headache, dizziness, and irritability reappear. If activity continues, fatigue grows at an increasing rate. To control the situation, the first move is to establish the maximum period of work that can be accomplished without bringing on symptoms. The target is to achieve this regularly each day, stepping up the target only when the patient can achieve a week at this rate with confidence.

Even in the best circumstances, this situation is fragile. One day the patient feels fine when reaching his or her target, and therefore decides to continue working and finish the job. Or, it may be the patient's own conscience—or his or her workmates, employer, or bank manager, on seeing a fit-looking person—who suggests that the patient can do that extra piece of work *if he or she really tries.* Pushed either internally or externally, the patient battles on, becomes fatigued, and experiences a recurrence of symptoms that had abated some time ago. He or she starts the next day without completely clearing the fatigue from the previous day. The patient now has to struggle to reach his or her target and finishes that day with an even greater debt of fatigue. Now caught in a vicious circle, the patient becomes progressively more exhausted over the next few days, until he or she is too tired even to begin the day. The trial has failed, and the patient must now return to the starting point, with a burden of depression and guilt adding to the stress and diminishing his or her capacity even further.

A warning of a regression of this sort will be evidenced by the patient's test results. These will have improved to a certain level before he or she was allowed to return to work, and the working hours will have been prescribed on this basis. If the patient holds to the prescribed hours, the test results usually continue to improve. If fatigue starts to accumulate, test scores fall off.

This process must be clearly explained to the patient; he or she must understand it and contract to accept responsibility for monitoring his or her own activity. If the patient manages successfully, so that symptoms do not return and test results remain good, the hours are increased slowly until a full day's work is achieved. The patient will, however, still be fragile, and difficulties at work, family stress, or a heavy social weekend can cause a setback. This may call for a reduction of working hours for a time, or even a few days of complete rest, to restore the patient's optimal level of functioning.

## SPECIAL CASES

### School Children

Traditionally there has been reluctance to ascribe longer-term changes in personality and school performance to the effects of mild head injury. Older studies, particularly in Newcastle and Sweden (Craft et al., 1972, and Rune, 1970, respectively) support this view, but more recent work, based on neuropsychological data, suggests that there may be important changes in the capacity to learn (Gulbrandsen, 1984). To us it has not seemed reasonable that children should be immune to the middle group of symptoms that we see in adults, and, allowing for the difficulties of neuropsychological testing in children, we have shown that they go through the same phases in the early weeks after injury (Ramsden, 1980). This places children at a special risk, because the fall in performance may earn them the label of "not trying." Though they may recover from their cognitive deficits, this label can become a self-fulfilling prophecy, especially in those who are already at a socioeconomic disadvantage. Long-term reduction of capacity after mild head injury, such as is seen in adults, has not yet been convincingly documented. Nevertheless, it is difficult to see why it should not occur, and it may be that problems are present but are masked by the great reserve of capacity that children possess.

It can be argued that children are at special risk of a more permanent deficit, different from that encountered by adults. The intensity of learning and the time factors of maturation may not have been sufficiently considered, especially in younger children. This problem is currently being studied by the author's colleagues, in a series of preschool children who have suffered a mild head injury (unpublished results). Tests that are known to be sensitive to head injury may show no initial defect, but six months or one year later, raw scores remain the same, indicating that capacities have failed to develop. Even if there is improvement later, the child may have missed a developmental step, and may not completely recover the lost ground.

When children are admitted to hospital after mild head injury, their parents should be seen, and these dangers explained. School teachers can be asked to watch for difficulties, and in many cases a follow-up psychometric assessment should be done one or two months later. There is particular concern about the children whose injuries have not been severe enough to require admission to hospital, whose parents have often escaped counsel. These children can come to light months later, with established problems, even though their original cognitive defect may have been slight.

### University Students

Young people in senior school and university depend on cognitive competence more than any other group, and mild head injury can have a catastrophic effect, especially if it comes at a critical time in the academic year. As a group they tend not to admit their deficiencies to begin with and often fail to take advice. When their problems become obvious, there may be a swing to depression and destructive decisions, causing them to abandon their studies. A counselor familiar with university requirements and a good liaison with the university authorities is needed. It may be possible to make allowances in examinations, either by allotting extra time or granting aegrotat (sick leave) passes.

### Executives and Professional People

Similar problems arise with executives and professional people. They need to make decisions based on multiple factors, to switch from problem to problem, to follow conversation around a group, and to work long hours under stress—classical areas of difficulty after a mild head injury. Often they return to work too soon, either not having had advice about the problems they may meet, or ignoring it. They find that they cannot cope, and neither they nor the people they work with understand what has happened. Destructive situations develop rapidly. They are often hard to counsel, resist advice, and do not fit in with the usual group sessions. The counselor should try to persuade them to follow the same course as other patients do: They should start with a period of rest, and return to work part-time, only when test results are satisfactory. A formal scheme of fatigue management should be followed. A rearrangement of the working day can be helpful, such as scheduling the most difficult decisions for the first few hours in the morning. The situation is, however, likely to be fragile and at the mercy of a business crisis, a late night, or a family argument, any of which can set them back weeks. They are particularly vulnerable to the "I can do it if I try harder" danger.

### Older People

Recovery will be much slower and less complete in older people, even for those in their 40s. Those who depend on cognitive function again are most affected. Fatigue is more of a problem. For patients in their late 50s or 60s, if there has been minimal progress over three or four months, the best advice may be to accept a long-term disability and to rearrange their life-style, with partial or complete retirement. It may make the change more acceptable if some of the positive features of the disability are emphasized: Experience, judgment, and wisdom are all intact; it is the demand for speed and endurance that cannot be met.

### Long-Term Reduction of Capacity

This is of course a familiar problem after severe head injury, but it can also follow minor injury, and some patients remain for long periods with a disability sufficient to prevent them from playing their full part. They may have been under observation from the time of their injury, or may have presented with the late group of symptoms described above, after a period in which the origin of their symptoms has been uncertain.

There may be deficits that make specific cognitive rehabilitation useful, but the important strategies for coping with everyday life are usually those of fatigue management. Provided these can be worked out, the patient can often live a reasonably productive life. An example of a typical case history follows.

> *Case.* A 24-year-old girl with a degree in economics worked as an actuary in an insurance company. After a mild head injury she tried to return to work but could not cope with her job because of fatigue and associated headache. The company agreed to let her work half-time to begin with. She could manage very well for four hours, but if she worked longer than this she would begin to make foolish mistakes. After the four hours she would drag herself home, sleep for two hours and then do little until an early bedtime. She had no social life, and if she was up late she could not cope with work at all the next day. Over two years she slowly increased her time at work. Now, three years after the injury, she works a full day but still has little energy left for social life. Throughout this time her employers have been very satisfied with her work, and her salary has been increased.

## SOURCES AND INCIDENCE OF MILD HEAD INJURY CASES

In the author's community there is no doubt that mild head injury results in substantial disability and economic loss. About 10% of people admitted to hospital for one or two nights of observation have symptoms that persist for two months, sufficient to impair their working capacity (Gronwall and Wrightson, 1974). Rimel et al. (1981), reporting on patients who had been in hospital for two nights, found that a third of those who had been employed before the injury were not back at work after three months.

Though it is established that these problems occur in people who are admitted to hospital for management of mild head injury, this is only part of the picture. Patients with skeletal and multiple injuries often have been concussed as well. This may be of little consequence in the acute stage, but the head injury may remain a problem when the other injuries have healed. Again, many patients with mild head injury are not admitted to hospital, and they too can develop late symptoms. In the literature there is no guide to the total inci-

**Table 16-1** Mild Head Injuries in an Eight Weeks' Sample of Four Hospitals (patients aged 15 years and over)

| | Eight Weeks | | | One Year[a] | | Rate Per 100,000[b] | |
|---|---|---|---|---|---|---|---|
| | Cases | CC[c] | % | Cases | CC | Cases | CC |
| Not admitted | 577 | 21 | 3.6 | 3750 | 137 | 439 | 16 |
| Admitted | | | | | | | |
| Primary HI (0–7 days' stay) | 22 | 3 | 14 | 143 | 20 | 17 | 2.4 |
| Associated with other injuries | 69 | 11 | 16 | 449 | 72 | 53 | 9.2 |
| Totals | 668 | 35 | 4.9 | 4342 | 229 | 511 | 27 |

[a]Obtained by multiplying the eight weeks' column by 52/8.
[b]The population of the area served is 850,000 (all ages).
[c]Attended concussion clinic.

dence; therefore, in 1986 over a period of eight weeks, the author's team recorded all accident department attendances in their area that had resulted from an injury above the level of the clavicles. The survey covered the four hospitals available to a population of 850,000. The nature of the injury, the management, and the outcome were noted. A year later, they studied the patients from this period who had presented to the concussion clinic with significant symptoms. Of course, there were other sources of care, and not everyone who had significant symptoms was identified, but what is probably a reliable lower limit of incidence was obtained.

The results are summarized in Table 16–1. Patients aged 15 and over are listed because it is this age range that is seen in the concussion clinic. Of the patients who were not admitted to hospital, all had complained of significant neurological symptoms after the injury, such as severe headache, giddiness, and nausea, and had been observed to be disorientated or ataxic; in 43%, a period of unconsciousness had been observed or there had been a substantial loss of memory typical of posttraumatic amnesia. It is evident that though the likelihood of significant symptoms is small after the more minor injuries, cases from this source provide the majority of the work of the clinic.

The cost of the disability in terms of lost wages, treatment, and insurance payments is not known; the study is continuing with the help of the accident insurers to try to quantify it. There is no doubt, however, that it is substantial and that it justifies a determined attempt to improve management.

## IDENTIFICATION AND COUNSEL OF PATIENTS AT RISK

To identify these cases, physicans and paramedical staff must be alert to the syndrome and know what services are available in their area. The public also must be educated. Few patients find that their workmates, or even their families, understand the nature of their problems. It is difficult for most people to accept that what seems a trivial injury can cause persisting symptoms—especially when the victim looks physically well. Many of the mild injuries result from sport, and thus clubs and controlling bodies should be encouraged both to make their sport safer and to understand and help players who have been injured. In the author's community, the accident insurers have distributed to these organizations a booklet on prevention and management, which has been well received.

The other arm of the approach is to educate patients themselves about the symptoms they may experience, about how to cope with them, and what to do if they persist. Though simple in concept, this requires considerable organization.

Patients who have been admitted to hospital can usually be seen, together with their relatives, and counseled. A permanent reminder however is useful, and it is the author's practice to give patients a small booklet that summarizes the situation. It is more difficult to help those who are not admitted. Few accident services have the staff to counsel everyone with a minor injury, and in any case shortly after the injury most patients are not in a state to benefit from it. Some services arrange a follow-up visit after two or three days, and the situation can be explained then. Others find this impossible; giving out a booklet before discharge can then be a useful substitute. In practice, patients seem to find this helpful. The incidence of symptoms remains the same, but patients feel more secure and escape some of the anxiety usually experienced (unpublished observations).

It would be ideal to follow all patients after a few weeks. Whether this is practical will depend on the facilities available and the compliance of the population. In the author's practice, the number of patients with minor injuries who will attend is small. For routine recall, patients are selected who are at special risk—for example, schoolchildren and older people. This practice may be more useful than trying to see everyone.

Are there risks in patient education, follow-up, and specialist treatment? Is a ready-made scenario being presented to the malingerer or the neurotic? This is possible, but the policy should have the advantage of bringing them under the care of an experienced team. With psychometric tests and access to a psychiatric opinion, the diagnosis should be clear and effective management possible.

## ORGANIZATION OF A CONCUSSION CLINIC

A clinic concentrating on the treatment of the effects of mild head injury has substantial advantages: The syndrome is not widely understood, and therefore, research and teaching are important. Several disciplines are involved and must be coordinated. Access to a variety of rehabilitation opportunities is essential. Finally, support of patients and families needs to be organized.

The team with which the author is associated sees about 350 new patients a year, two-thirds of them referrals after recent injury. The team consists of a full-time neuropsychologist who plays the major part in clinical diagnosis and management, and is assisted by a variable number of students from the university's department of psychology working for master's or doctoral degrees. Medical aspects, both clinical and medicolegal, are covered by a physician (the author) one day a week. A psychiatrist attends one morning a week. There is ready access to the occupational therapy department. The medical social worker plays a vital role, and the Accident Compensation Corporation sends a representative to help patients with claims half a day per week. Patient support is completed by the Head Injury Society, an organization set up by families, which meets in the clinic after working hours once a week.

As an experimental, research-based organization, the clinic has always been short of funds and staff, and the present facilities are less than the minimum desirable. Anyone planning to set up such a clinic should try to achieve a substantially higher staffing rate.

## SUMMARY

The policy used to manage mild head injury patients and in getting them to return to work involves encouraging the patient to rest in the early stage and to increase activity slowly, being guided by clinical observation and test results, while paying great attention to the limitations imposed by the fatigue syndrome. The symptoms that occur after mild head injury are threatening and alarming to most patients, and the resulting stress is a major factor in reducing their performance and in slowing recovery. It can be managed by support, counseling, and relaxation techniques. In some cases, specific cognitive rehabilitation is important in the later stages, with the patient working within the limits of fatigue. It is important to provide well-organized and expert facilities to manage this condition if both patient distress and the cost to the community are to be minimized.

### ACKNOWLEDGMENTS

Research and development of services described here were supported by the Medical Research Council of New Zealand, the New Zealand Neurological Foundation, the Auckland Hospital Board and the Accident Compensation Corporation.

### REFERENCES

Craft AW, Shaw DA, Cartlidge NEF. Head injuries in children. Br Med J 4:200–203, 1972.
Gronwall D. Rehabilitation programs for patients with mild head injury: components, problems and evaluation. J Head Trauma Rehab 1:53–62, 1986.
Gronwall D, Wrightson P. Delayed recovery of intellectual function after minor head injury. Lancet 2:605–609, 1974.
Gulbrandsen GB. Neuropsychological sequelae of light head injuries in older children 6 months after trauma. J Clin Neuropsychol 6:257–268, 1984.

Lidvall HF, Linderoth B, Norlin B. Causes of the postconcussional syndrome. Acta Neurol Scand 50 (Suppl 56) 1974.

Ramsden RW. An investigation of cognitive deficits after mild concussion in children. Unpublished MA thesis, University of Auckland, 1980.

Rimel RW, Giordani B, Barth JT, Boll TJ, Jane JA. Disability caused by minor head injury. Neurosurgery 9:221–228, 1981.

Rune V. Acute head injuries in children: a retrospective epidemiologic, child psychiatric and electroencephalographic study on primary school children in Umea. Acta Paediatr Scand [Suppl] 209, 1970.

Wrightsman LS. The effects of anxiety, achievement, motivation and task importance on intelligence test performance. J Educ Psychol 53:150–156, 1962. *Cited in* Lezak M, Neuropsychological Assessment. New York: Oxford University Press, 1976, p 111.

Wrightson P, Gronwall D. Time off work and symptoms after minor head injury. Injury 12:445–454, 1981.

# 17

# Mild Head Injury in Sports: Neuropsychological Sequelae and Recovery of Function

JEFFREY T. BARTH, WAYNE M. ALVES,
THOMAS V. RYAN, STEPHEN N. MACCIOCCHI,
REBECCA W. RIMEL, JOHN A. JANE,
AND WILLIAM E. NELSON

Almost 45 years ago, Holbourn (1943) postulated the existence of "shear strain" of axonal and dendritic tissue, secondary to what is now described as rotational, acceleration/deceleration head trauma (Gennarelli, 1986; Gennarelli et al., 1981; Ommaya and Gennarelli, 1974). Only in the past seven years, however, has this theory of neurological impairment been utilized to explain the symptoms of mild head injury (postconcussive syndromes) (Alves et al., 1986; Boll and Barth, 1983). The symptoms of mild head injury usually include headaches, dizziness, memory loss, nausea, diplopia, tinnitus, personality change (irritability), attentional deficits, and information processing impairment. Although factors affecting rate and extent of recovery and persistence of symptoms continue to generate scientific debate, the popular press has characterized mild head injury as a "silent epidemic," which has subsequently drawn more attention to the potentially devastating cognitive, emotional, and economic consequences of this trauma (Barth et al., 1983; Rimel et al., 1981). In general, the public and scientific community have been slow to react to this rather common pathology, which results in hospitalization of close to 300,000 patients per year in the United States alone. Moreover, many more mild injuries occur that do not require extensive medical observation and intervention (Kraus et al., 1984).

Similar to the general public, competitive athletes are at risk for head injuries, but the evolving field of sports medicine is usually ahead of the general public in recognizing potential health problems for athletes and implementing corrective or protective strategies. For example, professional race car drivers were the first to wear seatbelts, and professional motorcycle racers wore helmets long before the general public took advantage of these protective devices.

In most sports, great efforts are made to evaluate and eliminate the potential for what is viewed as *significant or severe* head trauma. This has not, however, been the case with most sports-related *mild* head injuries. Until recently very little has been written about mild head trauma in sports because it was not seen as a major problem. Athletes typically do not complain about "minor injuries" because doing so would be a sign of weakness, and worse, might result in elimination from participation in upcoming competition. The ramifications of admitting to any injury include the possibility of losing one's position and scholarship (in collegiate sports); letting down the team, coaches, school, and fans; missing an opportunity to display one's skills to the professional agents and scouts; and being seen as a failure by oneself and one's friends and family. Because of our somewhat controversial and still limited knowledge of the effects of mild head injury and the negative consequences of athletes' admission of such problems, it is not surprising that mild head injury has not been a principal concern of most athletes or their institutions and organizations.

## HEAD TRAUMA IN BOXING

Although the potential effects of head injuries have generated little attention in some sports, moderate and severe head trauma have been studied in some depth in sports such as boxing (Morrison, 1986). Most studies of sports-related head injury have focused on boxing because it stands alone among other contact sports in having as its goal rendering opponents unconscious and helpless through successive blows to the head (Council on Scientific Affairs [AMA], 1983; McCunney and Russo, 1984). The earliest description in the literature on neurological, cognitive, and behavioral impairment resulting from boxing was provided by Martland (1928). In an article entitled "Punch Drunk," he delineated various neurological symptoms that characterize the syndrome, including mild confusion and an unsteady gait early on, which progresses to increased speech and motor latencies as well as upper-extremity and head tremors. Martland has stated that eventually this syndrome is characterized by a movement disorder similar to that seen in Parkinsonian patients, usually involving an extremely unsteady gait and considerable mental decline. Diffuse cerebral atrophy often occurs and has been variously labeled as "chronic boxers' encephalopathy" (Serel and Jaros, 1962), "dementia pugilistica" (Lampert and Hardman, 1984), and "traumatic boxers' encephalopathy" (Mawdsley and Ferguson, 1963).

### Mechanisms and Neuropathological Consequences of Acute Brain Damage

Lamper and Hardman (1984) describe four basic mechanisms that account for the neuropathological changes evidenced in acute brain damage from boxing and other contact sports. These include (1) rotational acceleration; (2) linear acceleration; (3) carotid injuries; and (4) deceleration upon impact. The authors state that rotational or angular acceleration, poses the most danger to a fighter, and typically occurs when he is groggy and most vulnerable. This pathological mechanism involves sudden acceleration of the head with subsequent rotational movement of the brain inside the skull, leading to the stretching and snapping of blood vessels. Paradoxically, protective head gear, such as the type worn by amateurs, tends to increase the inertial force of angular acceleration by increasing the surface size around the head (Timperley, 1982). Complications and lesions such as diffuse axonal injuries, subdural hematomas, and intracerebral hemorrhages may result from rotational force, depending upon the characteristics of the impact.

The second mechanism described is that of linear or translational acceleration, which results in focal cerebellar ischemic lesions (Lampert and Hardman, 1984). These lesions "develop a few days after repetitive trauma and their severity increases proportional to the number of subconcussive blows" (p. 2678).

Carotid artery injury resulting from blows to the neck can cause reflex hypotension and a subsequent brief period of dizziness due to diminished blood flow to the brain. This is a dangerous state for the boxer, who then is more vulnerable to significant head acceleration from an opponent's blow.

The final mechanism described by Lampert and Hardman is that of impact deceleration, which can occur when the dazed or knocked-out boxer hits the canvas or rope posts. This typically can result in occipital coup and frontotemporal contrecoup lesions. Clinically though, whatever the injury mechanism may be, these types of neurotrauma are complicated by the body's natural responses such as edema, ischemia, and possibly herniation of brain tissue within the skull (Lampert and Hardman, 1984; Serel and Jaros, 1962).

### Severity and Long-Term Effects

An important factor contributing to the severity of head trauma in boxing, particularly as this relates to long-term residual deficits, is the cumulative effects of multiple blows to the head, not necessarily resulting in knockouts. Casson et al. (1982) studied 10 professional boxers shortly following a knockout with electroencephalography (EEG), computed tomography (CT), and neurological examinations. These professional athletes, 20–31 years of age, had engaged in anywhere from two to 52 bouts. According to these authors, "All the boxers had mild head injuries by clinical criteria, with duration of loss of consciousness and posttraumatic amnesia of less than two minutes" (p. 172). Testing results, however, indicated that one boxer had an abnormal neurological examination, another two had abnormal EEGs, and five evidenced clearly abnormal CT scans with mild to moderate cerebral atrophy. These authors suggested that abnormalities that they detected were not due to the number of knockouts because no boxer had even been knocked out more than twice. Instead, they indicated that multiple subconcussive blows to the head was a much more plausible etiology.

Kaste et al. (1982) in one of the few neuropsychological studies, examined eight amateur and six professional boxers. Results showed that 86% of these boxers performed in the mildly impaired range on the Trail Making Test from the Halstead–Reitan Neuropsychological Test Battery, and two professional boxers demonstrated more severe neuropsychological difficulties. One boxer obtained very poor scores on the Digit Symbol Test from the Wechsler Adult Intelligence Scale, the Benton Visual Retention Test, and the Trail Making Test, whereas the other had performed poorly on the Wisconsin Card Sorting Test and the association learning subtest of the Wechsler Memory Scale. CT scans revealed "brain atrophy in 3 of 6 professionals and 1 of the 8 amateurs" (p. 1187). The authors concluded that the effects of repeated concussions are cumulative, and beyond a yet to be determined number of concussions, the neuropathology is likely to be irreversible.

Casson et al. (1984) studied 18 active and former boxers who underwent neurological examination, neuropsychological testing, EEG, and CT. They excluded subjects with a history of neurological impairment, psychiatric difficulties, or drug and alcohol abuse. All fighters, in addition, were active in the post-World War II era, indicating that they fought during a time when increased medical supervision became an issue of public concern. However, subjects in this study were not selected at random, limiting the generalizability of the results. According to these authors, 87% of all boxers exhibited abnormal findings on at least two of the four examinations. Each boxer scored within the impaired range on more than one neuropsychological measure which included the Trail Making Test, Digit Symbol Test, Wechsler Memory Scale, and recall of the Bender Visual–Motor Gestalt figures. They found that the percentage of abnormal neuropsychological test scores correlated significantly with abnormal CT scans, age, and the number of professional fights. These authors concluded that their study lends "further support to the direct relationship between length of professional boxing career and the presence of brain damage" (p. 2666).

### Mild Head Injury in Boxing

Relatively little is known about *mild* head injury in boxers although some previously cited studies such as that by Casson et al. (1982) refer to such trauma. Amateur boxers have generally had fewer bouts, rounds, and knockouts, and they usually weigh less and are more closely supervised than their professional counterparts. Because these factors have been shown to be directly related to severity (as well as chronicity) of neurobehavioral trauma, amateur and young professional boxers are the main focus of such mild head injury studies.

An early investigation by Blonstein and Clarke (1957) examined athletes who were knocked out more than once, or suffered severe concussions in the London Amateur Boxing Association during a seven-month period. They found that only 58% (N = 29) of all boxers active at that time fit their criteria. EEG and neurological examinations did not detect abnormalities, although the theory "that deleterious cerebral changes may occur in amateurs after an interval is a possibility that has by no means been excluded by this study" (p. 363). They raised an additional point, however, which is of some interest: that is, the importance of assessing retrograde and anterograde amnesia in boxers who were not rendered unconscious. These authors suggested that a classification of boxing head injuries according to degree of amnesia was potentially useful. Duration and severity of traumatic amnesia proved helpful in understanding and predicting the sequelae of head injury, and might be particularly useful with regard to mild head injury in boxing.

A more recent study examined neuropsychological, neurological, and EEG results in 53 former amateur boxers and a control group of 53 former amateur soccer players (Thomassen et al., 1979). Significant differences were not found between soccer players and boxers in the EEG or neurological examinations performed. Neuropsychological data showed that boxers evidenced significantly more dysfunction than the control group on measures of left-handed motor function, visuospatial intelligence, expressive speech, logical memory, phonetic analysis of numbers, and synthesis of letters in simple and complex words. Yet, after results were statistically corrected for age, education, and vocabulary, the only significant differences remaining between boxers and controls concerned left-handed motor dysfunction.

CT scan, EEG, and neurological evaluations of professional boxers in Italy were completed to facilitate early detection of cerebral atrophy. This study found significant correlations between CT scan and EEG findings but no evidence that neurological assessment was of diagnostic benefit (Sironi et al., 1982). Young boxers' career successes and failures were directly related to CT scan and EEG results (i.e., the higher the number of knockouts, the more impairment on these tests). Years of boxing activity and number of matches did not predict cerebral dysfunction.

Three very recent studies of young amateur and professional boxers utilized standardized neuropsychological test procedures in addition to other medical procedures to determine the effects of what may be considered mild to moderate head trauma (Brooks, 1987; Levin et al., 1987a; McLatchie et al., 1987). In the McLatchie et al. study of 20 active boxers, 1 had an abnormal CT scan, 7 had impaired neurological exams, 8 demonstrated abnormal EEG, and 9 out of 15 had deficient neuropsychological examinations. Because the boxers performed significantly more poorly than controls on several neuropsychological measures, the authors concluded that neuropsychological assessment is the most sensitive measure of neurologic dysfunction.

Brooks et al. (1987) and Levin et al. (1987a) on the other hand, found no significant neuropsychological deficits in their samples of amateur and young professional boxers and matched controls. They suggest that their results should be intrepreted cautiously because absence of neuropsychological deficits could be due to such factors as low frequency and duration of ring exposure and knockouts as well as the possibility of the delayed appearance of degenerative disorders such as Alzheimer's disease.

It is unclear what effect mild head injury has on immediate and long-term neuropsychological functioning in amateur boxers. Longitudinal studies of a wide range of amateur boxers with varying skills, levels of success, frequency of ring exposure, head and neck contacts, and knockouts must be initiated to address this question. Johns Hopkins University, supported by the United States Olympic Committee, is presently carrying out such research and hopes to control for additional factors such as premorbid cognitive and psychosocial functioning.

## FOOTBALL

Empirical attention has also been paid to football-related head trauma; however, like boxing, few controlled prospective studies are available in the scientific literature. Epidemiological, descriptive, retrospective, and case studies provide the basis for most of our understanding of football head injury.

The mechanisms of these injuries are similar to boxing trauma described by Lampert and Hardman (1984), and severity of impairment often appears to be related directly to number and recency of previous blows to the head or acceleration/deceleration injuries. Case studies such as those reported by Harbaugh and Saunders (1984) and Schneider (1973) demonstrate devastating cerebral injury characterized by widespread edema, midline shift, herniation, hemorrhage, and anoxic changes secondary to what appears to be relatively mild trauma if such trauma follows closely on the heels of previous mild head injury.

A retrospective study by Gerberich et al. (1983) of 103 Minnesota high school football teams, comprised of 3,063 varsity players who responded to mailed questionnaires, revealed a 19% loss of consciousness or awareness rate during the 1977 season. Sixty-nine percent of these concussed players returned to athletic competition the same day, but postconcussive symptoms were reported by some players up to nine months post season. Permanent disability was noted in six cases and "players with a prior history of loss of consciousness had a risk of loss of consciousness four times that of the player without a prior history" (p. 1370).

In 1979, Torg, Truex, Quedenfeld, Burstein, Spealman, and Nichols published results from the National Football Head and Neck Injury Registry which began collecting data in 1971 on football injuries that involved "hospitalization for more than 72 hours, surgical intervention, fracture-dislocation, permanent paralysis or death" (p. 1477). There were 1,129 injuries that met these severe head and neck injury criteria, and over that time period the rate of intracranial hemorrhage decreased, presumably owing to the development of better head and face protective helmets. However, they also reported a concomitant increase in the number of cervical spine injuries due to a recently outlawed tackling technique known as *spearing,* involving use of the head and helmet to knock down a player.

A prospective study of head and neck injuries in 342 football players over an eight-year period at the University of Iowa (Albright et al., 1985) established an incidence of 175 injuries in 100 players during the length of the study.

> [Players with previous] histories of head or neck injuries or abnormalities of the cervical spine (on prescreening) were twice as likely to have head or neck injuries at some point in their college careers as those players with a normal screening examination, [and] . . . the probability of subsequent head or neck injury escalated sharply following a single incident. (p. 147)

According to Maroon et al. (1980), in their review of 47 years of National Collegiate Athletic Association and American Football Coaches Association data collection efforts, most severe football head injuries occur during defensive blocking or tackling maneuvers. They also point out, as do Harbaugh and Saunders (1984), that most team physicians apply what is referred to by Schneider (1973) as *Quigley's rule,* when evaluating potential dangers from cerebral insult. This rule proposes that athletes should discontinue active participation in sports after receiving three cerebral concussions. This rule is supported by data gathered by Gronwall and Wrightson (1975) as well as others, who contend that cognitive deficits are cumulative in successive concussions. Maroon et al. (1980) go on to underscore that neurological impairment that is documented by CT or other radiological measures "may be enough to strongly discourage or forbid further football participation" (p. 427).

## Mild Head Injury in Football

Mild head injury in football has only recently been considered a problem requiring scientific investigation. Most football players report having one or more mild concussions or "dings" over their careers. These injuries are often characterized by a change in (but not loss of ) consciousness, as well as confusion, retrograde or posttraumatic amnesia, or immediate memory loss, yet these athletes usually continue to play (Meggysey, 1970; Yarnell and Lynch, 1973). These symptoms are often complicated by headache and/or dizziness as well as other postconcussion symptoms (Cook, 1969).

Several attempts have been made to classify cerebral concussion in athletes; these systems have been summarized by Nelson et al. (1984). Torg (1982) has described four grades of mild and moderate head trauma which range from symptoms of having one's "bell rung" (i.e., short-term confusion, unsteady gait, being dazed, and mild posttraumatic amnesia), to immediate and transient loss of consciousness with the above symptoms. Nelson et al. (1984, p. 104) have argued for a concussion classification system for athletes that would focus on five grades of mild head injury, from grade 0, indicating no loss of consciousness but confusion and subsequent difficulty concentrating; to grade 4, characterized by loss of consciousness for more than one minute (yet no coma), headache, cloudy sensations, possible irritability, confusion, and dizziness during recovery.

Although there were no prospective neuropsychological studies of mild head trauma in football players until our own (described later), the recent surge of concern regarding mild head injury in the clinical population has generated interest in high school and college communities, with particular focus on early identification, recovery, return to practice and athletic competition, and improvement of equipment, rules, and coaching techniques. More recently, it has been proposed not only that team physicians implement Quigley's rule, but also that resumption of athletic activities after one mild head injury be predicated on a total resolution of postconcussive symptoms (Hugenholtz and Richard, 1982). In addition, Yarnell and Lynch (1973), in their article entitled "The 'ding': Amnestic States in Football Trauma," based on observations and case studies, concluded that evaluation of memory is a key aspect in the assessment of mild concussion. They refine this concept by suggesting that

> one should not ask [concussed players] questions requiring immediate memory or cognition (digit recall, simple arithmetic, reverse spelling, etc.). Rather, items concerning recently experienced or consolidated events are [more appropriate assessment strategies] ("Where did you go after you left the playing field? What are some of your plays and assignments for this game?"). (Yarnell and Lynch, 1973, p. 197)

## HEAD TRAUMA IN OTHER SPORTS ACTIVITIES

Although head trauma tends to occur more frequently as a result of participation in such sports as boxing and football, athletes who engage in a variety of other competitive physical activities are also at risk for sustaining craniocerebral injuries. Head trauma appears to be the most common, as well as the most severe, type of injury in the equestrian sports (Bixby-Hammett, 1983). Riders who do not wear helmets are at additional high risk for sustaining significant head trauma. Foster et al. (1976) describe five cases of brain damage in British National Hunt jockeys, one of whom died a number of days after being admitted to a neurological center in a coma. All of the jockeys had histories of previous concussive injuries sustained during race-riding. These authors conclude that "National Hunt jockeys are exposed to frequent and often severe unrecorded concussive head injury, and that this can result in brain damage and temporal-lobe epilepsy and the other features recognized as post-traumatic encephalopathy" (Foster et al., 1976, p. 983). As is the case for authors reporting on boxing in the United States, Foster and his colleagues call for stricter safety regulations in order to prevent individuals from sustaining repeated, and rather severe head trauma. Ilgren et al. (1984) reviewed a number of cases in which horse riding accidents resulted in neurotrauma. These authors have observed that this cumulative trauma effect occurs in equestrians as well and results in progressive encephalopathy.

Harris (1983) studied 126 winter sports injuries, occurring over a four-year period, at a neurosurgical medical clinic in an American winter resort area. The sample included 82 individuals who sustained concussions while skiing. The most severe neurotrauma appeared to result from one of four mechanisms of injury: (1) colliding with trees; (2) colliding with other skiers; (3) colliding with large boulders or ski-lift equipment; and (4) performing aerial maneuvers. Harris states that the most dangerous collisions occurred at high speeds, with the skier being abruptly decelerated upon impact. Consequently, the extent and nature of the neuropathology sustained typically fell more toward the severe end of the injury spectrum.

The literature on head trauma resulting from participation in other sports has typically described cases of significant and extensive neuropathology often leading to death (with little mention of mild head injury). These athletic activities include squash (Clement and Fairhurst, 1980), rugby (Roy, 1974), lacrosse (Rimel et al., 1983), and ice hockey (Fekete, 1968; Kraus et al., 1970). Many of these authors conclude that special safety helmets should be developed, and worn by players and that serial concussions should be avoided.

## MAGNITUDE OF THE SPORTS-RELATED HEAD TRAUMA PROBLEM

Although head trauma in sports is a serious problem (see further reviews by Kraus and Conray, 1984), it pales in comparison to head trauma unrelated to sports in the general clinical population. In fact, in one epidemiological study, only 2.7% of 1,900 significant head injuries over a five-year period in Glasgow, Scotland, were sports related (Lindsay et al., 1980). Within sports themselves, significant head injuries seem to occur quite infrequently, and only a small percentage of players suffer such trauma (Bruce et al., 1984). For example, only 1% of 19,413 high school football players in southern California sustained significant head injuries in 1961 (Alley, 1964), and the incidence of such injury appears to have decreased over time.

The incidence and outcome of sports-related mild head trauma have not been sufficiently investigated, and empirical examination of head injury in sports remains important in order to (1) continue reducing the rate and severity of head injury in this arena; (2) ensure rapid and complete recovery; (3) determine the seriousness of the mild head trauma and repeated injury in sports; and (4) utilize sports injury as a "laboratory" model for acceleration/deceleration mild head injury in the general population.

## THE UNIVERSITY OF VIRGINIA PROSPECTIVE STUDY OF MILD HEAD INJURY IN FOOTBALL

For the above reasons, in June 1982 we began a four-year prospective study of football-induced mild head injuries, which was sponsored by a grant from the Pew Memorial Trusts. The objectives of the study were to (1) estimate the incidence of football-induced head injuries and determine the extent and nature of neuropsychological and psychosocial deficits of injured players; (2) establish a recovery curve for players with mild head injury and develop guidelines as to when players can resume normal activities, including football; (3) identify the personal and football-related factors predisposing players to the risk of head injury; and (4) evaluate the longer-term neuropsychological and psychosocial consequences of sustaining more than one head injury during players' college careers.

Data were collected on a total of 2,350 players at 10 universities including the Ivy League (Brown, Columbia, Cornell, Dartmouth, Harvard, Pennsylvania, Princeton, and Yale), the University of Pittsburgh, and the University of Virginia. Players who sustained a mild head injury during this study were evaluated for cognitive and psychosocial dysfunction through the use of neuropsychological techniques and self-report questionnaires up to four times after injury. Mild head trauma was defined as a change in or loss of consciousness for less than two minutes and immediately demonstrating attentional/memory

**Table 17-1** Classification of Players Studied

| Total number of players | 2350 |
|---|---|
| Postinjury protocol: | |
|     Head injuries | 195 |
|     Orthopedic injuries | 59 |
| Student controls | 48 |

problems, as suggested by Yarnell and Lynch (1973). Team physicians and trainers documented 195 injuries involving 182 players during the study. Twelve players suffered two injuries, and one player sustained three injuries.

In addition to head-injured players, 59 players sustaining mild orthopedic injuries and 48 male college students were tested using the same protocol. These two control groups were employed to provide an estimate of the learning effects of repeated testing (normal testing behavior) and to assess the possible cognitive and psychosocial consequences of trauma per se as compared to head trauma.

The tables that follow present some of our initial data analyses. Tables 17–1 and 17–2 show the number of players tested and their characteristics, based on the entire population of football players studied. Of special note is section C of Table 17–2 which indicates that approximately 42% reported a history of at least one minor head injury prior to participation in the study. Over 11% reported two prior minor head injuries, and 11.6% had sustained three or more such injuries. The consequences of the history of previous head injury are currently being explored in our continuing analysis of the data.

**Table 17-2** Player Characteristics (N = 2350)

| | Mode | Percent |
|---|---|---|
| A. *Age and year in school* | | |
| Age | 19 | 48.4[a] |
| Year in school | Sophomore | 56.7[a] |
| | | |
| B. *Position Played* | | |
| Offensive line | | 23.01 |
| Receivers | | 10.18 |
| Running back | | 11.39 |
| Quarterback | | 5.72 |
| Defensive line | | 16.93 |
| Linebackers | | 11.89 |
| Defensive back | | 16.93 |
| Other (special teams) | | 3.95 |
| | | |
| C. *History of previous head injury* | | |
| None | | 57.54 |
| One | | 19.52 |
| Two | | 11.34 |
| Three or more | | 11.60 |

[a]Percent of total series who are at model age and year in school.

**Table 17–3**  Time When Injury
Occurred ($N$ = 195)

|                          | Percent |
|--------------------------|---------|
| *Game*                   |         |
| First quarter            | 15.4    |
| Second quarter           | 12.7    |
| Third quarter            | 14.3    |
| Fourth quarter           | 13.2    |
| Total                    | 55.6    |
|                          |         |
| *Practice*               |         |
| First session            | 33.2    |
| Second session           | 9.8     |
| Third session[a]         | 1.4     |
| Total                    | 44.4    |

[a]Only the University of Pittsburgh engaged in three daily practice sessions during the preseason practice period.

Table 17–3 indicates that there is no apparent game quarter in which players are at greater risk for mild head injury. Nearly 56% of the injuries occurred in the game situation, suggesting that players are at slightly more risk for injury during a game situation as compared to practice sessions. The vast majority of practice-related injuries occurred during the first practice session of the day. Our initial finding is that most practice injuries do occur during the preseason session and may be related to conditioning and/or coaching factors, whereas during the season most injuries occur in game situations.

Table 17–4 shows the injured players' positions. The only group of players that seem to be at somewhat greater risk appear to be those who perform special team functions (e.g., kickoff and punt return teams). The injury rates for other player positions seem consistent with the distribution of all players across the various team positions (see Table 17–2). We should point out, however, that it is possible that there is a differential risk to players in certain positions, depending on the number of plays in a game situation in which those specific positions may be involved. As expected, tackling and blocking are the primary activities of players when they are injured (see Table 17–5). There is

**Table 17–4**  Injured Player's Position ($N$ = 195)

| Position       | Percent |
|----------------|---------|
| Offensive line | 23.2    |
| Receiver       | 7.9     |
| Running back   | 12.9    |
| Quarterback    | 2.3     |
| Defensive line | 13.6    |
| Linebacker     | 10.7    |
| Defensive back | 15.8    |
| Other          | 13.6    |

**Table 17–5**  Injured Player's Activity ($N$ = 195)

| Activity                          | Percent |
|-----------------------------------|---------|
| Running and tackled               | 14.8    |
| Tackling opponent                 | 18.1    |
| Being blocked                     | 17.0    |
| Blocking opponent                 | 25.8    |
| Other (includes practice drills)  | 24.3    |

slightly more risk for the player who is blocking or tackling an opponent (nearly 44%), as compared to the player who is being blocked or tackled (nearly 32%). The majority of "other" activities (comprising 24% of injured players' activities) are largely special team functions as discussed above, and injuries occurring during practice drills.

Table 17–6 lists the primary mechanism of injury classified by impact to the head versus no apparent impact to the head. Over 54% of all injuries involved direct impact to the head, whereas 34.6% involved no impact to the cranium. In 10.8% of the cases, the mechanism of injury was unclear (i.e., there was no identifiable collision that could be identified). In injuries involving direct impact to the head, the majority were helmet-to-helmet impacts (21.1%). Almost 12% of trauma involved a collision to the head in which an opponent's torso or body struck the head, 9.19% of the players were kicked in the head, and 2.16% were kneed in the head. The primary nonimpact category was collision with another player, which did not involve direct impact to the head but which probably involved some form of rotational injury. We are currently reviewing the narrative descriptions of the injuries to see if we can provide more detail interpreting these broad categories of mechanism of injury.

Tables 17–7 to 17–9 present initial findings from our analyses of neuropsychological test scores which were gathered at preseason, 24 hours post injury, 5 and 10 days post trauma, and at post season. Assessment procedures included the Trail Making Test A and B from the Halstead–Reitan Neuropsychological Test Battery (Reitan and Davison, 1974), Aaron Smith's Symbol Digit Test (Smith, 1973), and the Paced Auditory Serial Addition Task (PASAT) (Gronwall and Sampson, 1974; Gronwall and Wrightson, 1980). The

**Table 17–6** Mechanism of Injury (N = 195)

| | |
|---|---|
| *Impact to head* | |
| Helmet-to-helmet | 21.08% |
| Collision to head | 11.89 |
| Kick to head | 9.19 |
| Head struck ground | 3.78 |
| Head first tackle | 3.24 |
| Knee to head | 2.16 |
| Head-to-torso | 2.16 |
| Forearm to chin | 1.08 |
| Total | 54.6 |
| | |
| *No impact to head* | |
| Collision with other player | 24.40% |
| Hard tackle | 4.86 |
| Hard block | 1.62 |
| Speared on ground | 1.62 |
| Speared in air | 1.08 |
| Total | 34.6 |
| | |
| *Unclear (no identifiable impact)* | |
| Total | 10.8% |

**Table 17-7** Changes in PASAT 4 Scores of Head-Injured Players and Student Controls (Mean Score and Percent Change)

| Time of study | Head injured | | Student controls | |
|---|---|---|---|---|
| | Mean score | Percent change[a] | Mean score | Percent change[a] |
| Preseason | 66.3% | | 66.8% | |
| | | 5.3% | | 17.7% |
| 24 hours | 69.8 | | 78.7 | |
| | | 14.8 | | 7.6 |
| 5 days | 80.1 | | 84.6 | |
| | | 6.5 | | 4.1 |
| 10 days | 85.3 | | 88.1 | |
| | | 0.7 | | 1.1 |
| Postseason | 84.7 | | 89.1 | |

[a]Percent change reflects the percent increase in PASAT 4 scores at the time of the study, compared to the score at the preceding time of study (e.g., 24 hours post injury compared to preseason; 5 days post injury compared to 24 hours, etc.).

Trail Making Test is a measure of sustained attention and concentration, which requires sequential problem solving and ability to keep two things in mind simultaneously. The Symbol Digit Test is an alternative to the Wechsler Adult Intelligence Scale Digit Symbol subtest and requires psychomotor problem solving and visual perceptual abilities. Gronwall's PASAT is a task involving rapid presentation of auditory numeric material for complex mental manipulation and requires a high level of attention, concentration, and immediate recall memory.

Table 17-7 shows the mean percentage of correct responses at each time of study and changes in mean scores of head-injured players and student controls on subtest 4 of the PASAT (1.2-second interval between numbers). These changes (reported as percent change) indicate increases in PASAT 4 at the time of study compared to the score at the preceding study time (e.g., 24 hours v. preseason, 5 days vs. 24 hours, etc.). Tables 17-8 and 17-9 present the ratios of average test score differences and their standard errors (average test score difference divided by standard deviation) for head-injured players (Table 17-8) and student controls (Table 17-9). The ratios shown in Tables 17-8 and 17-9 can be interpreted as statistically significant if their absolute value is greater

**Table 17-8** Ratios of Average Test Score Differences and Standard Error of Differences for Head-Injured Players

| Difference between:[a] | Trail A | Trail B | Symbol digit | Pasat 3 | Pasat 4 |
|---|---|---|---|---|---|
| Pre-Sn—24 hours | −2.39 | −2.46 | .54 | 1.13 | 1.93 |
| 24 hours—5 days | −5.04 | −5.29 | 6.39 | 4.44 | 5.73 |
| 5 days—10 days | −1.84 | −3.00 | 3.53 | 2.83 | 3.33 |
| 10 days—Post-Sn | −0.02 | 1.99 | −2.59 | 0.12 | 0.42 |

[a]*Later* score minus *earlier* score.

*Note:* Ratios refer to average test score difference as compared with previous examination (see column on left) divided by standard deviation.

**Table 17-9**  Ratios of Average Test Score Differences and Standard Error of
Differences for Student Controls

| Difference between:[a] | Trail A | Trail B | Symbol digit | PASAT 3 | PASAT 4 |
|---|---|---|---|---|---|
| Pre-Sn—24 hours | −3.79 | −2.55 | 2.46 | 3.04 | 4.04 |
| 24 hours—5 days | −1.47 | −2.59 | 2.97 | 1.73 | 2.19 |
| 5 days—10 days | −2.05 | −2.54 | 1.06 | 0.99 | 1.39 |
| 10 days—Post-Sn | −0.05 | 0.38 | −0.15 | 2.45 | 0.42 |

[a]*Later* score minus *earlier* score.

*Note:* Ratios refer to average test score differences divided by their standard deviation.

than or equal to 1.96. The changes in PASAT subtest 4 scores shown in Table
17–7 display a rather typical pattern when comparing head-injured players and
student controls. The change from preseason score to 24-hour score for the
head-injured players is not significant, whereas the comparable change for the
student controls is statistically significant. The student controls also showed
statistically significant improvement between 24 hours and 5 days, but showed
no significant differences in the 5- to 10-day interval and the 10-day to postseason interval. On the other hand, the head-injured players demonstrated statistically significant improvement between 24 hours and 5 days and between 5
and 10 days, with no significant improvement in the 10-day to postseason
interval.

To summarize these changes, we can say that the student controls displayed the normal testing behavior (i.e., there was an initial practice effect)
which we would expect in serial administration of the PASAT 4 tests, whereas
the head-injured players maintained a preseason baseline score (on average) in
the preseason to 24-hour postinjury period, and then displayed an apparent
recovery in the 24-hour to 5-day interval. These players continued to recover
in the 5- to 10-day interval, and then leveled off throughout the remainder of
the season to the post season. One sees the same pattern in Symbol Digit and
PASAT 3 test performance but not in the performance on Trail Making tests
A and B from the Halstead–Reitan battery (Tables 17–8 and 17–9). We are not
certain at present why we do not see the same pattern on the Trail Making
Test, but one possible explanation is that the practice effect for this test is so
strong as to dilute the consequences of the injury on test performance. This
hypothesis is being explored currently in further analyses.

Table 17–10 presents the percentage of head-injured players, players with
orthopedic injuries, and student controls who reported selected symptoms at
each assessment time. To summarize the table, we can state that there was a
considerable increase in symptom reporting 24 hours post injury, compared to
preseason symptom-reporting rates, for the head-injured players, which then
diminished over time to return to the preseason rate by 10 days post injury.
We do not observe the same pattern of symptom reporting for either the
orthopedic group or the student controls. This gives us rather considerable evidence that the sequelae of mild injury are unique to head injury and not a
consequence of general trauma or of population reporting rates for individuals

**Table 17-10** Percent Reporting Selected Symptoms at Each Assessment

| Symptom | Group | At Pre-Sn | At 24 hours | At 5 days | At 10 days | At Post-Sn |
|---------|-------|-----------|-------------|-----------|------------|------------|
| Headache | Head-injured | 27 | 72 | 55 | 27 | 17 |
| | Orthopedic | 37 | 21 | 14 | 27 | 15 |
| | Controls | 27 | 11 | 17 | 10 | 15 |
| Memory | Head-injured | 03 | 35 | 27 | 08 | 03 |
| | Orthopedic | 04 | 04 | 02 | 00 | 07 |
| | Controls | 02 | 02 | 02 | 02 | 04 |
| Nausea | Head-injured | 03 | 31 | 24 | 08 | 03 |
| | Orthopedic | 06 | 02 | 05 | 11 | 11 |
| | Controls | 08 | 07 | 10 | 06 | 07 |
| Dizziness | Head-injured | 03 | 38 | 23 | 10 | 02 |
| | Orthopedic | 06 | 04 | 02 | 07 | 07 |
| | Controls | 04 | 09 | 06 | 02 | 00 |
| Weakness | Head-injured | 13 | 28 | 20 | 08 | 05 |
| | Orthopedic | 06 | 10 | 07 | 09 | 02 |
| | Controls | 10 | 09 | 12 | 12 | 07 |

of similar age and sex. We are currently performing formal statistical tests to support these interpretations.

In a broad sense, our study suggests that single mild head injury in football players often causes cognitive/information processing deficits which can be documented on neuropsychological assessment within 24 hours of the insult, and that rapid, although perhaps incomplete, recovery may take place over the next 5–10 days. These findings demonstrate similarities to general population mild head injury studies by Levin et al. (1987b) and McLean et al. (1984), who reported mild neuropsychological impairment within days and weeks of mild head trauma with rather rapid recovery of function. Earlier studies by Barth et al. (1983) and Rimel et al. (1981), in contrast, suggest that cognitive and psychosocial problems following such injuries may persist beyond three months post injury in clinical populations. As Dacey and Dikmen (1987) explain, the differences between these studies in severity of deficit and speed of recovery may be due to a variety of sample selection factors such as previous head injury, multiple trauma, alcohol use, psychosocial problems, and low premorbid intellectual/cognitive functioning. The Levin et al. (1987b) and McLean et al. (1984) studies eliminated or controlled for such factors, and for that reason evaluated much "cleaner" patients who are similar to this population of intelligent (estimated mean IQs of well over 100) and healthy, young athletes. Unfortunately, the football study, as well as other similar investigations, begins to break down in generalizability to the overall clinical mild head injury population since such trauma in the latter is more likely to be sustained by individuals who may have had previous cerebral insult and dysfunctional psychosocial histories (Barth et al., 1983; Rimel et al., 1981).

Another difficulty in generalizing from these football findings to other mild head trauma is that most (over 90%) of the reported football injuries reflected very mild trauma or "dings." The major mechanism of mild head injury in the general population is acceleration/deceleration in automobile accidents, which often results in more severe cerebral insult due to rotation and shear-strain.

What can be gleaned from this football study relates first and rather specifically to football itself:

1. Approximately 10% of all college football players will experience mild head injuries over any given season.
2. Over 40% of these athletes will have at least one mild head injury in their high school and college careers.
3. The effects of mild head injury may be measured by neuropsychological assessment.
4. Significant neuropsychological recovery will often take place in this healthy, young population within 10 days of their injury.

Questions still remain regarding the full extent of recovery and compensation, the short- and long-term effects of multiple head trauma, and factors predisposing a player to the risk of mild head injury.

Through further data review and analysis, it is our hope that we can provide the football community, and sports medicine psychologists in particular, with a brief and easily administered set of neuropsychological assessment tools that will aid team physicians in determining level of preseason information-processing skills in individual football players so that recovery of function following mild head injury can be closely monitored (along with other factors such as type of injury, history of previous injury, and reported postconcussion symptoms) to best determine risk for return to competition. Until our data are completely analyzed and further research is completed, a conservative approach to the practical question of when a player may return to competition is suggested, which emphasizes individual evaluation of the head injury circumstances including severity of trauma, number of previous head injuries, length of time since last cerebral insult, premorbid and present neuropsychological functioning, and recovery from postconcussion symptoms. Studying other football teams and sports with differing premorbid characteristics and mechanisms of injury, as well as appropriate control groups, will undoubtedly contribute to our better understanding of what we have now come to view as the spectrum of mild head trauma.

## REFERENCES

Albright JP, Mcauley E, Martin RK, Crowley ET, Foster DT. Head and neck injuries in college football: An eight-year analysis. Am J Sports Med 13:147–152, 1985.

Alley RH. Head and neck injuries in high school football. JAMA 200:118–122, 1964.

Alves WM, Colohan A, O'Leary TJ, Rimel RW, Jane JA. Understanding post-traumatic symptoms after minor head injury. J Head Trauma Rehab 1:1–12, 1986.

Barth JT, Macciocchi SN, Boll TJ, Giordani B, Jane JA, Rimel RW. Neuropsychological sequelae of minor head injury. Neurosurgery 13:529–533, 1983.

Bixby-Hammett DM. Head injuries in the equestrian sports. Physician Sports Med 11:82–86, 1983.

Blonstein JL, Clarke E. Further observations on the medical aspects of amateur boxing. Br Med J 1:362–364, 1957.

Boll TJ, Barth JT. Mild head injury. Psychiatr Dev 3:263–275, 1983.

Brooks N. Neurobehavioral effects of amateur boxing. Presented at the European International Neuropsychological Society Meeting, Barcelona, Spain, 1987.

Brooks N, Galbraith S, Hutchinson JSF, McLatchie G, Melville I, Teasdale E, Wilson L. Clinical neurological examination, neuropsychology, electroencephalography and computed tomographic head scanning in active amateur boxers. J Neurol Neurosurg Psychiatry 50:96–99, 1987.

Bruce DA, Schut L, Sutton LN. Brain and cervical spine injuries occurring during organized sports activities in children and adolescents. Primary Care March 11:175–194, 1984.

Casson IR, Sham R, Campbell EA, Tarlau M, DiDomenico A. Neurological and CT evaluation of knocked-out boxers. J Neurol Neurosurg Psychiatry 45:170–174, 1982.

Casson, IR, Siegel O, Sham R, Campbell EQ, Tarlau M, DiDomenico A. Brain damage in modern boxers. JAMA 251:2663–2667, 1984.

Clement RS, Fairhurst SM. Head injuries from squash: a prospective study. NZ Med J 92:1–3, 1980.

Cook JB. The effects of minor head injuries sustained in sport and the postconcussional syndrome. In Walker AE, Caveness WF, Critchley M (eds), The Late Effects of Head Injury. Springfield, CC Thomas, 1969, pp. 408–413.

Council on Scientific Affairs (American Medical Association). Brain injury in boxing. JAMA 249:254–257, 1983.

Dacey RG, Dikmen SS. Mild head injury. In Cooper P (ed), Head Injury. Baltimore: Williams & Wilkins, 1987, pp. 125–140.

Fekete JF. Severe brain injury and death following minor hockey accidents: the effectiveness of the "safety helmets" of amateur hockey players. Can Med Assoc J 99:1234–1239, 1968.

Foster JB, Tilley PJB, Leiguarda R. Brain damage in national hunt jockeys. Lancet 1:981–983, 1976.

Gennarelli TA. Mechanisms and pathophysiology of cerebral concussion. J Head Trauma Rehab 1:23–29, 1986.

Gennarelli TA, Adams JH, Graham DI. Acceleration induced head injury in the monkey: I. The model, its mechanical and physiological correlates. Acta Neuropathol (Berl) [Suppl] 1:23–25, 1981.

Gerberich SG, Priest JD, Boen JR, Staub CP, Maxwell RE. Concussion incidences and severity in secondary school varsity football players. Am J Public Health 73:1370–1375, 1983.

Gronwall DMA, Sampson H. The psychological effects of concussion. Auckland, NZ: Auckland University Press/Oxford University Press, 1974.

Gronwall D, Wrightson P. Cumulative effect of concussion. Lancet 2:995–997, 1975.

Gronwall D, Wrightson P. Duration of post-traumatic amnesia after mild head injury. J Clin Neuropsychol 2:51–60, 1980.

Harbaugh RE, Saunders RL. The second impact in catastrophic contact-sports head trauma. JAMA 252:538–539, 1984.

Harris JB. Winter sports. Physician Sports Med 11:111–122, 1983.

Holburn AHS. Mechanics of head injuries. Lancet 2:438–444, 1943.

Hugenholtz H, Richard MT. Return to athletic competition following concussion. Can Med Assoc J 127:827–829, 1982.

Ilgren EB, Teddy PJ, Vafadis J, Briggs M, Gardiner NG. Clinical and pathological studies of brain injuries in horse-riding accidents: a description of cases and review with a warning to the unhelmeted. Clin Neuropathol 3:253–259, 1984.

Kaste M, Vilkki J, Sainio K, Kuurne T, Katevuo K, Meurala H. Is chronic brain damage in boxing a hazard of the past? Lancet 2(Nov 27): 1186–1188, 1982.

Kraus JF, Anderson BD, Mueller CE. The effectiveness of a special ice hockey helmet to reduce head injuries in college intramural hockey. Med Sci Sports 2:162–164, 1970.

Kraus JF, Conroy C. Mortality and morbidity from injuries in sports and recreations. Annu Rev Public Health 5:163–192, 1984.

Kraus JF, Black MA, Hessol N, Ley P, Rokaw W, Sullivan C, Bowers S, Knowlton S, Marshall L. The incidence of acute brain injury and serious impairment in a defined population. Am J Epidemiol 119:186–201, 1984.

Lampert PW, Hardman JM. Morphological changes in brains of boxers. JAMA 251:2676–2679, 1984.

Levin HS, Lippold SC, Goldman A, Handel S, High WM Jr, Eisenberg HM, Zelitt D. Neurobehavioral functioning and magnetic resonance imaging in young boxers. J Neurosurg, 67:657–667, 1987a.

Levin HS, Mattis S, Ruff RM, Eisenberg HM, Marshall LF, Tabaddor K. Neurobehavioral outcome following minor head injury: a 3-center study. J Neurosurg, 66:234–243, 1987b.

Lindsay KW, McLatchie G, Jennett B. Serious head injury in sport. Br Med J 281:789–791, 1980.

Maroon JC, Steele PB, Berlin R. Football head and neck injuries-an update. Clin Neurosurg 27:414–429, 1980.

Martland HS. Punch-drunk. JAMA 19:1103–1107, 1928.

Mawdsley C, Ferguson FR. Neurological disease in boxers. Lancet 2:795–801, 1963.

McCunney RJ, Russo PK. Brain injuries in boxers. Physician Sports Med 12:53–64, 1984.

McLatchie G, Brooks N, Galbraith S, Hutchinson JSF, Wilson L, Melville I, Teasdale E. Clinical neurological examination, neuropsychology, electroencephalography and computed tomographic head scanning in active amateur boxers. J Neurol Neurosurg Psychiatry 50:96–99, 1987.

McLean A, Temkin N, Dikmen S, Wyler A, Gale JL. Psychosocial functioning at one month after head injury. Neurosurgery 14:393–399, 1984.

Meggyesy D. Out of Their League. Berkeley, CA: Ramports Press, 1970, p 125.

Morrison RG. Medical and public health aspects of boxing. JAMA 225:2475–2480, 1986.

Nelson WE, Jane JE, Gieck JH. Minor head injury in sports: a new system of classification and management. Physician Sports Med 12(3):103–107, 1984.

Ommaya AK, Gennarelli TA. Cerebral concussion and traumatic unconsciousness: correlation of experimental and clinical observations on blunt head injuries. Brain 97:633–654, 1974.

Reitan RM, Davison LA. Clinical Neuropsychology: Current Status and Applications. Washington, DC: VH Winston, 1974.

Rimel RW, Giordani MA, Barth JT, Boll TJ, Jane JA. Disability caused by minor head injury. Neurosurgery 9(3):221–228, 1981.

Rimel RW, Nelson WE, Persing JA, Jane JA. Case report: epidural hematomas in lacrosse. Physician Sports Med 11(3):140–144, 1983.

Roy SP. The nature and frequency of rugby injuries: a pilot study of 300 injuries at Stellenbosch. S Afr Med J 2(7890):2321–2327, 1974.

Schneider RC. Head and Neck Injuries in Football: Mechanisms, Treatment, and Prevention. Baltimore: Williams & Wilkins, 1973.

Serel M, Jaros O. The mechanisms of cerebral concussion in boxing and their consequences. World Neurol 3:351–358, 1962.

Sironi VA, Scotti G, Ravagnati L, Franzini A, Marossero F. CT scan and EEG findings in professional pugilists: early detection of cerebral atrophy in young boxers. J Neurosurg Sci 26:65–168, 1982.

Smith A. Symbol Digit Modalities Test. Manual. Los Angeles: Western Psychological Services, 1973.

Thomassen A, Juul-Jensen P, Olivarius BDF, Braemer J, Christensen AL. Neurological, electroencephalographic and neurospychological examination of 53 former amateur boxers. Acta Neurol Scand 60:352–362, 1979.

Timperley WR. Banning boxing. Br Med J 285:289, 1982.

Torg JS. Athletic Injuries to the Head, Neck and Face. Philadelphia: Lea & Febiger, 1982.

Torg JS, Truex R, Quedenfeld PR, Burstein A, Spealman A, Nichols C. The National Football Head and Neck Injury Registry: report and conclusions 1978. JAMA 241:1477–1479, 1979.

Yarnell PR, Lynch S, The "ding": amnestic states in football trauma. Neurology (Minn) 23:196–197, 1973.

# 18

# Neurosurgeon as Victim

LAWRENCE F. MARSHALL
AND RONALD M. RUFF

There has been a surge of interest in the morbidity of mild head injury. From the pioneering works of Gronwall and Wrightson (1974, 1981), it became apparent that mild head injury was associated with objective disturbances of cognitive function, particularly in the area of memory, information processing, and attention. Confusion has arisen regarding the length of time that these sequelae persist. An initial report by Rimel et al. (1981) suggested that recovery was, in fact, delayed in many instances and that a significant number of patients had long-term sequelae. A more recent cooperative effort by Levin et al. (1987) indicates that most of the cognitive sequelae of head injury have abated by three months but that there are occasional patients who do not recover fully.

Because one of us (L.F.M.) was a victim of minor head injury, it seems appropriate to relate his experiences following the injury.

### CASE REPORT

This 42-year-old moderately coordinated neurological surgeon was in Vail, Colorado in 1984, for a meeting of the National Traumatic Coma Data Bank. Following the morning meeting, he spent the afternoon touring the mountains of Vail, and while descending one that had only a modest incline, he lost his balance and fell, striking his head. He was rendered immediately unconscious for a period of a few seconds—certainly no more than 10–15. Upon awakening, the world appeared upside down, with the sky below and terra firma above. This condition cleared, but a very modest vertigo persisted. This did not interfere in any way with descent from the mountain, and in fact did not interfere with further skiing activities. Neuropsychological testing was soon recommended by the neuropsychologists at the meeting, but was respectfully declined.

Upon returning home, the neurosurgeon noted that he was a bit more distractable than was his norm and that he had a great deal of difficulty remembering recent events, including particularly the location of objects necessary for work, such as a dictaphone, briefcase, and keys. List making in order to recall meetings scheduled and tasks to be performed became necessary, whereas they were not necessary before. Referencing articles from memory storage was difficult; authors were frequently transposed and dates incorrectly recalled. Information processing did not appear to be affected, but the ability to attend to a task required a higher level of energy expenditure than previously. These symptoms persisted, but they improved gradually over a period of approximately 18 months, and by the fall of 1985 they appeared to have reached their asymptote. Modest improvement in information storage retrieval has continued, indicating that neither Alzheimer's nor a presenile dementia was revealed by the head injury. Function as judged by others remains good, but is not optimal.

## DISCUSSION

The above description is an accurate recollection of the events that occurred, given the recent memory disturbance that accompanies this condition. What does such an injury illustrate? It illustrates first that recovery from mild head injury is a *gradual* process which, although it has a much steeper curve or slope initially, continues for many months. Second, in each instance, measurement against the individual's previous performance would be ideal but is usually unobtainable. The neurosurgeon in question here is certain, however, that had he been tested within one week of his injury, performance would have exceeded at least the average for national controls, if not for local controls in San Diego. Thus, frustration would have set in because clearly the individual was not functioning at this level after the injury.

This is a modest illustration of the need for physicians and neuropsychologists to listen to their patients when they describe symptomatology that cannot be detected by neurocognitive testing. The problem with testing performance in a laboratory setting is that the individual gears up or increases the level of intellectual energy expenditure to function, just as I do in an attempt to maintain a rather busy work pace. In addition, the introduction of significant distractors—for example, someone talking in the background—which had never been disturbing before, now became a major burden. Music on the other hand, which used to interrupt performance, seemed to have no effect. This clearly cannot be captured in a neuropsychological test mode, and I am not suggesting that it should. Rather, we need to think about the consequences of our conclusions when we indicate to the subject that everything is fine—when the subject continues to maintain that things are *not fine.*

For those who function at above-average levels of intellectual performance, neurocognitive testing is likely to leave significant unanswered questions. Perhaps the strategy of asking the patient to judge his or her performance, if and when the test results are also normal, might be a useful one. In such a strategy if the patient claims that his or her performance is normal and the test results support that, then one can assume that the patient has completely recovered. Thus I would not have been convinced if Dr. Ruff or his colleagues had told me that my performance was normal, because I knew that in fact it was *not normal,* and it now continues to be minimally impaired, although it has improved. The latter point is important, because one can begin to blame all dysfunction of recent memory on the aging process, whereas in my case, although it may have played a minor role, it certainly was not the major factor.

Has this discussion from a minimally brain-injured neurosurgeon been of any value? It is probably only of very limited value, but it does serve to make the point that perceptions of a disease by one who has not had the disease as a patient tend to be modestly inaccurate. Recovery from head injury appears to be a prolonged process, one requiring innumerable strategies for compensation. Neurocognitive testing will indicate part of the story *only if* the results are abnormal; it leaves something to be desired in predicting levels of performance for those who are adequate competitors in a modern society.

## COMMENTS BY A NEUROPSYCHOLOGIST

The insightful reflections of the neurosurgeon expressed here suggest a variety of conclusions regarding the sensitivity, if not validity, of neuropsychological assessment in those individuals who function somewhat above average. Although one might agree that conventional memory tests do have a ceiling effect, the neurosurgeon's challenge to the neuropsychologist should not go without reply. It is possible to develop memory measures that would more closely match individual potential as it is presently conceptualized in intelligence tests. Even for those who function at a superior level, anterograde memory can be assessed at an upper threshold. For example, one could determine the individual's span for immediately recalling words; that is, a word span for an individual could be established. In a second step, the lists to be learned could be double that of the individual's word span so that, for example, a patient who could recall only four words would have to learn a list of eight, whereas an individual who could immediately recall 12 would now need to recall 24 words.

Neuropsychological testing, therefore, could be made more sensitive to individuals who function at the higher level of performance if test measures were individualized with no absolute fixed end point. It is true, however, that such test batteries do not, in general, exist and would need to be developed and normed.

The neurosurgeon here also noted that referencing articles of scientific merit for testing remote memory was difficult. To some degree, recall of remote memory relies primarily on information stored prior to the minor head injury. However, retrograde memory measures are typically not standardized or clinically useful. However, Squire and Slater (1978) have described an empirically developed test to measure interference with retrograde memory in a more sophisticated fashion, and such a test might be applicable here.

The ability to focus on a task, the ease with which one is distracted, and alterations in specific features of attention have not received much investigation when one assesses minor head injury. Neuropsychological testing typically has lagged behind the more sophisticated investigations that are done, for example, in the selection of astronauts or pilots. In simulator environments, such individuals are asked to process multiple tasks—often four or five—concurrently, by selectively attending and prioritizing their information processing. Thus, similar to anterograde memory, attention measures need to be devised which can be individualized and which do not have ceilings.

The neurosurgeon who suffered this minor injury estimated that the duration of recovery was approximately 18 months, in spite of the fact that a variety of compensatory mechanisms, such as list making and an increase in the level of energy expended (using the term "energy" in a very global fashion) in order to improve function, were employed. In the absence of normative data, one could plot attention and memory recovery for such an individual. The availability of norms would be useful in teasing out the learning effect from repeated testing, and perhaps this brief chapter has adequately demonstrated the need for developing such norms.

What this case report illustrates is that individuals do in fact suffer long-term residua from head injury, and that it is dangerous to conclude from the recently completed group study that cognitive recovery per se occurs entirely within three months (Levin et al., 1987). In these group studies, the minor head injury subjects were matched to local control groups, and thus the comparisons merely take into account significant differences between the groups. Thus, if an individual were to have functioned at the 95th percentile level prior to injury and, as a result of the accident, dropped to the 60th percentile rank, the use of such group comparisons would be relatively insensitive, and conclusions based on them would in fact be misleading. However, if longitudinal testing were performed using instruments that had relatively high ceilings of performance, one could then argue that recovery or compensation for the injury is taking place.

This description of the course of head injury by a person who has had some experience in the field serves to emphasize the need for a continued search for test measures that not only describe reliably the varying aspects of brain function, but also relate closely to the day-to-day experiences of the individual patient.

## REFERENCES

Gronwall D, Wrightson P. Delayed recovery of intellectual function after minor head injury. Lancet 2:605–609, 1974.

Gronwall D, Wrightson P. Memory and information processing capacity after closed head injury. J Neurol Neurosurg Psychiatry 44:889–895, 1981.

Levin HS, Mattis S, Ruff RM, Eisenberg HM, Marshall LF, Tabaddor K, High WM Jr, Frankowski RF. Neurobehavioral outcome following minor head injury: a three-center study. J. Neurosurg 66:234–243, 1987.

Rimel RW, Giordani B, Barth JT, Boll TJ, Jane JA. Disability caused by minor head injury. J Neurosurg 9:221–228, 1981.

Squire LR, Slater RPC. Anterograde and retrograde memory impairment in chronic amnesia. Neuropsychologia 16:313–322, 1978.

# Index